ANATOMY FOR DENTAL STUDENTS

Third Edition

•

D. R. JOHNSON, B.Sc., Ph.D., D.Sc.
Centre for Human Biology
University of Leeds

and

W. J. MOORE, B.D.S., M.B., Ch.B., B.Sc., Ph.D., D.Sc.
Emeritus Professor,
University of Leeds

Illustrated by Ann Johnson, N.D.D.

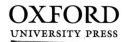
OXFORD
UNIVERSITY PRESS

OXFORD
UNIVERSITY PRESS

Great Clarendon Street, Oxford OX2 6DP
Oxford University Press is a department of the University of Oxford.
It furthers the University's objective of excellence in research, scholarship,
and education by publishing worldwide in

Oxford New York
Auckland Cape Town Dar es Salaam Hong Kong Karachi
Kuala Lumpur Madrid Melbourne Mexico City Nairobi
New Delhi Shanghai Taipei Toronto

With offices in
Argentina Austria Brazil Chile Czech Republic France Greece
Guatemala Hungary Italy Japan South Korea Poland Portugal
Singapore Switzerland Thailand Turkey Ukraine Vietnam

Published in the United States
by Oxford University Press Inc., New York
© D.R. Johnson and W. J Moore, 1997
The moral rights of the authors have been asserted
Database right Oxford University Press (maker)

First published 1983
Second edition 1989
Third edition 1997
Reprinted 1998, 1999, 2000 (twice),2003,2004,2005,2006

British Library Cataloguing in Publication Data
Data available

Library of Congress Cataloging in Publication Data
Data available

ISBN-13: 978-0-19-262673-8
ISBN-10: 0-19-262673-6
9 10
Printed in China

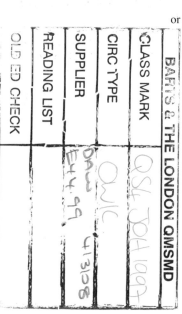

PREFACE TO FIRST EDITION

In recent years the teaching of anatomy to undergraduate students has been subjected to many changing fashions. We have seen the arrival of the integrated curriculum, an increasing reliance on audio-visual aids, and in some schools a trend towards using prosected parts instead of personal dissection in the teaching of topographical anatomy. Methods of examination have also changed with the widespread introduction of continuous assessment and multiple-choice questions. But perhaps the greatest change has been the reduction in the emphasis placed upon the teaching of topographical anatomy. The extent to which this has occurred varies from one centre to another, and has perhaps been more marked in medical than in dental courses, but nevertheless a substantial reduction in the time available for gross anatomy appears to be a widespread feature of modern dental curricula.

Despite these fashions, the value of many of which has yet to be proved, there are certain fundamentals which do not change. The most important to our mind are (i) the practical value of a sound working knowledge of the structure and function of the healthy human body for all directly involved in health care; (ii) that this knowledge, in the case of the dental student at least, is best obtained through dissection of the cadaver; and (iii) that anatomy, like the other preclinical subjects, has its own natural unity and that the losses outweigh the gains if this is obscured by obsessive attempts at integration with clinical subjects.

This book has been written with these three points in mind, our aim being to provide the dental student with a textbook containing all the gross and developmental anatomy—apart from that of the dentition itself—necessary for the practice of dentistry and its major specialities. We have assumed that the student will be receiving a practical course in topographical anatomy, preferably one based on dissection. We hope that the book may also prove useful for post-graduate dentists, especially those taking the Primary Examination of the Royal College of Surgeons or similar examinations.

A few words of explanation of certain specific points may be helpful. In selecting material for inclusion our criteria have been its clinical relevance and/or its importance in understanding structure and function in the dentally important regions. The emphasis is on head and neck, thorax, and nervous system. Apart from a description of the cubital fossa and gluteal region we have included no topographical anatomy of the limbs nor of the trunk below the diaphragm. We have excluded the dentition from our account because under-standing the gross and developmental anatomy of the teeth requires a detailed knowledge of the microstructure of the dental tissues and these topics are therefore better dealt with together as a separate and integrated subject. The dividing line between such 'dental anatomy' and general anatomy is, of course, artificial and the student must ensure that no gaps exist in knowledge in the two fields.

Throughout the book we have had in mind the eventual clinical needs of the dental student and of the practising dentist. In some cases the clinical applications of the anatomy are obvious and require no special emphasis. In other cases there are clinical aspects which may not be apparent to the preclinical student and here we have given short accounts of these aspects in the hope that they will emphasize the practical importance of the anatomy as well as add interest.

We have also tried to convey something of the scientific basis of anatomy by giving accounts of the evolutionary history and comparative anatomy of the structures being described where this seems likely to aid understanding.

In general we have not included references to the original literature because in our experience the busy undergraduate has neither the time nor the inclination to pursue these. Where the teacher wishes to encourage his students to use the original literature and to develop a critical approach, both excellent educational objectives, this can be more effectively achieved through reading directed towards clearly defined and circumscribed topics. Some additional reading has been suggested in the chapters dealing with mastication and growth because we believe that a satisfactory grasp of these important but still incompletely understood subjects requires a rounded view which can be achieved only by reading the accounts of several authors.

We have used an anglicized form of the terminology of the third edition of the *Nomina Anatomica* apart from a few instances where we believe alternative terms suit the purposes of the dental student better. Where older terminology is likely to be still in use by clinical dental teachers this has been indicated.

We should like to express our gratitude to Mr P. N. Hirschmann for providing us with radiographs. Our thanks are also due to Miss Lorraine Brooke, Mrs Celia Peters, and Miss Hilary Rogers for help with the preparation of the manuscript.

Leeds   D.R.J.
August 1982   W.J.M.

PREFACE TO THIRD EDITION

In preparing the third edition of this book we have made numerous changes to both the text and illustrations. Many of the changes to the text are to improve accuracy, remove ambiguities, and, we hope, enhance readability, but in the chapters on development and on the nervous system more extensive modifications have been necessary to take account of improving knowledge which stems from the rapidly advancing research in these fields. The changes to the illustrations are mostly of a minor nature and aimed at improving clarity although Fig. 4.24 is completely new. We have been pleased to learn that our textbook is being used by several other groups of students in the health care professions and, at the request of their teachers, we have included appendices on the development of the eye and ear.

Leeds
July 1996

D.R.J.
W.J.M.

CONTENTS

Section 1

Introduction

1

The study of anatomy

Human anatomy deals with the structure of the human body at the gross, cellular, and subcellular levels. It also deals with the way in which development and growth alter structure and with the relationships between structure and function. A knowledge of these topics is essential for anyone wishing to become a clinical practitioner and this is especially so for those whose practice is likely to be of a surgical nature. It is impossible to understand the effects of disease and its clinical manifestations without an understanding of healthy structure and function; nor is it possible to intervene effectively and safely with surgical procedures, in order to cure or ameliorate disease, without a good working knowledge of the anatomy of the relevant part of the body.

The principal aim of this book is to provide you with sufficient practical information about the gross anatomy of the human body to form a basis on which to build your clinical practice. Its main focus is the dental region – that part of the body in which are located, or through which pass, structures of importance to the dentist. This region stretches from the orbits above to the larynx below and reaches back to the base of the skull and the vertebral column. A second major topic is the anatomy of the thorax which is important for dental practitioners partly because diseases of the chest are common, and may have implications in the planning of dental treatment, and partly because some of the procedures carried out in the dental surgery, especially the giving of general anaesthetics and other systemically acting drugs, may have effects upon the thoracic viscera.

In clinical work it is often necessary to locate or to obtain information about internal structures without being able to gain access to them directly. A good example of this is the need to be able to locate the nerves supplying the teeth and the surrounding soft tissues in order to anaesthetize them with a local anaesthetic delivered through a syringe needle. Fortunately most structures have a sufficiently constant relationship to surface features to allow their position to be judged with considerable accuracy. The study of these relationships is called *surface anatomy*. Information about deep structures can also be obtained by the use of X-rays. These are absorbed to different degrees by the various tissues of the body, being absorbed most completely by bone and least by organs (such as lungs) containing air. After penetrating the body the X-rays are used to expose a photographic film which thus records in different shades, from black through grey to white, and in two dimensions, the structures through which the beam has passed. The exposed film is called a *radiograph*. The interpretation of radiographs requires a knowledge of the radiographic appearance of normal body structures, the study of which is called *radiological anatomy*. Surface and radiological anatomy are obviously of great practical importance and are accordingly emphasized in the sections on the dental region and thorax.

Congenital abnormalities of the oral structures are common and their treatment often involves the dental practitioner. To understand how these abnormalities occur requires a knowledge of the development of the dental region which, in turn, requires some knowledge of early general development. A further section of this book is therefore devoted to these topics. This section also includes an account of postnatal growth, again with special reference to the dental region.

The last section of the book deals with the central nervous system. Some knowledge of the structure and function of this important system is essential for anyone concerned with the diagnosis and treatment of disease. The account included here emphasizes those aspects of the brain and spinal cord which are of particular importance to the dental student, but also gives sufficient information about the remainder of the system to form a basis for a general understanding of its functioning.

Intravenously and intramuscularly administered drugs are now widely used in dental practice. The most popular routes for giving these agents are through the veins of the forearm and into the gluteal muscles of the buttock. An account of these structures is given in a short appendix.

No description of the teeth themselves is included. We strongly believe that the gross morphology of the dentition is best dealt with together with the microstructure of the dental tissues. It is only against such a background that the naked eye appearance of the teeth can be fully understood.

It will probably be obvious that gross anatomy can be studied in two ways. One method is to take each region of the body in turn and examine all the structures found there, together with their relationships to each other. This is *regional* or *topographical anatomy*. It is the anatomy that a surgeon needs to know so that he is always aware of the structures that lie adjacent to his instruments. The second method is to deal with all the ramifications of one system wherever they are found. This is *systemic anatomy*. It is also of practical value in that it allows the relationship of the part of the system under attention to the remainder of the system to be appreciated. This is perhaps most readily apparent in the case of blood vessels and nerves where it is obviously essential to know the origin, course, and distribution of a vessel or nerve before subjecting it to any surgical procedure. You must, therefore, build up in your mind a picture of both the topographical anatomy of the region you are studying and of the systemic anatomy of the systems you find there.

The emphasis in this book is on regional anatomy, as is appropriate in a work intended for men and women who will eventually be using their anatomy in a practical way. As a prelude to this, however, you will find it helpful to read the brief descriptions of the major systems which immediately follow this chapter.

There are several difficulties in studying gross anatomy which may be new to you. First the subject lacks the logical starting point and progressive build up which are such obvious features of most of the physical sciences. Wherever you begin you will find that information is immediately required about other, and frequently remote, structures or regions. Secondly there is a great deal of factual detail to be appreciated and memorized, much of it apparently lacking a reasonable explanation which would aid memory. Thirdly you will probably find anatomical terminology daunting, at least initially.

So far as the first of these difficulties is concerned there is little practical help that can be offered. However, it will probably be reassuring to know that it is a problem encountered by all when they first begin studying anatomy and that quite soon, as your circle of knowledge expands, you will find that individual items of information will begin to interlock and reinforce each other.

The best way of dealing with the second difficulty is a practical one. Nearly everyone finds that examining specimens, or much better still actually carrying out your own dissection, fixes detailed structure in the mind with an ease and security of recall which cannot be matched by any amount of reading or the studying of illustrations. If you are fortunate enough to have access to a dissecting room cadaver make full use of the opportunity you have been given. It is also helpful in memorizing factual detail if it can be given a logical basis. Frequently the arrangement of the structures of the human body, which may appear quite adventitious in itself, is explicable in evolutionary terms. Where we think it will be helpful we have included a brief, and often simplified, account of the evolutionary history of the structures concerned. Our aim in doing this is to help you understand human anatomy, not to teach comparative anatomy.

The third difficulty stems from the fact that the early anatomists used Latin, or sometimes Greek words to name the structures they encountered. This can in fact be helpful, for you will find that many anatomical terms have the same roots as words used in everyday English. Probably the most quoted example is the name 'vagus', given to the very long tenth cranial nerve, which has the same root as words such as vagrant and vagabond, but there are numerous others. The realization that a Latin or Greek term has an appropriate meaning aids understanding and memory. To help in this we have included a glossary of the derivations of the commoner anatomical terms likely to be encountered by dental students.

A final general point to be made concerns variation. Variation is a feature of all biological systems and you will encounter it continuously in every facet of your clinical career. Human beings, like all other organisms, vary in all aspects of their structure and function. We differ from each other in our external features, in the arrangement of our internal organs, in our physiology and biochemistry, in our reaction to disease agents and in our response to treatment. So far as gross anatomy is concerned you will find that all the structures of the body vary in size, shape, and arrangement. This means that no two dissecting room specimens are completely alike and that you will frequently find that the cadaver you are examining differs considerably from the textbook description. In general the arrangement of the nervous system is the least variable and that of the cardiovascular system, especially the venous side, the most variable. The descriptions given in this book are those that we have found to be the most usual or typical.

DESCRIPTIVE TERMS

The anatomical position

The body is always referred to as if it were in the **anatomical position.** This is defined as follows (Fig. 1.1):

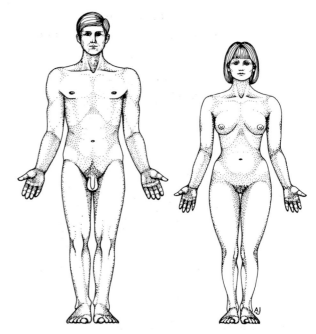

Fig. 1.1. The anatomical position.

The individual is standing erect.
The face and eyes are directed forwards.
The hands are by the sides with palms directed forwards.
The heels are together, the feet pointing forwards so that the great toes are adjacent.

It is important always to describe the cadaver or patient *as if in the anatomical position* and anatomical descriptions are always written in this way. There is a temptation to use the horizontal orientation of the cadaver on the dissecting table or the patient on the bed; this should be resisted as it may lead to serious confusion or error.

Planes

A body standing in the anatomical position can be divided by three planes mutually at right angles (Fig. 1.2).

The **median** or **sagittal plane** is the vertical plane which divides the body into left and right halves. The anterior and posterior margins of this plane reach the surface of the body along the median line or **midline.** Any plane parallel to the median or sagittal plane is **paramedian** or **parasagittal.** The term sagittal is derived from the fancied resemblence of the sagittal suture of the newborn skull (Fig. 2.41, p. 70) to an arrow.

A **coronal plane** is any vertical plane at right angles to the median plane. It is named from the coronal suture of the skull.

A **transverse** or **horizontal plane** is any plane at right angles to both median and coronal planes.

Any other plane of division is referred to as **oblique.**

Terms

Related to these planes are the following paired descriptive terms:
1. **medial** – closer to the midline of the body
   lateral – further from the midline of the body;

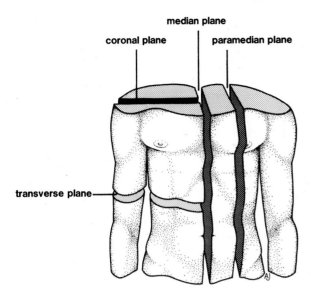

Fig. 1.2. Planes of section.

2. **anterior** – nearer the front surface of the body
posterior – nearer the rear surface of the body;
3. **superior** – nearer the crown of the head
inferior – nearer the soles of the feet.

Comparative anatomical and embryological terms

The system of nomenclature just outlined is inappropriate when describing the anatomy of mammals other than man. It is also unsuitable for describing the structure of the developing embryo. In both comparative anatomy and embryology the following synonyms are preferable:
1. **ventral** = anterior
dorsal = posterior;
2. **rostral, cranial,** or **cephalic** (towards the head) = superior
caudal (towards the tail) = inferior.
These terms are also frequently used in descriptions of the nervous system.

Specialized terms

In the limbs it is necessary to augment the usual terms as follows:
1. **proximal** = nearer the trunk
distal = further from the trunk;
2. **preaxial** = the lateral border (i.e. thumb or big toe side)
postaxial = the medial border (little finger, little toe side):
3. **flexor** = the anterior side of the upper limb, posterior side of the lower limb (see 'Terms of movement' below)
extensor = the other side of the limb.

Terms of movement

1. To **flex** is to bend or make an angle.
To **extend** is to straighten. Flexion and extension take place, for example, at the elbow and knee.
2. To **abduct** is to draw away from the median plane.
To **adduct** is to move towards the median plane.
A combination of abduction, adduction, flexion, and extension, such as can take place at the wrist, is called **circumduction.**
3. To **protrude** or **protract** is to move forwards.
To **retrude** or **retract** is to move backwards.
4. To **pronate** was originally to bow deeply; it is now a specialized term meaning to turn the hand so that the palm faces backwards from the anatomical position.
To **supinate** is the opposite of pronate.
5. To **medially rotate** is to turn a limb on its long axis, so that the palm, for instance, faces medially.
To **laterally rotate** is the opposite of medial rotation.

Other terms

Inside, interior, internal; outside, exterior, external are best reserved for bony cavities (like the thorax) or hollow **viscera,** like the gut.
Invaginations and **evaginations** are inward and outward bulges in the wall of a cavity.
Superficial and **deep** refer to proximity to the skin surface.
Ipsilateral means on the same side of the body; **contralateral** means on the opposite side.

Locomotor and nervous systems

The locomotor system comprises the skeletal elements, composed principally of bone and cartilage, the joints between them, and the muscles which move the joints.

SKELETON

Bone and bones

The greatest popular misconception about bone is that it is static and unchanging. This is not so. A bone has blood vessels, lymphatics, and nerves. It grows, is subject to disease, and, when broken, is self-repairing. It is constantly remodelled to preserve its mechanical efficiency. Unnecessary bone is removed. The walls of an empty tooth socket, for example, disappear after the extraction of a tooth. After a fracture, the temporary framework (or callus) which unites the broken ends is soon remodelled into a mechanically more efficient structure. In a paralysed limb the bone becomes thinner and weaker; in an athlete or an overweight person it may become stronger and heavier.

Bone tissue has two main parts: the bone cells, or **osteocytes,** and the **intercellular matrix.** The matrix is composed principally of **collagen** and inorganic crystals of **hydroxyapatite.** The collagen fibres give bone tissue its great tensile strength while the hydroxyapatite crystals provide its compressive strength. Bone is least strong when resisting forces of shear.

Because the osteocytes are surrounded by a rigid, mineralized matrix bone is incapable of growing **interstitially.** Instead it grows by **apposition** (or accretion) to its surfaces, both external and internal. In order that a growing bone preserves its proportions it is necessary that as bone is added to some surfaces it is simultaneously removed from others (Fig. 1.3). Bone deposition is brought about by **osteoblasts** (which become incorporated in the new bone as osteocytes) and resorption by multinucleated giant cells called **osteoclasts.** These two cell types are found in the **periosteum** and **endosteum** lining the external and internal surfaces, respectively, of bones.

In addition to the great intrinsic strength of bone tissue, further strength is given to the skeleton by the fact that the tissue is formed into structures in a manner resembling that seen in the best engineering practice. The shaft of a long bone, for example, is hollow like the frame of a bicycle giving a strong structure with an economical use of material. Within the ends of long bones and within short bones and irregular bones the cavity is filled with bony spicules arranged along the lines of the principal tensile and compressive stresses. Bones are yet further strengthened by the muscles attached to them contracting in such a way as to offset the applied force.

Functions of bone

Bone has the following functions.

   1. It forms a supporting framework for the body and provides the levers to which the muscles are attached.

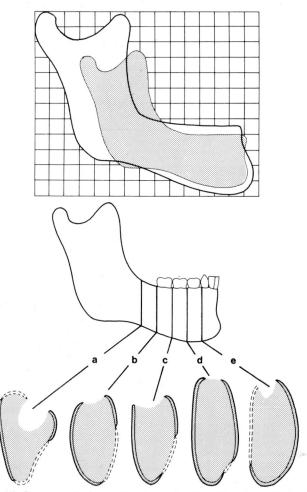

Fig. 1.3. Bone growth. Bones do not grow by deposition alone. Above, the outlines of a young (shaded) and an adult mandible are superimposed. Note that the anterior margin of the vertical ramus has to be resorbed in order for the adult proportions of the bone to be achieved. Below are shown the areas of deposition (solid line) and resorption (dotted line) involved in growth of the body of mandible.

2. It protects internal organs.

3. It acts as a calcium and phosphorous store; 99 per cent of the body's calcium is stored in bone from where it is easily mobilized.

4. Many bones are hollow and contain **marrow cavities.** During prenatal life most of the marrow is a site of formation of blood cells (**red marrow**) but during the growth period the areas of haemopoiesis become progressively restricted until, in the adult, red marrow is found only in the bones of the skull, the vertebrae, sternum, ribs, shoulder girdle, hip and the proximal ends of some long bones. Elsewhere the marrow becomes converted to fatty tissue (**yellow marrow**).

Types of bone

Bone may be of several types. First formed bone is often of the **fibrous** or **woven** variety, so called because it has a network of randomly orientated large collagen fibres in its matrix.

Woven bone is remodelled to form:

1. **compact bone,** which is strong, hard, and heavy, and forms the continuous outer layer, or **cortex,** of all bones;

2. **cancellous** or **spongy bone,** which consists of a network of spicules or **trabeculae;** it is lighter and less strong than the compact variety and is found in the ends of long bones and in the irregular bones.

Origin of bone

Bone has two main embryonic origins. **Cartilage-replacing** bone is formed by osteoblasts in the remains, usually calcified, of a cartilaginous model. **Membrane** or **dermal** bone is formed by osteoblasts in fibrous connective tissue without a preceding cartilage model. These two types of bone have a long evolutionary history. A skeleton based on calcium rather than silicon appeared in the Cambrian period (550 million years ago), presumably because of a change in the chemistry of the ocean or the physiology of the creatures which lived in it. The first vertebrates had an **exoskeleton** consisting of bony plates within the skin. It is presumed that the same creatures had **endoskeletons** of cartilage which were not preserved. In later vertebrates cartilage-replacing bone developed in the endoskeleton. The cartilage-replacing and dermal bones of modern vertebrates are believed to have been derived from these two sources. The postcranial skeleton (except the clavicle) and the base and sense capsules of the skull are formed of cartilage-replacing bones and represent the endoskeleton. The vault of the skull and most of the facial skeleton are composed of dermal bones which are derivatives of the exoskeleton. Some of the skull bones, which are partly in the skull base and partly in the vault, are of mixed origin being formed by fusion of elements from both the endoskeleton and the exoskeleton. The clavicle has a similar mixed origin.

Classification of bone

As well as classifying bones developmentally, according to whether or not they are preformed in cartilage, we can also classify them as **axial** (skull, vertebrae, ribs, sternum) or **appendicular** (shoulder and pelvic girdles, limb bones). A third classification is a rather arbitrary one, relying on shape:

1. long bones ⎫
   short bones ⎬ of the limbs;
2. flat bones ⎫
   irregular bones ⎬ of the axial skeleton and girdles;

3. pneumatic bones of the skull;

4. sesamoid bones.

Long bones

The long bones are typical of the limbs. They consist of a central tubular shaft, the **diaphysis,** and specialized ends, the **epiphyses.** Each epiphysis is joined to the diaphysis by a junctional region, the **metaphysis.** The diaphysis is filled with bone marrow (red in children, yellow and fatty in adults). The shaft walls are made up of compact bone and are thickest in the middle of the bone where transverse forces are greatest. The interiors of the epiphyses are occupied by cancellous bone and the marrow is restricted to the interstices between the trabeculae.

The long bones are preformed in cartilage. The diaphysis is ossified from an ossification centre which appears early in development in the shaft of the cartilage model. Bone from this ossification centre spreads until only the ends of the model remain unossified. In mammals one or more ossification centres later appear in each of these unossified regions. As the epiphysial ossification centre expands the cartilage is eventually restricted to the articular surface of the epiphysis, where it forms the **articular cartilage,** and to a zone in the metaphysis, where it forms the **epiphysial cartilage** sandwiched between the bone of the epiphysis and that of the diaphysis. The epiphysial cartilage subsequently provides the principal site of elongation of the long bone, the cartilage growing interstitially and being replaced by bone on the diaphysial side.

Short bones

These are confined to the wrist and ankle and tend to be cuboidal. They are made up of a cancellous interior with a cortex of compact bone. Of their six surfaces, four are usually articular, leaving two for the attachment of ligaments and for the entry of blood vessels and nerves. Short bones develop in cartilage and ossify in a fixed sequence after birth.

Flat bones

These are composed of two layers of compact bone separated by a layer of cancellous bone (the **diploë**) containing red marrow. Since these bones are often curved it is possible to term one cortical layer the **inner table** and the other the **outer table.** Developmentally flat bones may be cartilage replacing or dermal. At birth they consist of a single layer of bone, the diploë forming later.

Irregular bones

Irregular is the term used to describe the bones left when other types are excluded. They are, therefore, a very mixed group, including the bones of the skull (excluding the flat bones), the vertebrae and the pelvis.

Pneumatic bones

Evaginations of the mucous membrane lining certain cavities, especially the nasal cavity, invade the adjacent flat and irregular bones of the skull to form **air sinuses.**

Sesamoid bones

These form in certain tendons where they rub on a bony surface. The largest example is the **patella** or knee cap. The friction bearing surface of a sesamoid bone is covered with articular cartilage, the rest is buried in the tendon.

Markings on dry bones

The character of the surfaces of a dried bone gives us considerable information about the structures which were adjacent to it during life. Wherever fibrous tissue (ligament, tendon, fascia, aponeurosis) has been attached, the bone will be marked. Fibrous tissue markings are absent in the young, first seen at puberty and increase with age. These markings may take the form of roughened areas or elevations. Linear elevations are termed, according to size, **lines, ridges,** or **crests;** rounded elevations are called **tubercles, tuberosities,** or occasionally **trochanters;** sharp protrusions are called **spines** or **styloid processes.**

A depression in a bone surface is termed a **pit, fovea,** or **fossa** or, if elongated, a **sulcus.** Smooth areas are called **facets.** These may have been covered in life with articular cartilage or have been areas over which tendons played. Knuckle-shaped articular surfaces are called **heads** or **condyles.**

A **notch** or **incisure** is a depression in the margin of a bone. A **foramen** is a hole in a bone usually giving passage to nerves or blood vessels or both. An elongated foramen is termed a **canal** or **meatus.**

Clinical aspects

A bone which is subjected to too much force, especially of a shearing nature, may fracture. Young bones are pliable and fracture raggedly or partially (greenstick fracture), older bones are harder and fracture spirally or transversely according to the direction of the force applied. The broken ends of a bone ultimately reunite by the formation of a large callus of connective tissue and woven bone, most of which is eventually resorbed. It may be necessary to reduce or set a fracture in order to align the broken ends of the bone. Often this involves traction, pulling against the muscles crossing the break, and it may be necessary to maintain this traction, after the bone has been immobilized in a plaster cast, by means of weights and pulleys. The rapidity of bone healing depends on the blood supply of the particular bone fractured. This is notoriously poor in some cases, leading to long periods of recovery. The bone may, in fact, never recover but die (avascular necrosis) if the blood supply is very poor or was destroyed by the injury. Fortunately for the practice of dentistry the bones of the facial skeleton have an excellent blood supply. In a simple fracture the broken bone ends do not penetrate surrounding tissues. In a compound fracture they pierce the skin and precautions must be taken against infection. The broken ends of bones are sharp and may cut through nerves, muscles, blood vessels, or tendons, causing considerable damage.

Cartilage

Cartilage, unlike bone, grows **interstitially** (i.e. throughout its substance) as well as by **apposition** to its surfaces. It is thus an important skeletal material during fetal and postnatal life when rapid growth is taking place. Many cartilaginous elements, including the cartilaginous models of long bones, vertebrae, and the base of the skull, are later replaced by bone by endochondral ossification but others persist into adult life as structures, such as the tracheal rings, laryngeal cartilages, and costal cartilages, which do not ossify. Cartilage cells are termed **chondrocytes** and are surrounded by a **matrix.** Histologically, cartilage may be divided according to the type and number of the collagen fibres in its matrix into **hyaline cartilage, fibrocartilage,** which replaces hyaline cartilage in areas subject to

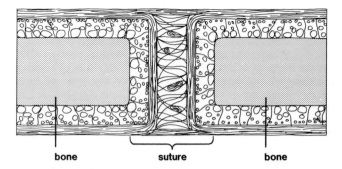

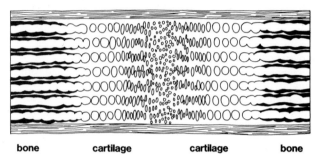

Fig. 1.4. Cross-section of a suture (above) and a synchondrosis of the cranial base (below)—see pp. 69–70 for an explanation of the growth mechanisms at these sites.

great stress, and **elastic cartilage,** a pliable tissue found in the walls of the external acoustic meatus and larynx.

Joints

A joint is a junction between two or more bones. This is obviously a very broad definition because the sites of union of bones can have very different properties. In some joints no movement is possible. In most cases such joints are sites of growth. In other joints movement is possible but the amount of movement permitted varies over a wide range. It is convenient to classify joints into immovable, slightly movable, and freely movable, since this classification correlates closely with their structure.

Immovable joints

Sutures (Fig. 1.4) occur between the dermal bones in the cranial vault and face. During the growth period the bones at a suture are separated by an active osteogenic membrane (p. 69) and much new bone tissue is added to their edges. As the amount of growth declines the adjacent edges of the bones become interdigitated or serrated, thus strengthening the joint. Once growth has ceased completely the sutures start to fuse. In the skull of an elderly person the sutures are usually obliterated. At birth the sutures are very wide and permit some movement. This is important in allowing the head to **mould** as it passes through the maternal birth canal during birth.

Gomphoses are the membranous peg and socket joints between the teeth and the alveoli of the jaw bones. They allow a slight degree of movement, for the purpose of shock absorption, when the teeth are biting.

Synchondroses (Fig. 1.4) are joints of hyaline cartilage formed between cartilage replacing bones. They are found between the bones of the cranial base where they provide the principal sites of growth (p. 70). The epiphysial cartilages of long bones are also synchondroses. If movement occurs here (slipped epiphysis) the growth in length of the bone will be severely deranged. Like sutures, synchondroses usually fuse after they have ceased growing.

Slightly movable joints

Symphyses are joints where the two bony surfaces are faced with hyaline cartilage and united by fibrocartilage. The joint is usually supported by copious ligaments. Symphyses are found in the midline of the body. The symphysis pubis uniting left and right pubic bones is this type; it gives a little in childbirth under the influence of mechanical stress and relaxing hormones. The joints between adjacent vertebral bodies (the **intervertebral discs**) are also symphyses although complicated by the presence of a **nucleus pulposus,** a central mass of fluid (p. 80). The amount of movement at each disc is small but over the total length of the vertebral column adds up to an appreciable amount.

Syndesmoses are joints where bony surfaces are united by ligamentous fibres. Between adjacent vertebrae are two types of syndesmosis. The **ligamentum flavum** uniting the laminae has many elastic fibres. The **interspinous ligaments** and **supraspinous ligaments,** joining the spines, are less elastic.

Freely movable joints

Most **synovial joints** (Fig. 1.5) permit a wide range of free movement. The articulating surfaces are coated with a layer of smooth hyaline cartilage which has a low coefficient of friction. They are recipro-cally curved and are lubricated by synovial fluid, essentially a dialysate of blood plasma. The bones are united by a fibrous capsule arranged like a cuff around the joint. The capsule is often thickened locally to form **intrinsic ligaments.** The synovial fluid is secreted and resorbed by the **synovial membrane** which lines all the intracapsular surfaces except those that are weight-bearing. It is a richly vascular sheet of connective tissue, covered by a layer of flattened synovial cells, and is often folded to increase its effective area. The **synovial cavity** (i.e. the space enclosed by the synovial membrane and articulating cartilages and which is filled with synovial fluid) is often of very small volume. In many cases it is continuous with a **bursa,** a cavity resembling a very slightly inflated balloon with walls formed from synovial membrane. Bursae are not part of a synovial joint but are usually adjacent to one where they form antifriction devices, preventing the rubbing of tendons as they pass over the joint.

Within the synovial cavity are found various inclusions, mainly concerned with improving the fit of the articular surfaces.

Fat pads (covered by synovial membrane) occupy the gaps between bone ends which open up in some positions of the joint. They are readily compressible when the joint moves.

Pieces of fibrous cartilage may appear as **labra, menisci,** or **discs.** A **labrum** is a ring of fibrous cartilage which deepens a bony socket by forming a lip around it. The shoulder joint has a well-developed labrum. A **meniscus** is an incomplete disc or crescent of cartilage which increases the area of the articular surface in a similar fashion. The knee has medial and lateral menisci (Fig. 1.6). A fibrocartilaginous **disc** may completely or almost completely separate a joint cavity into two compartments. Each cavity is then equivalent to an individual synovial joint and the bones involved in these joints may

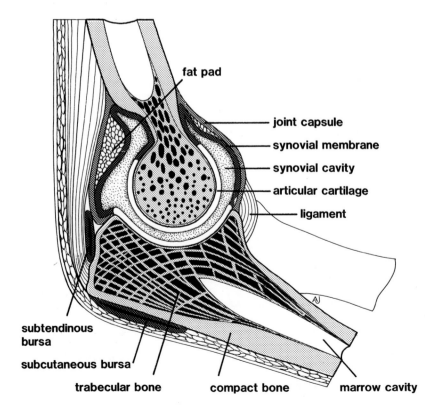

fat pad

joint capsule

synovial membrane

synovial cavity

articular cartilage

ligament

subtendinous bursa

subcutaneous bursa

trabecular bone

compact bone

marrow cavity

Fig. 1.5. Section through a synovial joint. For clarity the distance between the articular cartilages has been exaggerated.

move independently in different axes at the same time. The temporo-mandibular (jaw) joint is subdivided in this way (Fig. 1.6). The weight-bearing parts of a meniscus or disc are not covered by synovial membrane.

Tendons may pass through a joint space, enclosed in their own lubricating sheath. The tendon of one head of biceps brachii passes through the cavity of the shoulder joint in this manner.

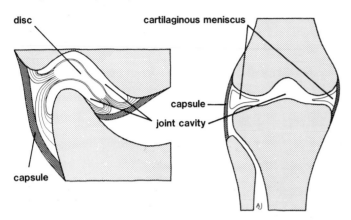

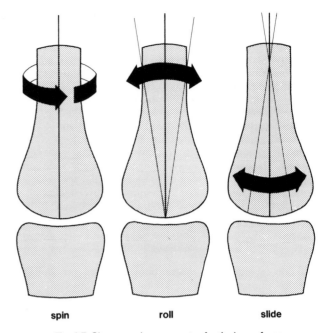

Fig. 1.6. Sections of synovial joints to show a disc (left) and menisci (right).

Fig. 1.7. Shapes and movements of articular surfaces.

Movements at synovial joints

There have been numerous attempts to classify synovial joints, and the movements which can take place at them, on the basis of the shape of their articulating surfaces. This has led to joints being compared to hinges, ball and sockets, and other mechanical devices. Such descriptions are inaccurate and hide the essential unity of synovial joints and the way they move.

In fact, all synovial articular surfaces are sections of ovoids (egg-shaped bodies). One surface is usually convex and the other concave, although in some joints the surfaces may be concave in one direction and convex in the other. The surface which is convex, or predominantly convex, is larger than that which is concave (Fig. 1.7).

The movements which can take place between the articular surfaces are: (i) spin, in which one bone rotates, about its long axis, relative to the other bone; (ii) roll, in which one articular surface moves over the other, rather like a car wheel rolling on the road; and (iii) slide, in which one articular surface slides against the other. These movements are often combined. If the convex surface is moving relative to the concave, it can be seen from Fig. 1.7 that rolling and sliding take place in opposite directions whereas when the concave surface moves relative to the convex, rolling, and sliding take place in the same direction.

Since the articulating surfaces are sections of ovoids, it is obvious that there will be one position of the joint where they fit best (Fig. 1.8). In all other positions the area of contact between the articular surfaces will be less. The position of best fit is called the **close-packed position** and is usually at the end of the range of habitual movement in the position of full extension. As the joint approaches this position, the ligaments of the capsule are stretched and often some spin is imparted to 'screw' the joint home. The close-packed position is thus one of maximum stability. In practice this is closely approached but not achieved so as to avoid stretching the ligaments and

damaging articular surfaces. A joint can be held in the close-packed position (for instance, the extended position of the knee joints) for long periods without discomfort because little muscular effort is necessary to maintain it.

All other positions of the joint are **loose-packed.** The loosely fitting surfaces will allow spin, roll, and slide; the area of contact is reduced, and so is the friction. The continually changing wedge-shaped gaps between the articular surfaces force the synovial fluid to circulate and lubricate the joint. Considerable muscular effort is required to maintain a loose-packed position (compare how much more tiring it is to stand with the knees flexed rather than extended).

Limitation of movement at a joint is necessary if damage is to be avoided. This is controlled in several ways. Ligaments and joint

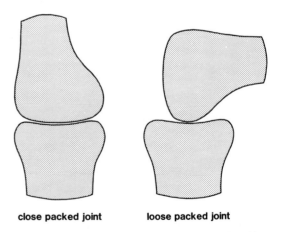

Fig. 1.8. To show the close-packed and loose-packed positions.

capsules contain stretch receptors which feed data into the nervous system about their degree of tension. The tension or tone in the muscles around a joint offers passive resistance to stretch and reflex contraction occurs in response to stimulation of the stretch receptors of the ligaments and capsule. Joint movement is also limited by the extent of the articular surfaces and by the approximation of soft parts, e.g. the arm and forearm when the elbow is flexed. The ligaments and joint capsules contain pain receptors which are stimulated by excessive movement of the joints.

Ligaments

Ligaments are well-defined bands or cords of fibrous tissue usually connecting two bones. Most are developed to resist or limit the movement of a joint in a certain direction. **Intrinsic** ligaments are local thickenings of the joint capsule, **extrinsic** ligaments are completely isolated from the capsule. In some cases ligaments are thought to be laid down by fibroblasts in response to stresses tending to pull bones apart; other ligaments merely close over a notch, converting it to a foramen or join two parts of the same bone and therefore cannot be under stress. You will also come across structures termed ligaments which are no such thing because in the past the term has been loosely applied to tendinous muscle attachments, remnants of embryonic structures, and peritoneal folds connecting viscera.

Clinical aspects

When a joint moves beyond its normal range, so that the articular surfaces are no longer in their normal relationship, it is said to be dislocated. Some joints (e.g. temporomandibular and shoulder) are particularly susceptible to dislocation because of poor support by ligaments, poor fit of articular surfaces, and weak supporting musculature. Dislocations are reduced by performing manoeuvres designed to relocate the joint without causing damage to surrounding structures. Dislocation of the temporomandibular joint is usually a sequel of yawning, when the mouth is opened very wide. It is reduced by pressing the lower molar teeth down and then back (taking care to avoid being bitten by the patient).

Cartilaginous menisci in a joint are liable to damage, especially if the joint is weight-bearing like the knee. Tears in the menisci allow portions to be caught and ground between the bones which increases the damage and may lock the joint. In the well-known 'cartilage operation' of professional sportsmen, the damaged meniscus is removed from the knee joint, often with little or no subsequent disability.

In certain diseases of the nervous system (e.g. syringomyelia) pain sensation from a joint may be lost and no message is received when a joint is overextended. The resulting abuse may severely damage the joint.

Synovial joints may become infected (arthritis) following trauma or due to the spread of micro-organisms from a nearby focus or from a distant lesion through the bloodstream.

A common disorder of synovial joints in the elderly, especially of those joints that bear much stress, is osteoarthrosis. In this condition the articular cartilage is destroyed and movement at the joint becomes restricted and painful. Its cause is unknown.

Irritation of the synovial membrane is usually followed by rapid production of large quantities of synovial fluid causing painful swelling of the joint (as in a sprain) or bursa (bursitis) concerned.

MUSCLES

Types of muscle

Muscle is a contractile tissue and is divided into three types according to its histological appearance. **Striated** or **skeletal muscle** makes up the large muscle masses of the body which are attached directly or indirectly to the skeleton. **Smooth** or **visceral muscle** is found in the walls of hollow viscera, such as the gut and blood vessels. **Cardiac muscle,** also striated but histologically distinguishable from skeletal muscle, is confined to the heart. Skeletal muscle is often termed voluntary because it is usually under the control of the will. This is not always the case however. The diaphragm, for example, is made up of skeletal muscle but does not normally function under voluntary control. Smooth muscle is not generally under conscious control and is often referred to as involuntary.

Smooth muscle

Smooth muscle is usually found in sheets, either flat or rolled into a cylinder as part of the wall of a hollow tubular viscus. Alternatively, it may form a sphincter which closes off the end of the viscus. In many sites smooth muscle occurs as two concentric cylinders with differing fibre orientation, often spoken of as the circular and longitudinal muscle layers. Smooth muscle contracts relatively slowly, but is able to maintain a contracted state over long periods without fatigue.

Striated muscle

Striated muscle is usually attached to bone, although not always directly. Muscles pass from one bone to another across a movable joint (sometimes more than one) so that contraction of the muscle results in movement at the joint. The nerve to a muscle usually gives a sensory branch to the joint which the muscle moves and another to the skin over the joint (**Hilton's law**).

Skeletal muscles are attached at **origins** and **insertions.** It is conventional to call the more proximal end of the muscle, or the end that moves least, the origin and the other end the insertion. In fact, a muscle may act from origin to insertion or vice versa. Within the muscle distinct regions can often be recognized. The **fleshy belly** is made up of contractile fibres which are well-vascularized and have a high metabolic rate. They are, however, poorly adapted to resist pressure or friction. The remainder of the muscle, the **tendon,** is made up of non-contractile inelastic, poorly vascularized connective tissue, which is excellent in resisting friction.

The attachment of a muscle may, therefore, be of two types. A **fleshy** attachment is large in area and the pull acting through such a large area is diffuse. A **tendinous** insertion is much smaller in cross-sectional area and thus the pull exerted is more localized. Because of this localization tendinous attachments often raise crests or ridges on the bones to which they attach. Tendons are made up of collagen fibres which resist stretch but are flexible so that they are able to pass around pulley arrangements to change direction. Because of their low vascularity they appear white and take the form of cords or strips or of laminated flat sheets termed **aponeuroses.** The fibres of a tendon are arranged in bundles, often large enough to be seen with the naked eye. They are not strictly parallel but intertwine, so that a single area in the fleshy muscle body is represented everywhere in the tendinous insertion. As the angle of a joint changes, different parts of the tendon take the pull; this arrangement ensures that full muscle power is available at all times. Tendons are functionally continuous with the outer layer (periosteum) of the bone to which they are attached, often passing through a pad of fibrocartilage *en route*.

When a tendon must move independently of surrounding tissues it is enclosed in a **synovial sheath**. A synovial sheath is structurally similar to the synovial bursa already mentioned in connection with joints. A bursa can be pictured as a slightly inflated balloon but containing a small quantity of lubricating synovial fluid instead of air (Fig. 1.9). If this is interposed, as bursae often are, between a tendon and a bone at a point of potential friction, the friction will be considerably reduced. The friction-reducing properties of such a system can be improved in two ways. First the bursa may be enlonged so that it separates tendon and cause of friction over a considerable length (often a matter of several centimetres). Secondly the bursa may be wrapped around the tendon so as to protect it on all sides. Such a wrapped and elongated bursa is a synovial sheath. The gap between the two adjacent edges of the bursa provides a line of entry for blood vessels and nerves supplying the tendon.

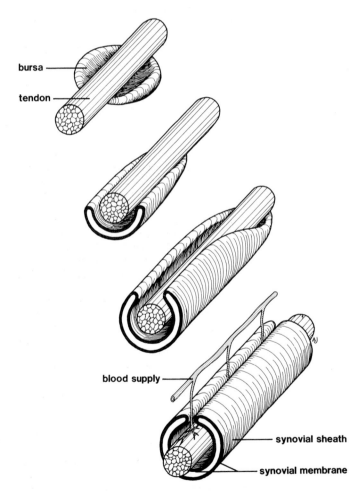

Fig. 1.9. Development of a synovial sheath around a tendon.

Form and function in striated muscles

There is a wide functional variation in the size and shape of muscles and in the arrangement of their constituent fibres. The size of muscle fibres ranges from 10 to 100 μm in diameter and their resting length up to 30 cm. Precision muscles, such as those controlling the fine movements of the hand or eye, have many fine fibres per unit mass; power muscles, such as those of the lower limb or buttock, have fewer coarser fibres in each unit of mass. In precision muscles the **motor unit** (the number of muscle fibres innervated by a single nerve fibre) is small; in power muscles the motor unit is large. Hence, precision muscles, as their name indicates, are under fine control whereas power muscles can generate plenty of power, but with little precision. Motor nerve fibres end on muscles fibres at **motor end plates,** accumulations of muscle cytoplasm rich in mitochondria and nuclei upon which the terminal branches of the nerve fibre ramify.

When muscle fibres contract they shorten by between one-third and one-half of their resting length. The degree of shortening of a whole muscle belly is determined by the **length** of its individual muscle fibres. The power of a muscle belly, on the other hand, is dependent upon the **mass** (number and diameter) of the muscle fibres it contains.

The simplest fibre arrangement is found in the **strap muscles** (Fig. 1.10). The strap may be broad or narrow and its fibres may run from end to end of the muscle, or there may be intermediate tendinous regions. Strap muscles generally have a good range of contraction

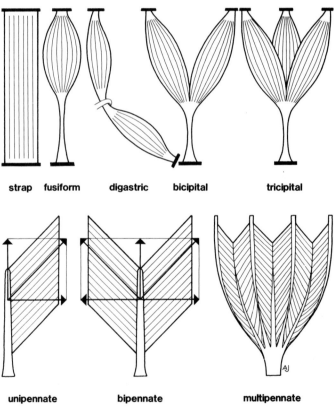

strap   fusiform   digastric   bicipital   tricipital

unipennate   bipennate   multipennate

Fig. 1.10. Types of muscles and arrangements of fibres. The force vectors are indicated for the unipennate and bipennate arrangements.

but their power is limited because of the relatively small number of fibres which they incorporate. The fibre mass is increased in **fusiform** muscles. Such muscles often have a large number of fibres converging at one end into a tendon. Sometimes there are two fusiform muscle 'bellies' connected with each other by an intermediate tendon (**digastric** muscles); sometimes muscle bodies from two or more origins are attached to a single tendon of insertion (**bicipital** or **tricipital** muscles).

Another way in which the mass of muscle fibres can be increased is by the fibres being inserted into the side rather than the end of a tendon. This arrangement is called **unipennate** because of its resemblance to a feather. Many more fibres can be packed in by this arrangement but the resultant force along the tendon is composed of two vectors because of the angulated pull. This means that (a) some force is wasted and (b) the wasted force is directed at right angles to the tendon making it pull off line. If fibres are attached in equal numbers on each side of the tendon (**bipennate**), the unwanted components cancel each other out. Often bipennate units are joined together to form a **multipennate** muscle. Pennate muscles are powerful but because the length of the individual muscle fibres is short they have a limited range of contraction.

Muscles do not suddenly snap from a state of relaxation to a state of contraction. At any given time some of the motor units will be contracting, some relaxing, some at rest and some under stimulation. The net result of this continuous activity is **muscle tone** and, if the proportion of units in each state does not change, muscle tone will be constant although individual units will be cycling constantly.

When an individual motor unit contracts, it tends to approximate its ends, but whether or not this results in muscle contraction depends on the magnitude of the force relative to the forces opposing contraction. The latter comprise (i) the passive internal resistance of the muscle itself; (ii) the resistance of articular tissues; (iii) opposing muscles (if a flexor is to contract, extensors must relax); (iv) opposing soft tissues; (v) inertia of the segment to be moved; (vi) load on the segment to be moved; (vii) gravity. If the force generated when a number of units contracts exceeds the sum of these opposing forces, then the joint is accelerated from rest. Once accelerated to the necessary velocity, a smaller number of units will produce enough force to maintain the movement just as accelerating a car requires firm pressure on the accelerator and heavy fuel use, while once the required speed is reached the pedal can be partially released and the fuel consumption lowered.

Most movements are thus produced by throwing a greater number of units into contraction in a **prime mover** or **agonist** and relaxing any opposing muscles or **antagonists.** When a prime mover contracts, its antagonists undergo a variable brief twitch, then remain passive until movement is almost completed, when they contract strongly to end the movement. This is equivalent to a boatman allowing a rope to run freely round a bollard, then immobilizing it once the boat is in the required position. If prime mover and antagonist act together across a joint, they will lock it solid, or **stabilize** it. This may be used when stabilization cannot be achieved by close packing of the joint or by gravity which are preferred as energy conserving measures. Movements are always helped or hindered by gravity and this is turned to advantage when possible. In lowering a weight on to a table, the extensor of the elbow is not triceps but gravity, the movement being controlled by slow 'paying out' of the flexors of the elbow.

Because of the complexity of joint shapes and of the mechanical and topographical factors governing muscle insertions, the prime mover often generates a little spin or other unwanted movement. This is opposed by **synergists,** muscles helping other muscles during the course of a movement. Obviously a single muscle may be involved in several movements and play different roles; it may be a prime mover, synergist, fixator, or antagonist at different times.

Innervation of striated muscles

About 60 per cent of the fibres in a nerve supplying a muscle are motor. The remaining 40 per cent are sensory.

Many of the motor fibres are the large diameter, heavily myelinated axons of the **alpha motor neurons** whose cell bodies are located in the ventral grey horn of the spinal cord. Within the muscles these axons divide into a number of branches, each of which ends on an individual muscle fibre at a **motor end plate.**

Scattered within the muscle belly are the **neuromuscular spindles.** These consist of a small number of fine **intrafusal** muscle fibres enclosed within a connective tissue capsule and lying parallel to the extrafusal fibres making up the main bulk of the muscle. The intrafusal fibres are innervated by the small diameter, myelinated axons of the **gamma motor neurons** whose cell bodies are again located in the ventral grey horn.

Many of the sensory fibres to the muscle end in the neuromuscular spindles. The endings are of two types: (i) *annulospiral endings* arranged around the equator of the spindle; and (ii) *flower-spray endings* arranged in a band either side of the equator. The function of the neuromuscular spindles is to supply the central nervous system with proprioceptive information about the state of contraction of the muscle.

Simple muscle mechanics

Consider a simple flexor muscle acting on a joint (Fig. 1.11). If one bone is fixed, contraction of the muscle will move the other. Now suppose that the distal attachment or insertion of the muscle is a little off-centre. The pull exerted by the muscle can be resolved into three components: (i) swing – tending to move the mobile bone; (ii) shunt – tending to stabilize the joint; and (iii) spin – rotating the mobile bone.

The relative size of each component can be varied by moving the attachments of the muscle. A muscle attached close to the joint on the mobile bone but remote from the joint on the stable bone (a **spurt** muscle) maximizes swing and is best for the initiation of movement. Conversely a muscle attached remote from the joint on the mobile bone but close to the joint on the stable bone (a **shunt** muscle) maximizes compression of the joint and hence stability. A muscle producing spin may be used either as a prime mover (e.g. in pronation or supination of the forearm) or as a synergistic force.

It is, of course, a great oversimplification to think about muscles one at a time. Most movements which we perform are a result of the concerted actions of groups of muscles. These groups may be physically close together and act over the same joint or they may be separate and help to control different phases of a complex of movements involving several joints.

Clinical aspects

Because of their poor blood supply, tendons heal slowly when damaged. Thus a severed Achilles tendon in the heel (usually caused by exertion of too much force) is a serious injury. A torn tendon requires prompt attention because immediately after the injury the

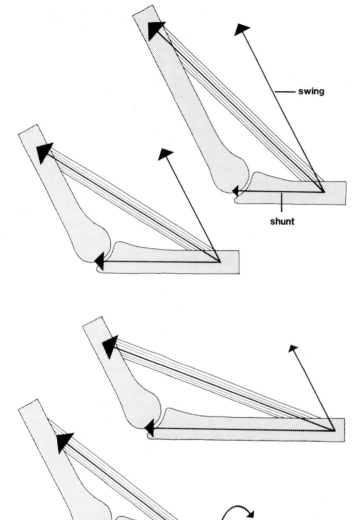

Fig. 1.11. Muscle mechanics.

THE NERVOUS SYSTEM

Our remote ancestors were probably a type of segmented worm. Each segment, a repeat of the one ahead and the one behind, was a fairly self-contained slice of the body. The muscle of each such segment is termed a **myotome,** the skeleton a **sclerotome,** and the skin a **dermatome.**

Since then, much modification has occurred. The presence of a head at the anterior end of the body, the part that enters a new environment first, has meant a concentration of sense organs there and an accumulation of nervous tissue, the **brain,** to deal with information received from them. In order to link the segmental nerves of the trunk with the brain, a large nerve cord (the spinal cord) has developed along the dorsal aspect of the trunk. Despite the modifications consequent upon the development of the head and also of limbs and tail, the legacy of segmentation persists in all modern vertebrates. The trunk, for example, still contains segmental structures, such as vertebrae, ribs, and segmental muscles, and the arrangement of the spinal nerves still clearly reflects the segmentation of our ancestors (as is most readily apparent from the dermatome pattern, the areas of skin supplied by particular spinal nerves – Fig. 1.12).

The principal function of the nervous system is conduction, and its basic cell unit, the **neuron,** is well adapted for this function. Neurons have a **cell body,** a **dendrite** or **dendrites,** processes transmitting impulses towards the cell body, and an **axon,** a process transmitting impulses from the cell body (Figs. 5.1 and 5.2, p. 222). The processes may be extremely long. Neurons are very active cells and accordingly have large energy requirements. These, and other requirements, are served by the **neuroglia,** the supporting cells of the nervous system.

The nervous system may be divided into the **central nervous system,** comprising the brain and spinal cord, and the **peripheral nervous system,** the rest. A cross-section through the thoracic spinal cord (Fig. 1.13) shows two main tissue types. In the centre is an

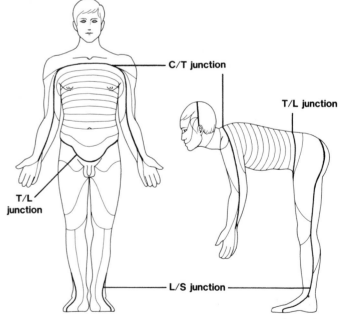

Fig. 1.12. Dermatomes (C = cervical; T = thoracic; L = lumbar; S = sacral).

severed ends move away from each other and are resistant to being replaced. Infection of a bursa (bursitis) or a tendon sheath (tenosynovitis) is accompanied by pain due to swelling of the sheath. Inflammation of tendinous sheaths may also occur without infection following a period spent doing an unaccustomed repetitive task where a sheath is in continual use.

A muscle which is paralysed by loss of its nerve supply will become flaccid and undergo irreversible atrophy. Muscles which are not used (as in the bed-ridden) will also atrophy but in this case the atrophy is potentially reversible. Muscles which are much used tend to increase in size and power. This is caused by hypertrophy of the individual muscle fibres, not by an increase in their number.

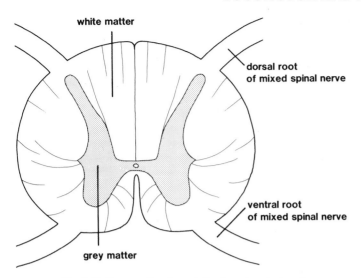

Fig. 1.13. Cross-section through the thoracic spinal cord.

H-shaped mass of **grey matter** continuous along the length of the cord and made up of accumulations of cell bodies. Around the periphery of the H is **white matter** made up largely of nerve fibres wrapped in **myelin** which reflects the light and makes the fibres appear white. Confusingly, some neurological stains turn this myelin black.

The brain is the expanded head end of the spinal cord. The arrangement of the grey and white matter seen in the cord can be traced upwards into the brainstem, the most caudal part of the brain, for a short distance but then becomes obscured by the development of new structures peculiar to this part of the nervous system. The rostral part of the brain has become greatly expanded, especially in man, to form the cerebral hemispheres. These structures play a major part in higher functions of the brain.

The two types of fibres connecting the central nervous system with the remainder of the body, **afferents** (or sensory fibres) coming in and **efferents** (or motor fibres) going out, are anatomically separated. In each segment of the spinal cord and brainstem the dorsal part of the grey matter is associated, on each side, with an afferent, or **dorsal**

root, containing fibres entering the cord. The ventral part of the grey matter is associated with an efferent, or **ventral root.** Each pair of dorsal and ventral roots in the spinal region unites to form a **mixed** (because it is both afferent and efferent) **spinal nerve.** In the cranial region the dorsal and ventral roots do not unite but remain as separate structures, the **cranial nerves.**

A simple illustration of the co-ordination of the sensory and motor sides of the nervous system is provided by a three-neuron reflex arc (Fig. 1.14). The peripheral process, or dendrite, of the sensory neuron runs from a receptor organ in the skin of the dermatome via the mixed spinal nerve to the point where dorsal and ventral roots are joined. The dendrite passes into the dorsal root to reach a swelling, the **spinal** or **dorsal root ganglion.** Here is located the cell body of the neuron. The dendrite and the axon of the sensory neurons are fused for a short distance close to their attachment to the cell body (the **pseudo-unipolar** arrangement). The impulse leaves the cell body via the axon which runs into the dorsal part of the spinal cord where it may terminate in a variety of ways. One route for the impulse to travel is through a **synapse** (a junction between two nerve processes across which the impulse can pass) to a **connector neuron.** The dendrites of the connector neuron are adjacent to the axon of the sensory neuron. Its cell body is in the dorsal horn and its axon passes to the ventral horn. Here are further synapses with the dendrites of the third link in the chain, an **alpha motor neuron,** whose cell body is in the **ventral horn** and whose axon passes out via the ventral root to the mixed spinal nerve and finally terminates in a muscle derived from the myotome of the segment. Our chosen sensory imput was in the skin of the trunk, but a similar pathway could also be traced from a receptor in a muscle, a tendon, or a joint capsule. In some cases the sensory neuron may connect directly with the motor neuron to form a monosynaptic reflex arc. In other cases the reflex arcs contain numerous connector neurons which pass between several segments of the central nervous system. In addition reflex arcs are acted upon by tracts of nerve fibres descending from centres in the brain and which may modify the reflex response greatly.

Autonomic nervous system

So far we have dealt principally with the part of the nervous system concerned with responses to external stimuli. A major part of the nervous system, however, is concerned with the control of the internal environment. This is the autonomic division and consists of efferent pathways from the central nervous system to the viscera (i.e. the cardiovascular, respiratory, alimentary, and urogenital systems) and a number of other structures (see p. 26) and also of centres and pathways within the brain and spinal cord. It can be divided into two parts, the **sympathetic system** and the **parasympathetic system,** on anatomical and functional grounds. The sympathetic system leaves the central nervous system in the central part of the body between the first thoracic (T1) and the second or third lumbar segments (L.2, L.3) of the spinal cord. The parasympathetic system leaves from the brain (in certain of the cranial nerves) and from the sacral part of the cord. There are also afferent fibres supplying the viscera but the term autonomic is usually restricted to just the efferent fibres defined above.

In both autonomic divisions the efferent neurons which leave the central nervous system synapse in a peripheral autonomic ganglion with a second neuron which passes from the ganglion to the organ being supplied. These two efferent fibres are called respectively **pre-**

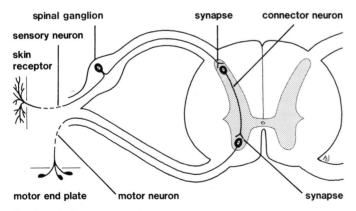

Fig. 1.14. A three-neuron reflex arc. The dendrites of the connector and motor neurons are not shown.

ganglionic and **postganglionic.** Many of the sympathetic ganglia are arranged in two chains, the **sympathetic trunks,** situated on the posterior wall of the trunk, one either side of the vertebral column. The parasympathetic ganglia are situated in an irregular fashion close to the viscera being supplied.

Stimulation of the sympathetic nervous system prepares the body for an emergency. It accelerates the heart, constricts the peripheral blood vessels and raises the blood pressure, thus bringing about a redistribution of the blood so that it leaves the skin and intestines and becomes available to the brain, heart, and skeletal muscles. It also inhibits peristalsis in the digestive tract and closes the sphincters. The parasympathetic nervous system reverses these trends to conserve and restore energy. It slows the heart, increases peristalsis and glandular activity and opens sphincters. Because of these essentially opposite effects, we often find dual innervation to a structure (for example, the heart) from sympathetic and parasympathetic systems. Under normal circumstances the two systems act in concert to maintain an appropriate level of visceral activity.

Clinical aspects

In the trunk the dermatomes overlap considerably, so that complete anaesthesia of a skin area often involves the interruption of sensory pathways in two or three nerve roots. With the help of a pin or cotton wool the function of a particular nerve can be checked if the dermatome pattern is known. Most muscles are innervated segmentally by fibres from two or three segments of the spinal cord. These fibres, although of different segmental origin, commonly run together as the 'nerve' of the muscle. To paralyse a muscle completely it is necessary for several segments of the spinal cord to be damaged. The integrity of segments of the cord can be tested by eliciting simple reflex response from a limited number of muscles (the well-known knee jerk, for instance, tests the second to fourth lumbar segments).

Severing of a spinal nerve will produce anaesthesia of the skin innervated by that nerve, complete paralysis, with wasting and absent reflexes, of the corresponding muscles and loss of sympathetic effectors to such structures as sweat glands. In all cases regeneration is possible from the sections of the nerve fibres still attached to their cell bodies. The regenerative nerve processes grow along the myelin sheaths vacated by degenerating cell processes isolated from their cell bodies. Regeneration is unselective and only successful if the regenerating processes reach the right kind of end organs. A dendrite growing back to the skin will not be able to function if it is re-routed to a muscle, for instance. Regeneration is thus always less than perfect.

The autonomic nervous system is open to modification by drugs and surgery. Blood pressure may be lowered by the administration of drugs which affect the functioning of the sympathetic ganglia and lead to vasodilation of the peripheral blood vessels. Sectioning the sympathetic nerve supply to a limb will have the same effect, and may increase blood supply sufficiently to compensate for the obstruction of an artery due to disease.

3

Circulatory system

The circulatory system has two interrelated but distinct parts, the cardiovascular system which circulates blood around the body and the lymphatic system which returns excess fluid from the tissues to the heart.

CARDIOVASCULAR SYSTEM

The blood vascular system comprises the heart, a muscular pump, and the blood vessels (arteries, capillaries, and veins). The circulatory system probably exhibits more variability than any other. In the embryo, after the stage of blood formation, the tissues resemble a blood-filled sponge, an intricate network comprising many vessels. During development this is reduced to form fewer vessels but exactly which vessels are preserved and which are eliminated is by no means constant. There is also a good deal of relative movement of structures during development; the plasticity of the vascular system is indicated by the fact that a structure on the move obtains its blood supply locally and may have several blood supplies *en route*. Its nerve supply, by contrast, is never altered; wherever the organ migrates it takes its original nerve supply with it. The kidney is a good example of this, being supplied by ever more dorsal branches of the dorsal aorta as it 'ascends' during development. One or more of these embryonic supplies may persist as 'abnormal' renal arteries.

Heart

The heart comprises two muscular pumps arranged in parallel and beating in unison. The right side of the heart receives deoxygenated blood from the body and transmits it to the lungs; the left side receives oxygenated blood from the lungs and transmits it to the body. The blood, therefore, passes alternately round a lesser **pulmonary circulation** and a greater **systemic circulation** (Fig. 1.15). To serve these circuits each side of the heart has a thin-walled receiver, the **atrium,** and a thick-walled dispatcher, the **ventricle.** The pulmonary circuit comprises right atrium → right ventricle → pulmonary arteries → pulmonary capillaries → pulmonary veins (→ left atrium); the systemic circuit comprises left atrium → left ventricle → aorta → arteries → capillaries → veins → venae cavae (→ right atrium). Over a period of time the right atrium receives the same volume of blood as the left ventricle supplies to the aorta. Although the capacity of the two ventricles is similar (60–70 ml), the resistance offered by the pulmonary circulation is less than that offered by the systemic. The wall of the right ventricle is, therefore, considerably thinner than that of the left.

Systemic circulation

The main systemic artery, the **aorta,** is about 30 mm in diameter. It gives off numerous branches which, in turn, branch repeatedly, the

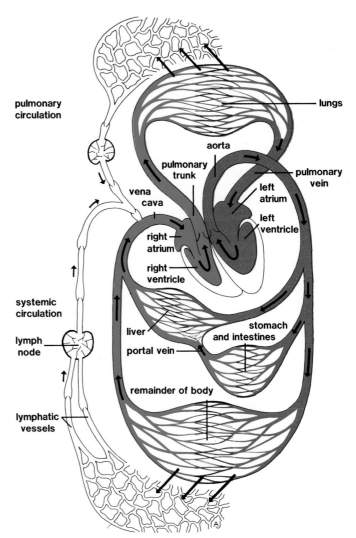

Fig. 1.15. Diagrammatic view of the blood and lymph circulation.

branches becoming progressively smaller in diameter as they become more numerous. The smallest vessels visible to the naked eye (**arterioles,** about 0.3 mm diameter) break up into **capillaries** 0.5–1 mm long and each wide enough to admit a single file of red blood cells (7 μm). The capillaries reunite to form **venules** which in turn are tributaries of **veins.**

The larger arteries form a low-volume, high-pressure **distributing system.** Arteries have smooth muscle and elastic connective tissue in their walls. Very large arteries near the heart have a very high proportion of elastic tissue which allows some distension as each gout of blood is pumped out of the heart and then recoils, so helping to even out the pressure in the great vessels. Smaller arteries further from the heart have a greater proportion of smooth muscle. The diameter of these muscular arteries is accurately monitored by sensors in their walls and controlled by the autonomic nervous system so as to regulate blood flow according to temperature, body activity, etc. Blood flow at a more intimate level is controlled by **resistance vessels,** muscular arterioles ending in **precapillary sphincters** of smooth muscle, which provide the chief resistance to blood flow. The blood then enters a reticulum of **exchange vessels,** the **capillaries** and **postcapillary venules.** Capillaries may be **plain** with complete walls, **fenestrated** with incomplete walls (allowing the passage of white blood cells) or **sinusoidal** with a tortuous course which slows down the flow of blood allowing maximum opportunity for the exchange between blood and tissues of oxygen, carbon dioxide, nutrients, water, inorganic salts, vitamins, hormones, and immunological substances. The venules unite into a network of low-pressure, high-volume **capacitance vessels,** the veins, through which blood returns to the heart. Veins are larger in cross-sectional area than arteries and have a correspondingly lower rate of flow. Veins accompanying an artery, **venae commitantes,** are often paired so as to provide sufficient cross-sectional area and to allow for the fact that they are easily compressed by surrounding tissues. For this reason venae commitantes or a network of anstomosing veins are common on the flexor side of joints where a single vessel would be particularly liable to interruption during postural changes. Because of their compressibility veins are absent from the superficial tissues in areas subjected to pressure. Compare the venous network on the back of your hand with the palm where no veins are visible.

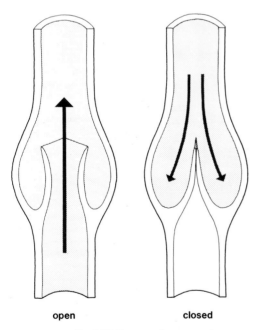

open   closed

Fig. 1.16. Venous valves.

Veins are often surrounded by a dead space occupied by a little connective tissue into which they can expand when full of blood. Venous pressure is so low that even gravity can interfere with the flow of blood back to the heart. In areas where the venous return is against gravity, reverse flow is presented by the presence of venous valves (Fig. 1.16). These simple pocket valves allow flow towards the heart but fill with blood and occlude the lumen of the vessel if reverse flow starts. Venous return is aided by the 'milking action' produced by the contraction and relaxation of the muscles around the vessels. Clearly the presence of valves is essential if this milking action is to move the blood in the required direction only. Valves are plentiful in the veins of the limbs but are few in number in the head and neck.

Portal circulation

A portal circulation differs from that already described in having two capillary beds. The main portal system in the body, the **hepatic portal system,** drains the stomach, small and large intestine (except the anal region), pancreas, spleen, and gall bladder. Blood which passed through the capillary beds of these organs drains into the **portal vein** which enters the liver. Here the blood passes through a second capillary bed before returning to the heart. The system allows the transfer of the products of digestion, absorbed in the first capillary bed, to the liver. A second portal system serves the pituitary gland.

Anastomoses

Arteries do not always end in capillaries. They often unite at **anastomoses,** which may occur between branches of equal or unequal size. Anastomoses increase in frequency with increasing distance from the heart and decreasing arterial diameter. In fact, they are so common in the smaller arteries that the latter form a branching network. Anastomoses provide for equalization of pressure and allow an alternative source of supply. They are especially common around joints where postural changes might occlude a single artery. If an artery is slowly blocked by a disease process other pathways may form a **collateral circulation** which is adequate to prevent tissue damage. A sudden blockage may cause **avascular necrosis** if the collateral circulation is inadequate or non-existent. **End arteries** have no anastomoses. The central artery of the retina and the arteries of the kidneys are end arteries. The **coronary arteries** supplying the muscle of the heart wall have **potential anastomoses** between them which are capable of opening up to some degree if the blockage of a major vessel takes place slowly but not if it occurs suddenly.

Vascular shunts

In many areas blood may be routed from artery to vein without passing through part or all of the capillary bed. Capillaries may be arranged as branches from a main channel which links terminal arterioles with venules. Each side branch has a precapillary sphincter. At times of low demand most of these sphincters will be closed and only a small part of the capillary bed irrigated. With increasing demand more and more sphincters will be opened. A main channel and its tributaries constitute a **microcirculatory unit.** In other cases a direct **arteriovenous anastomosis** between the smaller arteries and veins may be present, often coiled and with a thick muscular coat and a narrow lumen. The lumen may be closed off completely by the muscle of the wall, thus forcing blood to pass through the capillary bed. When open much of the blood flows directly from artery to vein, bypassing the capillary bed. The anastomoses in the skin play an important part in temperature regulation. These devices are few and poorly developed in the newborn and atrophy during old age, accounting for the poor temperature control in people at the extremes of life.

Pulmonary circulation

The general arrangement and structure of the pulmonary circulation are similar in essence to those of the systemic circulation. The principal difference, of functional significance, is the absence in the lung of vessels corresponding to the arterioles of the systemic circulation, the terminal arteries opening directly into the capillary bed. This is reflected in the limited capacity for controlling the distribution of blood flow within the lungs.

Clinical aspects

One of the commonest diseases of the circulatory system is hypertension or raised blood pressure. Blood pressure depends on the balance between the output of the heart and the peripheral resistance. In the healthy it is increased on exercise by increased cardiac output. In essential hypertension the cardiac output is normal but peripheral resistance increased. The condition is often difficult to diagnose due to the wide range of normal blood pressures found in a sample of healthy people of the same age and sex. Many patients diagnosed as hypertensive die from old age or other causes after a long and healthy life. Blood pressure can be controlled by supplying drugs which interfere with the autonomic nervous system, thus dilating blood vessels. Features of untreated hypertension can include enlargement of the left ventricle, which has more work to do, increase in size and thickening of the walls of blood vessels, headaches from thickened blood vessels in the brain, and eventual damage to kidney tissue which is fatal if untreated. It is also associated with an increased risk of stroke and heart attack.

The commonest cause of death in developed countries today is atherosclerosis, a degenerative change in the vessel wall which may lead to partial or complete occlusion of the lumen. This disease may attack any artery but is particulary prevalent in the coronary arteries. The resulting diminished blood supply to the heart muscle causes severe cramp-like pains, called angina, or, if the blockage is complete, death of a segment of the heart wall (myocardial infarction, usually known as a 'heart attack' or 'coronary', see p. 98). The causes are unknown but there is evidence that too much animal fat in the diet and smoking may be implicated. The symptoms are usually, though by no means always, confined to those over 50 but fatty streaks are often present in the arteries of the newborn. Blockage of the cerebral arteries may lead to dementia if gradual or a stroke if rapid.

Veins may be blocked by thrombi (clots). In superficial veins they cause phlebitis, inflammation of the vessel walls; in deep veins they are potentially more serious because of the risk of the clot breaking up and being transported elsewhere (notably to the lungs, brain, or heart). These thrombi are most common in the large venous sinuses of the soleus muscle in the calf in immobilized subjects such as patients in bed. Anticoagulants are often given after operations to decrease the risk of thrombosis occurring.

Varicose veins are a common, painful, and disfiguring condition in which the vessels become irregularly dilated, tortuous, and lengthened. The condition is commonest in the lower limb due to incompetence of venous valves allowing reflux and stasis of blood. This stasis may lead to ulceration.

LYMPHATIC SYSTEM

The tissue fluid which bathes the cells and fibres of the body is a clear fluid formed from the plasma of the capillary blood. The cells obtain their nutrients from the tissue fluid and excrete their waste products into it. There is a constant turnover of metabolites between the tissue fluid and the blood in the capillaries. Most of the tissue fluid returns to the capillaries and venules, but 10–20 per cent does not, and remains in the tissues. As fluid is constantly leaving the circulatory system and entering the tissues, the latter would rapidly become water-logged were the excess fluid not drained away. This excess fluid is collected by **lymph capillaries** which co-exist with blood capillaries in the capillary beds. They are especially plentiful in the skin and mucous membranes. Lymph capillaries drain into larger lymph channels which are thin-walled vessels, 0.5–1 mm in diameter, and beaded by frequent valves. Although more numerous than veins, the lymph channels tend to follow the same course and drain the same territories.

All the lymph vessels, except those from the right side of the head, neck, and thorax, and from the right upper limb, eventually drain into the **thoracic duct.** This begins below the diaphragm and ascends through the thorax to empty into the junction of the left internal jugular and subclavian veins (Fig. 3.34, p. 100). Lymph from the right side of the head, neck, thorax, and right upper limb drains into the **right lymphatic duct** which opens into the junction of right internal jugular and subclavian veins.

Lymph is usually colourless. However, the lymph vessels draining the gut may be white with emulsified fat and those draining the lungs may be black with carbon particles. Lymph vessels commonly contain phagocytic cells which enter tissue spaces from the bloodstream and return via the lymphatics. These will ingest bacteria and other foreign bodies *en route*. Lymph flow is normally maintained by a mixture of active contraction of the smooth muscle in the walls of the lymph vessels and intermittent muscular pressure exerted on

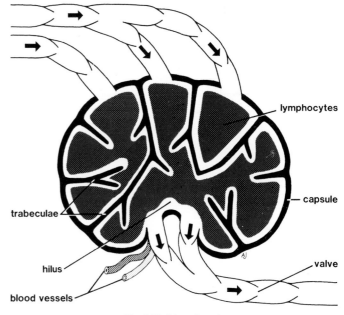

Fig. 1.17. A lymph node.

the valved vessels during movement. Negative or positive pressure generated in the thorax and abdomen during breathing may also play a part.

Along the course of lymphatic vessels are numerous **lymph nodes** (Fig. 1.17), so arranged that lymph traverses at least one set of nodes between capillary bed and bloodstream, although exceptions occur (e.g. the thyroid and oesophagus where some lymph drains directly into the thoracic duct). Nodes are small, bean-shaped bodies. One side has a slight depression, the **hilus,** through which blood vessels enter and efferent blood and lymph vessels leave. Afferent lymph vessels enter around the periphery of the node. The node is surrounded by a fibrous capsule which sends radial trabeculae into its substance. Between these trabeculae are masses of densely packed dividing lymphocytes. Lymph is thus exposed to lymphocytes on a large scale before it regains the circulation.

Clinical aspects

Paradoxically the lymphatic system, as well as being a site of phago-cytic and immune response, can also act as a distributor of disease throughout the body. Malignant cells may spread (metastasize) from a primary tumour to other areas, especially the lymph nodes, where secondary tumours may be formed. Carcinoma cells may spread, for example, from a primary tumour in the breast via the lymphatic drainage to the lymph nodes of the axilla and neck as well as to the contralateral breast. The lymphatic system itself may become the primary site of malignant disease (e.g. leukaemia and Hodgkin's disease).

An infected puncture wound to the skin of a finger or elsewhere is commonplace. The infection may spread through lymphatic channels, which become inflamed (lymphangitis) and reddened and hence visible, to lymph nodes which become inflamed (lymphadenitis), swollen, and palpable.

Lymph vessels can also be blocked by parasitic infection. *Microfilaris nocturna* is a tropical nematode worm whose hosts are man and mosquito. The adult worm thrives in the protein-rich, well-buffered, warm lymph and lays numerous eggs in the lymphatics, blocking them and causing gross swelling of affected parts (elephantiasis).

4

Respiratory and digestive systems

RESPIRATORY SYSTEM

Air passages

Air enters the body through the nose, where it is warmed by the copious blood supply of the nasal mucosa and filtered by hairs. It then passes via the **pharynx** to the **larynx** which guards the entrance to the lower respiratory tract. The narrowest part of the larynx lies between the vocal folds. These can be moved together or apart and their length and tension changed. Originally evolved as a sphincter, they have taken on the additional function of sound production.

The larynx opens below into the **trachea,** a tube kept open by incomplete rings of cartilage and lying immediately in front of the oesophagus. The trachea divides into right and left **main bronchi.** These enter the lung (the right bronchus dividing into two before doing so) where they undergo repeated branching. The final and smallest branches, the **bronchioles,** connect with extremely thin-walled sacs, the **alveoli** (Fig. 1.18). Cartilaginous elements are found in the walls of all branches of the respiratory tree greater than about

1 mm in diameter. Smaller branches have walls of smooth muscle with no cartilaginous components. The alveoli are interconnected by pores and are intimately related to a rich capillary network fed by branches of the pulmonary circulation. The blood in the capillaries is separated from the alveolar air by only the thin walls of the air sacs and the endothelial linings of the capillaries (together less than 0.6 μm in thickness) which allow the ready passage of oxygen and carbon dioxide.

As we breathe 15 times or more every minute, considerable quantities of detritus find their way into the respiratory tract, even in the most rural areas. Air is cleaned first by the hairs in the nose and the mucus secreted by the nasal epithelium. This removes the largest foreign bodies. Smaller particles settle in the trachea, bronchi, and bronchioles. They are removed by the action of the microscopic cilia on the surface of the cells lining the air passages. The cilia beat rhythmically with a wave-like motion, forcing particles, trapped in the mucus secreted by the epithelial lining of the respiratory tract, upwards to the throat, where they are eventually swallowed. Sensory receptors in the air passages triggered off by copious or irritant particles may initiate the more drastic measures of coughing and sneezing.

Some of the smallest particles eventually reach the alveoli which have no cilia or mucus producing cells. These particles are consumed by the phagocytic cells of the lymphatic system and removed or deposited in the tissues of the lung. The lungs of city dwellers and smokers are usually blackened by soot and tar.

Lungs

The bronchi, bronchioles, alveoli, and their nerves, blood vessels, and lymphatic vessels, together with a certain amount of connective tissue, form the substance of the left and right **lungs.** The lungs are cone-shaped structures with a spongy consistency due to the presence of the contained air. They are situated in the thoracic cavity being separated from each other by the structures, principally the heart and great vessels, occupying the middle part (or **mediastinum**) of the thorax. On the medial aspect of each lung is an oval area called the **hilus** through which the main branches of the air passages and pulmonary blood vessels pass.

The lungs can be subdivided into a number of **bronchopulmonary segments,** each a separate respiratory unit with its own bronchus and almost independent arterial supply, and venous and lymphatic drainage. The segments are separated from each other by thin layers of connective tissue.

Pleura

Each lung is wrapped in two layers of **pleura.** The outer layer is called the **parietal pleura** and the inner layer the **visceral pleura.** The two

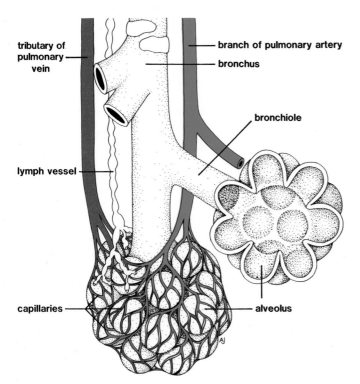

tributary of pulmonary vein

branch of pulmonary artery

bronchus

bronchiole

lymph vessel

capillaries

alveolus

Fig. 1.18. Alveoli of the lung.

layers are continuous with each other around the hilus which is itself not covered by pleura. The narrow space between the two layers of pleura is called the **pleural cavity.** In healthy subjects it contains just a very small quantity of **pleural fluid** which acts as a lubricant.

Breathing

The lungs are ventilated by variation in the size of the chest cavity brought about by the muscles of the chest wall and diaphragm. This process is described further in the section on thorax.

Control of breathing is normally automatic, but may be overridden at will to a certain extent (as in holding the breath or deep breathing exercises). When breathing is inadequate the concentration of oxygen in the blood falls and that of carbon dioxide rises. Either will increase the breathing rate. Reduced oxygen stimulates chemical receptors in the aorta and the carotid arteries (which supply the brain). Increased carbon dioxide has a direct influence on respiratory centres in the brain. Certain narcotic drugs have an inhibitory effect on these centres. A patient suffering from an overdose of these drugs breathes only because of the stimulus provided by the reduced blood oxygen level; administration of oxygen can be lethal because it abolishes the only remaining stimulus for breathing.

DIGESTIVE SYSTEM

The first parts of the digestive system, the mouth and pharynx, are principal areas of professional interest to the dentist and are fully described in Section 4. The anatomy of the remainder of the system is of limited vocational interest and will be described only briefly.

In essence the digestive tract is a long tube continuous at both ends with the skin covering the body surface. It consists of **mouth, pharynx, oesophagus, stomach, small intestine, large intestine,** and **anal canal** (Fig. 1.19). It is lined throughout by epithelium which shows marked structural differences from one region to another in association with functional requirements. Along most of its length the wall of the digestive tract is formed by layers of smooth muscle.

The principal functions of the digestive tract are the intake, digestion, and absorption of food. Food is ingested through the mouth and then divided and mixed with saliva by the chewing action of the teeth. Saliva has both a lubricative and digestive function. The food is then transferred to the pharynx and on to the oesophagus by **swallowing,** a complex, largely reflex mechanism involving the muscles of the tongue, pharynx, and soft palate. The passage of food along the remainder of the digestive tract is achieved by regular contractions (peristalsis) of the smooth muscle layers in its walls.

Oesophagus

The oesophagus is a tube, some 25 cm in length, which traverses the neck and thorax and is continuous with the pharynx above and the stomach below. It is lined by stratified squamous epithelium and its wall contains striated muscle in its upper two-thirds and only smooth muscle in its lower one-third. Towards its lower end the oesophagus passes through the muscular part of the diaphragm. The diaphragmatic muscle fibres, when they contract, act as a 'pinchcock' which prevents gastric contents from regurgitating into the oesophagus.

Stomach and small intestine

The stomach is a dilated part of the digestive tract. It lies immediately below the diaphragm within the abdominal cavity. It is lined by a mucous membrane which secretes hydrochloric acid as well as enzymes and mucus. The stomach opens through the **pyloric orifice,** guarded by the **pyloric sphincter,** into the first part of the small intestine or **duodenum.**

The duodenum forms the first 20 cm of the small intestine, the remainder being termed **jejunum** and **ileum.** Digestion is usually complete by the time food has reached the halfway point of the six metres of tubing which comprise the small intestine. Because of its great length the small intestine is much convoluted and occupies a large part of the abdominal cavity. Much of the jejunum and ileum is concerned with absorption rather than digestion. The folded wall of the small intestine is covered by minute finger-like processes, the **villi,** which are in turn covered by microscopic **micro-villi.** This produces an enormous surface area for absorption. Sugars, amino-acids, fats, and glycerol (products of digestion) are absorbed into the bloodstream from the small intestine. The venous drainage of the stomach and small intestine forms a major part of the **hepatic portal system** which drains into the liver, where storage and further metabolic processes occur.

As food passes through the stomach and small intestine it is acted upon by a large variety of enzymes and other digestive substances secreted by the glands of the lining mucosa and by the pancreas. Many of the enzymes are secreted in the form of inactive precursors, which are harmless to the cells which secrete them, and which are activated in the lumen of the digestive tract. The intestinal wall is itself protected by the copious secretion of mucus. Fats cannot be digested until emulsified with water. The necessary emulsifying agent is **bile,** secreted by the liver and liberated into the duodenum through the **bile duct.**

Large intestine

The small intestine is continuous with the large intestine on the right side of the abdominal cavity. The first part of the large intestine is called the **caecum.** Attached to its posterior wall is the vestigial **appendix** which can become inflamed and may have to be surgically removed. From the caecum the **ascending colon** passes up the right side of the abdominal cavity where it turns (the **right flexure)** to cross beneath the stomach, as the **transverse colon,** and then turns again (the **left flexure)** to descend, as the **descending colon,** on the left side and become continuous with the **sigmoid colon** which, in turn, is continuous with the **rectum.** The rectum opens into the anal canal. The colon resorbs water and ions. About 500 ml of intestinal contents enter the colon each day, of which 350 ml are resorbed. This resorption is linked with the ability of the cells of the colon to transfer sodium from intestinal contents to the blood. The volume of water which can be resorbed depends on the rate at which contents pass through the colon. If the rate is rapid, resorption is low and diarrhoea ensues. This is a response to certain foods and bacteria which stimulate peristalsis. Apart from inherent unpleasantness, diarrhoea can cause dehydration and upset ionic balance.

Faeces are stored in the rectum and sigmoid colon and ultimately voided via the anus. They contain indigestible components of food (roughage) and bacteria (one-third by weight) together with epithelial cells sloughed from the gut, bile pigments (which colour faeces brown), and small quantities of digestive enzymes.

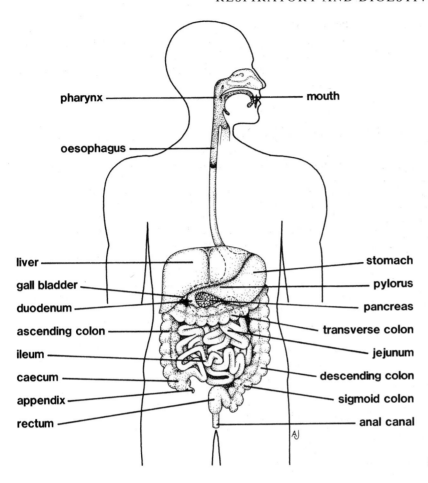

pharynx ——————— mouth

oesophagus ——————

liver ——————
gall bladder ——————
duodenum ——————
ascending colon ——————
ileum ——————
caecum ——————
appendix ——————
rectum ——————

stomach
pylorus
pancreas
transverse colon
jejunum
descending colon
sigmoid colon
anal canal

Fig. 1.19. The digestive system.

Liver

The liver is a large, solid viscus which occupies the upper part of the abdominal cavity on the right side. It lies immediately adjacent to the lower surface of the diaphragm and is protected by the lower ribs. It develops as an outgrowth of the duodenum.

The **portal vein** and **hepatic artery** enter the liver through a cleft on its undersurface called the **porta hepatis**. The portal vein conveys blood which has previously passed through the capillaries of the intestines and which contains the products of absorption. The hepatic artery is a branch of the coeliac trunk, a main branch of the aorta.

The liver consists of a large number of lobules, each of which receives blood from both the portal vein and the hepatic artery. The liver cells making up the lobules serve numerous functions including metabolic activities concerned with the products of absorption from the gut, the manufacture of plasma proteins, the synthesis of bile salts, the conversion of the breakdown products of haemoglobin into bile pigments, and the detoxification of substances (for example, alcohol) circulating in the blood.

The venous blood from the lobules passes into the hepatic veins, which open into the inferior vena cava. The bile pigments and bile salts pass into the bile canaliculi, small vessels lying close to the liver cells. The bile canaliculi unite to form ductules which unite further to

eventually form the **right** and **left hepatic ducts**. These leave the liver through the porta hepatis and join together to form the **common hepatic duct**. The common hepatic duct receives the **cystic duct** from the **gall bladder** and is then called the **bile duct.** The bile duct opens into the duodenum. When the connection between bile duct and intestine is closed, bile backs up and is stored in the gall bladder in preparation for the next meal.

Pancreas

The pancreas is a soft, glandular structure lying on the posterior abdominal wall behind the stomach. It consists of a **head, body,** and **tail**. The head is situated within the curve of the duodenum and the head and tail pass towards the left. The pancreatic cells produce numerous digestive enzymes. These pass into the pancreatic duct which traverses the gland and opens, in company with the bile duct, into the duodenum. The pancreas is also an endocrine (ductless) gland producing insulin; defective insulin production causes diabetes mellitus.

Blood and nerve supply of the digestive tract

The blood supply of the digestive tract, from the lower end of the oesophagus to the rectum, is by three main branches of the abdominal aorta. The **coeliac axis** supplies the lower end of the oesophagus, stomach, and first few inches of the duodenum, as well as the liver, spleen, and pancreas. The remainder of the small intestine and the large intestine as far as the transverse colon is supplied by the **superior mesenteric artery**. The large intestine from the transverse colon to the rectum is supplied by the **inferior mesenteric artery**. The oesophagus, apart from its lower end, receives its principal blood supply through branches of the thoracic aorta.

Venous blood from the abdominal part of the digestive tract drains into the **hepatic portal system**. From the oesophagus venous drainage is into the **azygos system**. Blood from the rectum and anal canal drains into the internal iliac veins as well as into the portal system. At either end of the abdominal part of the digestive tract, therefore, is a junctional zone between the portal and systemic venous drainages.

The digestive tract receives a rich autonomic innervation. The parasympathetic supply as far as the left flexure of the large intestine is through the **vagus** (tenth cranial) **nerves**; below this level it is through the pelvic splanchnic nerves from the sacral part of the spinal cord. The sympathetic supply is through branches of the sympathetic trunks.

Peritoneum

The abdominal cavity is lined by a serous membrane called peritoneum. Some parts of the abdominal digestive tract (the duodenum, ascending and descending colon) lie behind the peritoneum and are referred to as being **retroperitoneal**. The remaining parts are attached to the abdominal wall by two-layered folds of peritoneum called **mesenteries**. The fold of peritoneum associated with the stomach is called the **lesser omentum**. After being reflected around the stomach the two layers of peritoneum hang down, in front of the lower abdominal viscera, as a large apron-like fold called the **greater omentum**.

The space enclosed within the peritoneum is called the **peritoneal cavity**. In the healthy person it is very small and contains only a little lubricating **peritoneal fluid**.

5

Fascia and skin

FASCIA

Fascia is an anatomical term used in the dissecting room for a sheet of fibrous connective tissue large enough to be seen with the naked eye. The number of named fasciae rose abruptly with the use of formalin as a dissecting room fixative; formalin fixes connective tissue particularly well.

During development the mesoderm which gives rise to muscle, cartilage, and bone also forms less specialized connective tissue which 'fills in' spaces and accumulates between groups of muscles, viscera, and other large structures. The arrangement of this tissue is varied. On the surface of muscle it forms a visible layer or sheath; between muscles it is of the loose (**areolar**) variety and allows relative movement; between bones it may form stout fibrous **interosseous membranes**. Many larger blood vessels (e.g. the carotid artery and internal jugular vein in the neck) are invested by dense fascial sheaths whose functions are not clear. They may help venous drainage by binding large veins to pulsating arteries.

Superficial fascia

Superficial fascia, or **subcutaneous tissue,** is found between muscles and overlying skin. This is the site for the largest accumulations of body fat. Body fat is of variable thickness with regional distribution according to age and sex (Fig. 1.1) as well as diet. Branches of nerves and vessels run in this fascia, but the larger ones are usually deeper and better protected. The superficial fascia contains a few muscles (e.g. the muscles of facial expression), the remnants of a subcutaneous muscle sheet present over most of the body in other mammals (think of a horse or cow shrugging off flies). Fat is more abundant and more generally distributed in the adult female, producing rounded contours. In the male it is less abundant, especially towards the extremities. Fat becomes more noticeable in both sexes towards middle age ('middle-age spread'). It is thickest and most conspicuous on the anterior abdominal wall and thinnest on the dorsum of the hand and pinna of the ear.

In areas where relative movement between skin and underlying structures is undesirable (scalp, sole of foot, palm of hand) dense bands of connective tissue unite the surface layers and deeper structures.

Local subcutaneous infections, such as abscesses and boils, are relatively painless in areas where superficial fascia is abundant but become very painful where the superficial fascia is meagre because of the distortion of the surrounding tissues.

Deep fascia

Deep fascia has many collagen fibres arranged compactly, often in uniform directions so that it may be indistinguishable from aponeuroses. In limbs, where it is especially well-developed, its fibres are arranged longitudinally and circularly so forming a tough inelastic sheath for the musculature. Muscles are attached to this sheath in both the upper and lower limbs. In the lower limb it is particularly dense as it passes down the outer side of the thigh where it forms the iliotibial tract through which most of the pull of the gluteus maximus muscle is transmitted to the tibia.

In the neck and limbs, laminae of deep fascia run inwards between groups of muscles to connect extensively with bone, often separating different muscle groups with different functions as well as increasing the area of attachment of the muscles.

At wrist and ankle fascia is specialized to form **retinaculae** which retain tendons running deep to them which would otherwise bowstring out on flexion. In one or two cases (e.g. the **digastric muscle**) fascia forms a sling which alters the direction of muscle pull even more drastically.

SKIN

Skin is a specialized boundary tissue which forms virtually the entire external surface of the body, being continuous with the mucous membranes lining the respiratory, alimentary, and urinogenital tracts at their respective openings. The skin has many functions. It minimizes mechanical, thermal, osmotic, chemical, and photic stress, forms a barrier against micro-organisms, regulates heat exchange, and forms a sensory surface equipped with touch, pressure, temperature, and pain receptors. It has good frictional resistance useful in locomotion and handling objects, allows a certain amount of absorption and excretion and serves as a pathway for communication, as in blushing, facial expression, and tactile communication. Vitamin D is synthesized in the skin.

Skin is divided into two distinct parts, the superficial **epidermis** and the deeper **dermis**. The epidermis is a keratinized epithelium of varying thickness, thickest and most heavily keratinized on the sole of the foot and the palm of the hand. Habitual activity, such as holding a pen, digging with a shovel or using scissors, may produce localized thickenings of thick skin called calluses. In other areas, such as the face and the back of the hand, the epidermis is much thinner and less well keratinized. The dermis is made up of connective tissue containing numerous blood vessels, lymphatics, and nerves and is also of variable thickness. Generally the skin is much thicker and tougher on dorsal than on ventral surfaces. Leather (epidermis + dermis) for shoe soles comes from the back of a cow, glove leather and suede from the belly. In the dermis the bundles of collagen fibres are mostly arranged in parallel rows whose direction is seen as **skin creases** on the surface. These may be **tension lines** which are small, irregular furrows dividing the skin into a series of lozenges (easily seen on the back of the hand), or **flexure lines** which are associated with regular movements and are conspicuous opposite joints, especially on the palms and soles, where they indicate the points of attachment of the skin to the underlying deep fascia. **Papillary ridges** (friction ridges) are confined to the hands and feet where they form distinct parallel grooves in arrays determined by underlying dermal papillae. The arrangement of these ridges is under very strong genetic control, as indicated by hereditary disorders such as Down's syndrome, where a chromosomal anomaly leads to consistent alterations in their pattern.

An incision made in the direction of a skin crease will cut few collagenous fibre bundles and heal with a minimum of scarring; a cut across the skin creases will leave an unsightly, bulky mass of scar tissue.

Papillary ridges on the fingers are the basis of dermatoglyphics (fingerprinting) of forensic importance in identifying individuals. Patterns on the palm and sole of the foot may also be used in this way, although these are obviously less convenient.

Appendages

The skin bears nails, hair follicles, sebaceous glands, and sweat glands. **Nails** are keratinized plates on the dorsum of fingers and toes. The nail is surrounded on three sides by folds of skin, the nail folds. **Hairs** grow from follicles, invaginations of the epidermis into the dermis. The follicle is connected to the dermis by an **arrector pili** muscle, smooth muscle innervated by the sympathetic nervous system. Contraction of the muscle makes the hair 'stand on end' in response to cold or fright. The skin is disturbed by this manoeuvre to form **gooseflesh**. Distribution of hair over the body surface is dependent on race, age, and sex. **Sebaceous glands** associated with hair follicles secrete **sebum** onto the shafts of hairs, maintaining the flexibility of the hair and helping to waterproof the surrounding skin. **Sweat glands** are found all over the body except the vermilion border of the lips and the skin beneath the nails. Sweat is a watery fluid, hypotonic to plasma with about 0.5 per cent solids, the chief one of which is sodium chloride. If exposed to a warm atmosphere, we sweat over the whole body surface. Sweating in response to fear or anxiety (a cold sweat) occurs chiefly on palms, soles, and axillae, and is produced as a result of stimulation of the sympathetic nervous system which innervates the sweat glands. At rest the skin leaks water slowly (insensible perspiration); this loss is by osmosis and not through the sweat glands.

Clinical aspects

Nail folds, hair follicles, and sebaceous glands are commonly infected. Infection beneath the nail is called paronychia; infection of a hair follicle is termed a boil. A carbuncle is an infection of the superficial fascia which usually spreads from an infected hair follicle or group of hair follicles.

A burn which destroys the superficial part of the skin will heal from its edges and also by proliferation of the cells of the sweat glands. Healing of a burn which has penetrated deeper can be aided by a skin graft. A split thickness graft removes most of the epidermis from the donor site, leaving the dermis *in situ* to repair the damage there. A full thickness graft includes the dermis and will slough off if a new circulation is not rapidly established. The donor site of a full thickness graft is usually covered by a split thickness graft.

Skin colour is determined by at least five pigments, melanin (brown), melanoid (similar to melanin, but differently distributed), carotene (reddish), haemoglobin, and oxyhaemoglobin (purple and pink respectively). Pigmentation in pale-skinned individuals is variable within certain limits, being influenced principally by exposure to sun and wind. Melanin helps to protect the deep layers of the skin from the carcinogenic effects of ultraviolet radiation. This is probably the reason why the natives of sunny climates are often dark-skinned. It is possible that the pale skin of Northern Europeans is an adaptation to low levels of sunlight in allowing such small amounts of ultraviolet light as fall upon the skin to penetrate to the sites where vitamin D is manufactured.

Section 2

Developmental anatomy

1

Introduction and the first three weeks

INTRODUCTION

Embryology is a fascinating subject but one which often causes students difficulty. This seems to be inherent in the nature of the subject which involves descriptions of structures turning into other structures of quite different shape or folding themselves in a way that rivals origami.

The fact that the authors are aware of these difficulties (having experienced them ourselves) does not necessarily mean that we can offer an easy solution; some concepts in embryology require the student to read a text several times with full concentration before a picture emerges in his or her mind of what exactly is going on. This is not a fault of the student nor, we hope, of the text but is a consequence of the difficulty most people have in trying to picture, in the mind's eye, structures which are constantly changing in shape and size.

This is not a textbook of embryology. What we have tried to achieve in this section is an account of the development of the embryo from fertilization to the end of the third week followed by a series of detailed descriptions of the areas which we believe should be more fully understood by the dental student – the head and neck, nervous system, and circulatory and respiratory systems. A conventional text would also include gametogenesis and the development of areas which we have omitted – the gut and urinogenital system, for example. We cannot recommend too strongly that you read an account of these topics in a textbook of embryology.

FIRST THREE WEEKS OF DEVELOPMENT

First week

Life is conventionally described as beginning at the moment of fertilization which occurs up to 12–24 hours after ovulation. The fertilized egg or **zygote** has 22 pairs of autosomal chromosomes and one pair of sex chromosomes (i.e. 46 chromosomes in all – the diploid number). One member of each pair is derived from the egg and the other from the sperm (the **gametes** each containing only 23 chromosomes – the haploid number). At fertilization the zygote is stimulated to commence a series of mitotic cell divisions (**cleavage divisions**) which will finally result in the formation of a new individual. The sex of the zygote depends on whether the sex chromosome of the fertilizing sperm was an X or a Y.

During cleavage the original single cell of the zygote divides into two, four, eight, then 16 cells. The two-cell stage is reached in about 30 hours from fertilization, the four-cell stage after 40–50 hours, and the 12–16-cell stage at about three days. During this period the

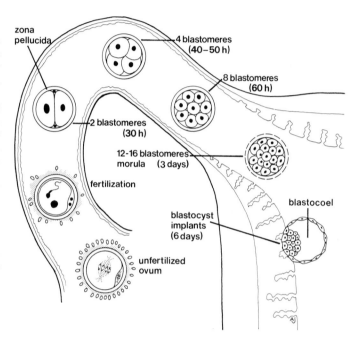

Fig. 2.1. Fertilization and cleavage. Times given are from fertilization.

cells (**blastomeres**) are surrounded by a membrane (the **zona pellucida**, Fig. 2.1) which originally encompassed the egg. The 16 blastomeres therefore occupy no more space than did the original egg.

Fertilization occurs in the distal third of the oviduct. By the time the 16-cell stage has been reached, the ball of blastomeres, now called a **morula,** has reached the uterus. The morula can be thought of as being made up of two types of cell, those on the surface, the **outer cell mass** (the future **trophoblast**) and those in the centre of the ball, the **inner cell mass** (from which the embryo proper will form). Uterine fluid passes into the spaces between the cells of the morula which become confluent to form a single cavity, the **blastocoel** (Fig. 2.1). The structure is now known as a **blastocyst**. By this stage it contains 100–150 cells and the zona pellucida has disappeared.

At about 5½–6 days after fertilization the blastocyst becomes attached to the uterine wall. Proteolytic secretions from the trophoblast erode the lining of the uterus (Fig. 2.2A) and the blastocyst thus becomes embedded or **implanted** in the uterine wall.

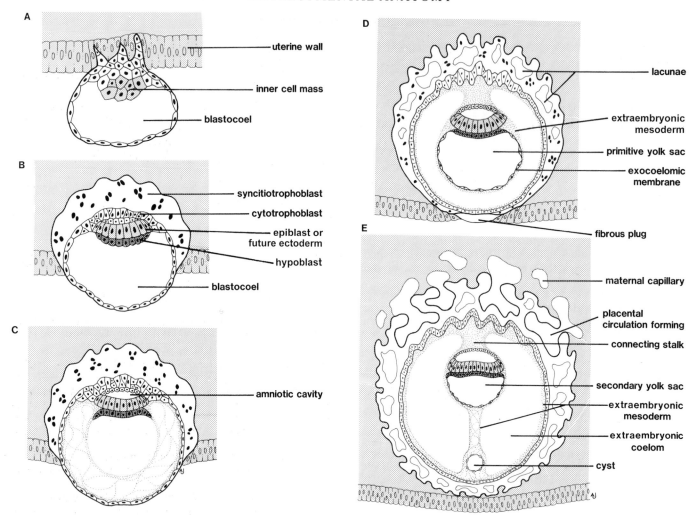

Fig. 2.2. Further development of the early embryo.

Second week

Once implanted the distinction between the trophoblast and the inner cell mass becomes more distinct. The former continues its lytic action so that by the eighth day of development the blastocyst has become firmly embedded in the uterine wall. The trophoblast has by now differentiated into two parts: adjacent to the embryo are the distinct cells of the **cytotrophoblast** and adjacent to the uterine tissue is a multinucleate syncitium, the **syncitiotrophoblast.** The inner cell mass has also divided into two layers (Fig. 2.2B). A layer of small, flattened cells facing the blastocoel is the **hypoblast**, while a layer of columnar cells, the **epiblast** or future **ectoderm,** faces the cytotrophoblast. The embryo is thus, briefly, in the form of a two-layered disc.

A small cavity now appears in the ectoderm, formed by the coalescence of fluid filled spaces which develop between the ectodermal cells. It enlarges to become the **amniotic cavity** (Fig. 2.2C).

Over the walls of the blastocoel not occupied by the embryo a single, flattened layer of cells, the **exocoelomic membrane,** can be made out (Fig. 2.2D). This is continuous with the hypoblast at the margins of the embryo. The cavity enclosed by the exocoelomic membrane and the hypoblast is the **primitive yolk sac** or **exocoelomic cavity**.

By the ninth day of development the blastocyst is deeply embedded in the uterine wall and the mouth of the cavity which it occupies is closed by a fibrous plug, rather as a cork closes a bottle. The syncitiotrophoblast now surrounds the blastocyst completely and is becoming vacuolated, especially over the embryonic pole. These vacuoles tend to coalesce into larger **lacunae.**

By the tenth day the trophoblastic lacunae have made contact with the maternal sinusoidal blood vessels, so forming the basis of the placental circulation (Fig. 2.2E). Between the cytotrophoblast and the exocoelomic membrane a loose, vacuolated tissue, the **extraembryonic mesoderm,** forms whose vacuoles later unite to become the **extraembryonic coelom.** The embryo remains united with the rest of the trophoblast by a non-vacuolated area of extraembryonic mesoderm, the **connecting stalk.**

At this stage the embryo proper is growing much more slowly than the tissues surrounding it. The primitive yolk sac becomes divided into a smaller secondary yolk sac united with the embryo and one or more cysts lined by what appears to be exocoelomic membrane. How this happens is uncertain, but whatever the mechanism the secondary yolk sac has been formed by 13 days.

Third week – primitive node and streak

By the beginning of the third week a slight thickening of the hypoblast, the **prochordal** (or **cephalic**) **plate** (Fig. 2.3) is present at one end of the embryonic disc. The prochordal plate indicates the future head end of the embryo and gives the embryonic disc a bilateral symmetry about a midline axis through the plate. Given this axis and the future head end, we can also locate the future **caudal** or tail end. Attached to this end is the connecting stalk.

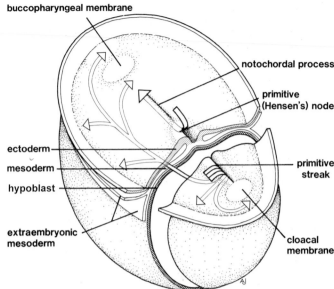

Fig. 2.4. Formation of intraembryonic mesoderm. The arrows show the spread of the intraembryonic mesoderm between ectoderm and hypoblast.

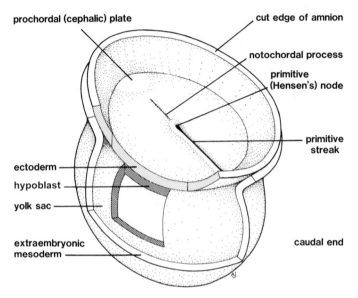

Fig. 2.3. Formation of the primitive node and streak.

It is at the future caudal end that the next major change takes place, resulting in the formation of the third embryonic layer, the **intraembryonic mesoderm**.

Formation of intraembryonic mesoderm

Ectodermal cells at the caudal end of the embryo tend to round up, divide and move towards the midline (Fig. 2.4). When they reach the midline, these cells seem able to break away from the ectodermal plate and pass downwards into the plane between ectoderm and hypoblast where they spread outwards to form a third embryonic layer, the **intraembryonic mesoderm**. The midline groove in the ectoderm caused by the process, the **primitive streak,** is clearly visible in the 15–16-day-old embryo extending over approximately the caudal one-third of the embryonic disc. The cephalic end of the streak is known as the **primitive** (or **Hensen's**) **node**. Here the same process of cell migration is taking place but the invaginated cells, instead of spreading out, stay together to form a blind-ended tube, the **noto-**

chordal process, which pushes gradually cephalad in the midline towards the prochordal plate, which it reaches on day 17.

The spreading mesoderm has meanwhile formed a layer separating ectoderm and hypoblast and has reached the edges of the embryonic disc where it encounters the extraembryonic mesoderm and fuses with it. The sheet of mesoderm is complete except in three areas:

1. the midline axis occupied by the notochordal process;
2. the prochordal plate which later forms the **buccopharyngeal membrane;**
3. a similar caudal area which forms the **cloacal membrane**.

Some of the ectodermal cells migrating through the primitive streak invade the hypoblast and displace its cells so that eventually the hypoblast is replaced by a new layer of cells, the definitive **endoderm**.

The process of migration and invagination which leads to the formation of the intraembryonic mesoderm and the endoderm is called **gastrulation**. Note that the three definitive layers of the embryo—the ectoderm, mesoderm, and endoderm— are all derived from the ectoderm or epiblast.

Further development of the notochord

On about the eighteenth day the notochord begins to undergo a series of changes, the net result of which is the abolition of its central canal. The process is complex and comprises the following stages:

1. the ventral aspect of the notochordal process fuses with the underlying endoderm;
2. the fused notochordal–endodermal plate disappears, establishing contact between the notochordal lumen and the secondary yolk sac;
3. the notochord rounds up and loses contact with the endoderm.

Mainly as a result of cell migration, allied to some growth, the initially almost circular embryonic disc has now become pear-shaped, widest at its cephalic end. The primitive node and streak do not change in size and become relatively ever more caudal in position during this process, although still supplying cells to the mesoderm (especially caudally) until the end of the fourth week of development.

FURTHER DEVELOPMENT OF THE GERM LAYERS

By the middle of the third week the embryo consists of three layers of cells. The ectoderm is continuous with the wall of the amnion above, the endoderm with the wall of the yolk sac below. The mesoderm is continuous with the extraembryonic mesoderm peripherally and separates the ectoderm and endoderm, except along the midline where it is interrupted by the notochord centrally, the buccopharyngeal membrane rostrally, and the cloacal membrane caudally.

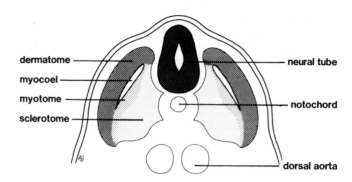

Fig. 2.5. Differentiation of somites.

Mesoderm

The intraembryonic mesoderm initially forms a thin sheet of tissue on either side of the midline. By day 17 the mesoderm on either side of the notochord begins to proliferate and thicken to form a mass of tissue, the **paraxial mesoderm.** Lateral to this the mesoderm is styled **intermediate mesoderm** and more laterally still **lateral plate mesoderm.**

Paraxial mesoderm – the formation of somites

At the end of the third week of development the paraxial mesoderm forms two solid rods of tissue, one on each side of the central notochord. Starting at the cephalic end, adjacent to the tip of the notochord, these rods undergo segmental condensation to form bilaterally paired, cuboidal masses, the **somites**. The process is referred to as **segmentation** or **metamerism**. From studies in non-human embryos it appears that the somites are preceded by, and formed from, whorls of cells in the paraxial mesoderm. These whorls are called **somitomeres**. The somites mould the surface of the overlying ectoderm into clearly visible humps, the number of which is often used as a measure of the age of the embryo. By the end of the fifth week of development 42–45 pairs of somites may be distinguished. These are classified, according to their later fate, into four occipital (or metotic), eight cervical, 12 thoracic, five lumbar, five sacral, and 8–10 coccygeal.

Further differentiation of the somite (Fig. 2.5)

During the fourth week of development the somites begin to differentiate further. Initially each somite has a vertical, slit-like cavity, the **myocoel,** which is obliterated by cell division as the somite grows, but which forms a useful marker so long as it persists. The somite tissue lateral to the myocoel, the **dermatome,** will eventually spread out beneath the ectoderm to become part of the dermis of the skin. The somite tissue medial to the myocoel has two divisions. The medial division, or **sclerotome**, differentiates into young connective tissue, or **mesenchyme,** and migrates to form a mass of tissue around the notochord and developing neural tube (see below) which will eventually form the vertebral column, ribs, and sternum. The sclerotomes of the metotic somites are believed to contribute to the skull. The lateral division becomes the **myotome** which spreads out to produce the flexor and extensor muscles of the vertebral column, the intercostal musculature, and, at least in part, the limb muscles.

Intermediate mesoderm

The intermediate mesoderm lateral to the developing somites differentiates cranially into segmentally arranged groups of cells but caudally persists as two unsegmented rods of tissue, the **nephrogenic cords.** The latter give rise to most of the urinary system. The adrenal cortex and much of the reproductive system (but not the germ cells) also arise from the intermediate mesoderm of the caudal region.

Lateral plate mesoderm

This, the most lateral of the three divisions of the mesoderm, is continuous with the extraembryonic mesoderm surrounding the amniotic cavity and yolk sac. Further development of the lateral plate involves the formation of a new cavity, the **intraembryonic coelom.**

Intraembryonic coelom

The intraembryonic coelom is formed by the coalescence of a series of vacuoles which appear in the lateral plate mesoderm. When the primitive mesoderm migrates from the primitive streak, it completely infiltrates the potential space between ectoderm and endoderm with three exceptions, the notochordal region, buccopharyngeal membrane, and cloacal membrane. The somites are confined to the region of the embryo between buccopharyngeal and cloacal membrane but lateral plate mesoderm is more widespread (Fig. 2.4). The vacuoles which appear form a U with its base passing in front of the buccopharyngeal membrane and its arms down each side of the paraxial mesoderm. The cavity formed by the coalescence of these vacuoles assumes a similar U shape. The anterior part of the intraembryonic coelom is the primitive pericardial cavity and the lateral parts are the primitive pleural and peritoneal cavities (Fig. 2.6). Lateral to the arms of the U the mesoderm breaks down, so that over a certain distance intraembryonic and extraembryonic coeloms are continuous. The formation of the new cavity within the lateral plate mesoderm splits it into two layers, a **somatic** layer adjacent to the ectoderm and a **visceral** or **splanchnic** layer adjacent to endoderm. These layers form the serous membranes lining the pericardial, pleural, and peritoneal cavities as well as contributing mesodermal elements to the body wall and to the heart, respiratory system, and gastrointestinal tract. The lateral plate mesoderm cut off ahead of the intraembryonic coelom at the cephalic end of the embryo will become the **septum transversum** in which the liver later develops.

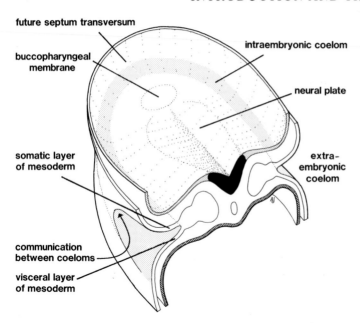

Fig. 2.6. Formation of the intraembryonic coelom.

Ectoderm – development of the neural tube

While we have been following the fate of the mesoderm, changes have also been taking place in the ectoderm. Shortly after the development of the notochord, and under its influence, the central part of the ectodermal disc (the neurectoderm) begins to differentiate as the **neural plate** overlying the notochord and paraxial mesoderm (Fig. 2.7). It quickly becomes much wider anteriorly, in the region of the future brain, than posteriorly where it will form the spinal cord. At the begin-

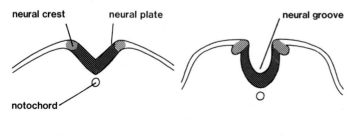

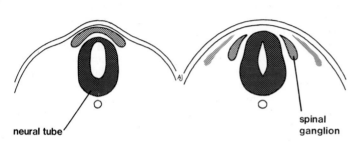

Fig. 2.7. Formation of the neural tube.

ning of the fourth week of development the neural plate becomes depressed along its midline, forming the **neural groove**. This converts the flate plate initially into a gutter and then, as the groove deepens, into a shape which, in cross-section, resembles a horseshoe. At the junction of neural plate and ectoderm a new tissue, the **neural crest,** becomes distinguishable. The edges of the neural plate approach each other and eventually fuse in the midline to form the **neural tube.** Closure of the tube begins opposite the fourth metotic somite and proceeds anteriorly and posteriorly almost, but not quite, to the ends of the neural plate. Two apertures, the **anterior** and **posterior neuropores,** persist here until the fourth week. The central nervous system then consists of a cylindrical posterior portion – the future spinal cord, and a broader tube anteriorly – the future brain.

The **neural crest** tissue is not incorporated into the neural tube but is pinched off to form a plate between the dorsal part of the neural tube and overlying ectoderm. The neural crest gives rise to **ectomesenchyme** which migrates widely to form, or contribute to, the dermis in the head region (cf. the rest of the dermis which we have already seen to be derived from the somites), the meninges surrounding the brain, the skeleton and connective tissue component of the musculature of the branchial arches, probably much of the rest of the skull, cells of the spinal and cranial nerve ganglia, the sympathetic and parasympathetic nervous systems and the adrenal medulla, the Schwann cells (which provide the myelin sheaths of peripheral nerves), and pigment cells, including those of the skin.

Endoderm

The fate of the endoderm can be understood only if we realize that the embryo does not remain a flat disc: it becomes folded. Let us look at the folding first.

FOLDING OF THE EMBRYONIC PLATE AND ITS CONSEQUENCES

We have so far considered the embryo as a flat plate. Above it lies the amniotic cavity, below it the secondary yolk sac. We have noted the growth of the ectoderm and mesoderm but have not considered the consequences of this growth. Because most of the growth takes place on its upper surface, the principal effect is that the embryo bulges upwards into the amniotic cavity. The resulting curvature, often referred to as folding or flexion of the embryo, is not confined to one axis but occurs in all directions, converting the formerly flat disc into a portion of a spheroid. It is best understood if we look at the process in two selected planes of section, longitudinal and transverse.

Longitudinal section (Fig. 2.8)

A longitudinal section through the midline of the flat embryonic disc presents the following features from before backwards: (i) converging layers of ectoderm and endoderm; (ii) the region of lateral plate mesoderm which will become the **septum transversum;** (iii) the intraembryonic coelom (primitive pericardial cavity); (iv) the buccopharyngeal membrane; (v) a region rather like a sandwich, with neural plate above, notochord between, and endoderm below; (vi) the cloacal membrane; (vii) a region of lateral plate mesoderm; (viii) diverging layers of ectoderm and endoderm.

As a result of the increasing longitudinal curvature of the embryo the buccopharyngeal and cloacal membranes become folded under the cephalic and caudal ends respectively of the embryo and in the process rotate so that their originally ventral surfaces come to face

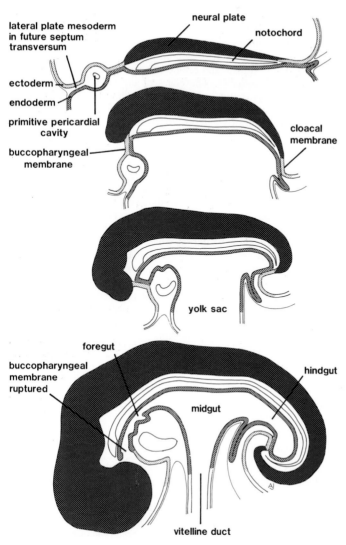

Labels on figure:
lateral plate mesoderm in future septum transversum
neural plate
notochord
ectoderm
endoderm
primitive pericardial cavity
buccopharyngeal membrane
cloacal membrane
yolk sac
foregut
buccopharyngeal membrane ruptured
hindgut
midgut
vitelline duct

Fig. 2.8. Embryonic folding in longitudinal section.

dorsally. A further consequence of this folding is that part of the yolk sac becomes incorporated into the embryo where it is known as the gut. The communication between the gut and the yolk sac becomes progressively constricted by the folding of the embryo and is eventually reduced to the narrow **vitelline duct.** The part of the gut in communication with the yolk sac is known as the **midgut,** that part extending towards the buccopharyngeal membrane is the **foregut,** and that part extending towards the cloacal membrane is the **hindgut.** The primitive pericardial cavity now lies beneath the foregut in the future chest region. The area of lateral plate mesoderm which was originally located in front of the pericardial cavity now lies caudal to it where it forms the septum transversum. The attachment

of the connecting stalk to the caudal end of the embryonic disc is similarly brought on to the ventral aspect of the folded embryo where it lies in front of the reversed cloacal membrane.

Transverse section (Fig. 2.9)

A transverse section through the midgut region of the flat embryonic disc presents the following layers from above downwards: (i) the ectoderm, thickened centrally to form the neural plate; (ii) a middle region with the central notochord flanked by blocks of mesoderm; this mesoderm splits laterally to form two layers continuous with the extraembryonic mesoderm and separated by the coelom; (iii) the endoderm.

The greatest growth is in the neural plate. As this increases in size, it causes the lateral margins of the embryonic disc to rotate downwards about an axis approximating to the notochord. This movement, together with the longitudinal folding, incorporates part of the yolk sac into the embryo as the gut.

In the central region of the embryo the lateral margins of the folding disc do not come into contact but remain separated around the vitelline duct and the attachment of the connecting stalk. The vitelline duct eventually becomes incorporated into the connecting stalk which is now called the **umbilical cord.** Continued folding of the embryo increasingly constricts off the vitelline duct from the yolk sac. The mesoderm dorsal to the gut becomes thinned to form the dorsal mesentery which persists along the entire length of the gut. A ventral mesentery is also formed, but is limited to the region of the foregut.

Clinical aspects

Accidents of fertilization are common but their causes are poorly understood. It has been estimated that one out of two zygotes has an abnormal chromosome number. Most of these abort so that by birth only some six per 100 000 individuals have detectable chromosome abnormalities. Probably the best known of these is Down's syndrome (mongolism) in which there are three instead of the usual pair of 21st chromosomes.

Twins are of two kinds. Fraternal or dizygous twins result from the fertilization of two separate eggs by two sperm. They are no more alike than brothers and sisters. Identical or monozygous twins are the result of the splitting of one zygote into two individuals who are, of course, of the same sex and genetically identical. About 70 per cent of twins are fraternal (seven per 1000 births) and 30 per cent (three per 1000) identical. Some idea of the time of splitting of the zygote is given by the structure of the fetal membranes. The rarest kind, with two entirely separate sets of membranes, results from a split at the two-blastomere stage. The commonest type, with a common placenta but separate amnion, is due to splitting at the inner cell mass stage. A third type with completely common membranes indicates that the embryo split later, after implantation.

Ectopic pregnancy is produced when a blastocyst implants outside the normal area of the uterine mucosa. Sites where this may occur are the oviducts, ovary, cervix of the uterus, and the abdominal or pelvic cavities. Such pregnancies almost invariably fail to go to term and may produce serious haemorrhage as they burrow into the surfaces of abdominal viscera.

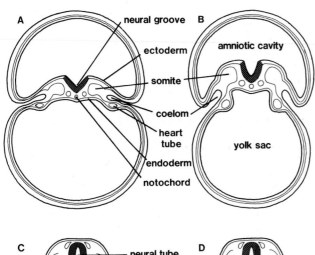

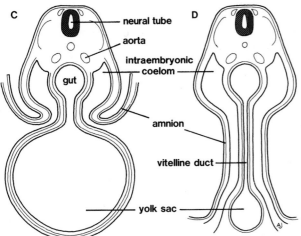

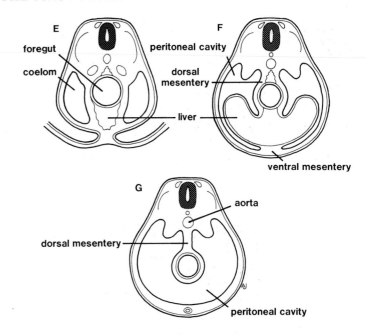

Fig. 2.9. Embryonic folding in transverse section. Early stages in the region of the heart tube (A, B); later stages at the umbilicus (C, D), through the foregut (E, F), and through the hindgut (G).

2

Development of heart, circulatory, and respiratory systems

HEART AND CIRCULATORY SYSTEM

The vascular system begins to appear at the start of the third week of development when the embryo reaches such a size that diffusion alone is no longer adequate to cope with its nutritional requirements.

The first sign of the developing system is the appearance of **angioblasts.** These are seen in presomite embryos as groups of cells in the mesoderm of the anterior margin of the embryonic disc and of the yolk sac wall. The angioblasts occur in isolated clusters or cords termed **blood islands.** The intercellular spaces within the blood islands increase in size and the peripheral angioblasts flatten to form the endothelial walls of the first blood vessels. Angioblasts located more centrally float free to become the first red blood cells. These early vessels increase their size by sprouting of the flattened wall cells and soon make numerous communications with each other to form a plexus. The angioblasts in the posterior wall of the yolk sac spread into the connecting stalk mesoderm and come into close association with maternal capillaries to form the **placental** and **umbilical vessels.** In other parts of the yolk sac they form a second network (**vitelline vessels**) which serves as a transient means of maternal–fetal exchange before regressing at eight weeks. These extraembryonic vessels are continuous with those formed within the embryo.

Heart

One group of angioblasts of special importance is that which will be incorporated into the future heart. These cells develop in the lateral plate mesoderm ventral to the primitive pericardial cavity and by a process similar to that just described for angioblasts elsewhere give rise to a U-shaped tube lined by flattened endothelial (endocardial) cells and containing red blood cells. The next stage of the development of this **endocardial tube** is brought about by the embryonic folding process which we have already discussed.

As a result of this folding relationships change. The heart tube has rotated through 180° and now lies caudal, instead of rostral, to the buccopharyngeal membrane and dorsal, instead of ventral, to the primitive pericardial cavity. Because of these changes the process is sometimes known as **reversal.**

The adjacent parts of the endocardial heart tube fuse. With continued growth the single heart tube so formed bulges more and more into the pericardial cavity (Fig. 2.10). It remains surrounded by a thin layer of mesoderm and attached to the dorsal wall of the pericardial cavity by a fold of mesoderm called the **dorsal mesocardium.** The mesoderm enveloping the heart tube proliferates to form an outer layer, the **myoepicardium,** and an inner layer, the **cardiac jelly.** The

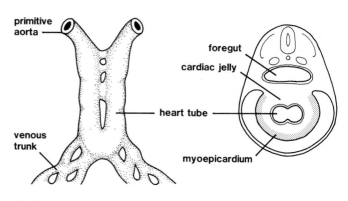

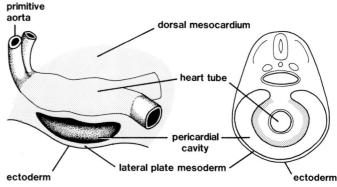

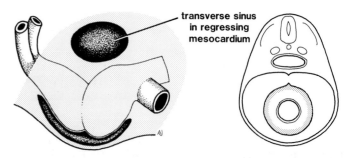

Fig. 2.10. Formation of the heart, early stages. Upper = formation of single heart tube in ventral view and cross-section; middle = single heart tube at later stage, viewed from left and in cross-section; lower = heart tube folding, viewed from left and in cross-section.

dorsal mesocardium then regresses, leaving the heart tube, enclosed in cardiac jelly and myoepicardium, suspended in the pericardial cavity at only its anterior and posterior extremities. The regression of the dorsal mesocardium leaves a passage, the **transverse sinus**, dorsal to the heart tube. From the myoepicardium and cardiac jelly develop the muscle (myocardium) of the heart and the inner (visceral) layer of the pericardium. The fibrous and parietal pericardia are formed from the lateral plate mesoderm lining the pericardial cavity. Visceral and parietal layers are continuous at the anterior and posterior extremities of the heart tube.

The cardiac loop

During the next stages (22–26 days) the heart develops rapidly. It differentiates into several distinct regions and enlarges considerably. The differentiation can be seen externally as the heart tube is divided into several regions by the appearance of transverse grooves. The first division is into cephalic **bulbus cordis** and caudal **ventricle** by the **bulboventricular sulcus**. The ventricle is then further subdivided by a second transverse groove which separates off the **common atrium** caudally. The atrium becomes continuous on each side with a short venous trunk draining vitelline and umbilical veins from the membranes and the **common cardinal vein** from the embryo proper.

The growth which accompanies this differentiation renders the heart tube too long to fit into the pericardial cavity without folding. As the arterial and venous ends of the heart tube are fixed the tube becomes bent in the region of the bulboventricular sulcus into a U-shaped loop with its convexity forwards (i.e. ventrally) and to the right. A second folding at the junction between ventricle and atrium renders the heart S-shaped (Fig. 2.11).

By the time folding is complete the following chambers can be distinguished. Most caudally is the **sinus venosus**, receiving venous blood from the vitelline, umbilical and cardinal veins of each side into its **right** and **left horns.** The sinus opens into the atrium which tends to bulge around either side of the adjacent bulbus cordis as left and right **auricles.** The ventricle descends on the left to the flexion at the bulboventricular sulcus from where the bulbus ascends on the right to drain into the paired dorsal aortae, continuations of the limbs of the original U-shaped heart tube. The bulbus cordis at this stage is dividing into three parts, a **trabecular** part which becomes incorporated into the right definitive ventricle, the **conus cordis** which will form the common outflow for the developing ventricles, and the **truncus arteriosus** which forms the root of the aorta and pulmonary trunk.

Development of the definitive heart

Between the fourth and eighth week the heart undergoes a massive reformation. At the beginning of this period the heart possesses a single continuous lumen throughout with blood flowing from sinus venosus to aortic roots (Fig. 211F). By eight weeks it is four-chambered and much more complex. Although changes occur in all chambers simultaneously, the easiest way to appreciate what happens is to look at each chamber separately.

Sinus venosus

The left horn of the sinus venosus is made redundant during the period under consideration. The veins draining into it are obliterated one by one, the left umbilical and the left vitelline veins during the fourth or fifth weeks and the left common cardinal vein at 10 weeks. The remains of the left horn form the **oblique vein of the left atrium** (a small coronary vessel) distally and the **coronary sinus** (which receives much of the blood returning from the coronary veins) proximally.

As the vessels draining into the left horn close down, more blood is diverted to the right, resulting in an increase in size of the right horn. When the atrium splits into two parts (see below), the right horn is incorporated into the right atrium as the smooth-walled **sinus venarum.** The primitive valve guarding the sinus–atrium division merges with the atrial wall on the left, whilst on the right it is incorporated into the valves guarding the inferior vena cava and coronary sinus.

As a consequence of the reduction of the left horn and enlargement of the right, the sinus–atrial opening is displaced to the right.

Septum formation in the atrium

Division of the common atrium into left and right chambers begins during the fifth week with the development of the **septum primum** (Fig. 2.12). This is a sickle-shaped ridge growing forwards, in the sagittal plane, from the posterior wall of the common atrium towards the atrioventricular opening. As the points of the crescentic septum approach this opening the latter is narrowed in the plane of the developing septum by the growth of **endocardial cushions** on anterior and posterior walls. These unite ahead of the arms of the crescent dividing the common orifice into a left and right opening. As the septum primum continues to grow, the communication between left and right halves of the atrium, the **ostium primum**, becomes rapidly smaller in diameter and eventually closes. The two halves of the common atrium can now be called the right and left atria. Communication between the two atria is maintained by a number of small openings which appear in the dorsal part of the septum primum and unite to form the **ostium secundum.** To the right of the rather thin septum primum a second stouter crescentic fold, the **septum secundum,** grows down from the roof of the right atrium during the seventh week. The septum secundum is never complete. Its free border overlaps the ostium secundum, leaving an opening, the **foramen ovale,** connecting the two atria which allows blood to flow from the right to the left atrium. The foramen persists until just after birth when it closes by fusion of the septa primum and secundum, leaving a relic, the **fossa ovalis,** on the completed atrial septum. The left atrium becomes connected with the developing lungs by the **pulmonary veins** which bud out from its posterior surface.

Atrioventricular valves

Fusion of the endocardial cushions divides the atrioventricular canal into the left and right orifices. The tissue surrounding each orifice becomes thickened to form a primitive atrioventricular valve. Below the newly formed valve lies the muscle of the ventricular wall. This gradually becomes perforated by many lacunae which combine to form larger apertures, leaving the valves attached to the ventricular wall by cords of muscle only. The part of each cord nearest the valve is replaced by connective tissue to form the **chorda tendinae** while the lower muscular parts persist as the **papillary muscles.**

Septum formation in the ventricle

Septum formation in the ventricle, which occurs in the fifth week, is by a different mechanism from that seen in the atrium. The right and left ventricles develop from the primitive single ventricle by the expansion of the right and left halves of the latter. The central band, which does not expand, is left behind as a cresent-shaped septum of cardiac muscle partially dividing the two newly formed ventricles.

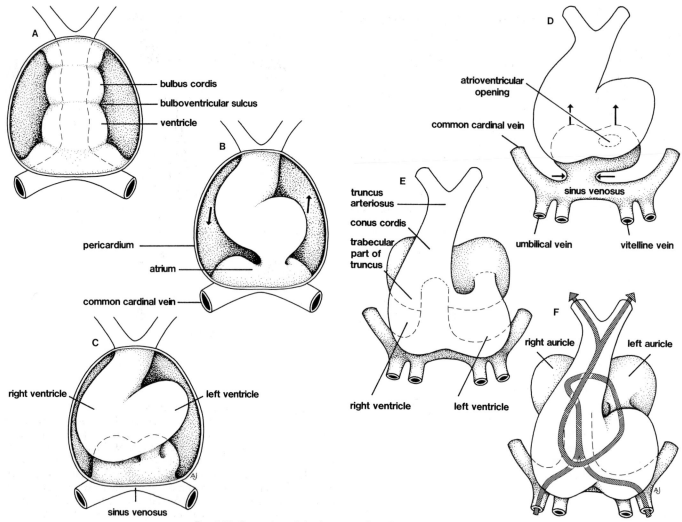

Fig. 2.11. Formation of the heart, continued. Ventral views. In F (about 4 weeks), the direction of blood flow is indicated.

The septum does not grow into the ventricle; the ventricles expand on either side of it. An aperture, the **interventricular foramen,** remains between the free margin of the muscular septum and the **septum intermedium** formed by the fusion of the endocardial cushions in the atrioventricular orifice. This foramen is later closed by proliferation of tissue from the endocardial cushions and bulbar ridges (see below) to form the membranous part of the ventricular septum. The right ventricle also incorporates the proximal (trabecular) part of the bulbus cordis.

Partitioning of the conus cordis and truncus arteriosus

At first the conus and truncus form a common outlet for the developing ventricles. Eventually they must divide to form systemic and pulmonary outlets so that the left ventricle discharges into the aorta and the right ventricle into the pulmonary arteries. This occurs in a way which appears complex at first sight, but which makes good sense on hydrodynamic grounds.

The ventricles lie side by side, with the right slightly anterior to the left. Because of this the stream of blood ejected from the right ventricle enters the anterior part of the bulbus and the stream from the left ventricle enters the posterior part. We know from the study of fluids in tubes that two jets ejected in parallel into a single tube will spiral round each other in a clockwise direction. It seems that the spiral path of the two streams of blood moulds the cardiac jelly to form two **bulbar ridges** which ascend on the walls of the conus and truncus, spiralling around each other in a clockwise direction as they do so (Fig. 2.13). The ridges eventually unite to form a continuous septum termed the **conus septum** in the conus and the **aorticopulmonary septum** in the truncus. In the ventricles the bulbar ridges unite with the arms of the crescentic ventricular septum, helping to close the interventricular foramen. The bulbus is thus divided into two parts, an outflow tract for the right ventricle and an outflow tract for the left ventricle.

Completely separate channels now exist for blood passing from the

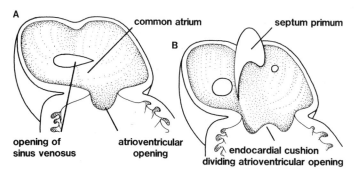

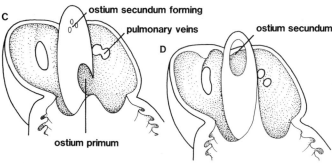

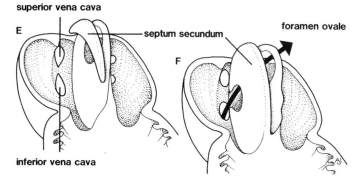

Fig. 2.12. Division of the common atrium. The anterior wall of the atrium has been removed to show the development of the septum. In F, the flow of blood through the foramen ovale is shown.

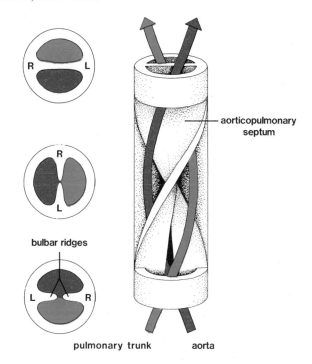

Fig. 2.13. Formation of the aorta and pulmonary trunk.

right ventricle to the pulmonary trunk and for blood passing from the left ventricle to the aorta. As the channels ascend they spiral around each other. The channel from the right ventricle begins anterior to that from the left and, as it ascends, passes to the left and then behind the aortic channel.

Development of semilunar valves

These are developed from thickenings in the cardiac jelly at the level of junction of conus and truncus which are, of course, covered by a layer of endocardium. These thickenings gradually become hollowed out on their upper surface to form the semilunar valves guarding the outflow tracts of the ventricles.

Development of the conducting system

Peristaltic movement of the developing heart begins in the absence of both a specialized conducting system and autonomic nervous input, the sinus venosus acting as the pacemaker and the impulse spreading along what is at this stage a simple tube. After 30 days of development the folding and rearrangement of the heart tube renders this arrangement inadequate and a conducting system composed of specialized muscle fibres develops. This specialized tissue is arranged to form the sinuatrial and atrioventricular nodes and the atrioventricular bundle (see p. 97).

Clinical aspects (Fig. 2.14)

The possibility of carrying out corrective surgery has led to increasing interest over the last 30 years in congenital defects of the heart. Many of these involve the septa.

Atrial septum

Normally the septum primum and septum secundum fuse at about the time of birth so that there is no opening between left and right atria. In some 25 per cent of individuals, however, fusion is incomplete and a narrow communication remains between the two atria. In most cases this does not allow any significant passage of blood. Serious leaks between the atria may be associated with an ostium secundum defect. In this condition a large opening between the two atria is left as a result of inadequate development of the septum secundum.

The foramen ovale may close prematurely during prenatal life, causing massive overdevelopment of the right atrium and ventricle and underdevelopment of the left heart. This is usually fatal.

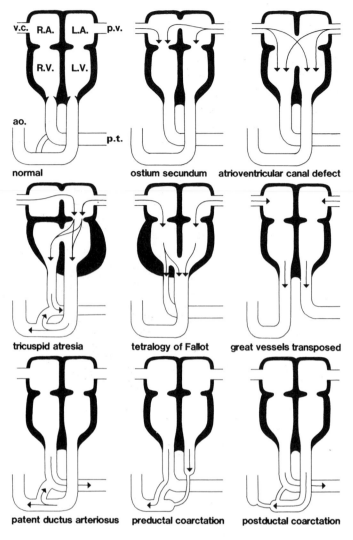

Fig. 2.14. Congenital defects of the heart and great vessels.

normal

ostium secundum

atrioventricular canal defect

tricuspid atresia

tetralogy of Fallot

great vessels transposed

patent ductus arteriosus

preductal coarctation

postductal coarctation

Ventricular septum

Defects are usually seen in the fibrous part which has a complex embryological development, although the muscular part is sometimes also involved. Because the left ventricle pumps at a higher pressure than the right, blood passes from left to right through a ventricular septal defect, so increasing the flow of blood to the lungs. The resulting pulmonary hypertension, if long continued, will lead to progressive thickening of the walls of the pulmonary arteries which will eventually increase the pulmonary blood pressure still further. Sooner or later a point will be reached when the pressure at which the right ventricle has to pump exceeds that of the left ventricle and blood starts to flow from right to left. Deoxygenated blood will then enter the systemic circulation and the patient will develop a bluish tinge (cyanosis).

The truncus and conus

The classic abnormality of this region is the tetralogy of Fallot. The four defects are: (i) pulmonary stenosis (reduction in calibre of the pulmonary trunk); (ii) ventricular septal defect; (iii) overriding aorta; (iv) hypertrophy of the right ventricle. All these defects arise from an unequal division of the conus, so that the septum is displaced. This narrows the output channel of the right ventricle, causing pulmonary stenosis and leading to a septal defect. The aorta is positioned directly above this defect and thus receives blood from both ventricles. The abnormally high pressure on the right side of the heart, resulting from the pulmonary stenosis, produces hypertrophy of the right ventricular wall. Since deoxygenated blood enters the overriding aorta from the right ventricle, a baby suffering from this defect will be cyanosed but usually survives, at least for a few years.

If the bulbar and truncus ridges of the two sides fail to fuse, a persistent truncus arteriosus is formed with the pulmonary artery arising from the aorta and a ventricular septal defect. The aorta again receives blood from both ventricles.

The bulbar and truncus ridges do not always spiral but may be straight. If so, transposition of the great vessels results.

The semilunar valves

The semilunar valves of the aorta and pulmonary artery may fuse to a variable extent, at best restricting the blood flow, at worst preventing it altogether. Pulmonary stenosis will lead to a narrow or even obliterated pulmonary artery with a patent foramen ovale draining blood from the right to the left side of the heart. Aortic stenosis and aortic valvular atresia may lead to underdevelopment of the aorta, left atrium and ventricle.

Position of the heart

Gross abnormalities of the position of the heart may also occur. The commonest of these is dextrocardia when the heart is located on the right side of the chest and the arrangement of the chambers is a mirror image of that usually found. It is often associated with situs inversus of the viscera, a more or less complete reversal of all asymmetrical organs in the abdomen.

Arterial system

The early development of the great vessels resembles that of the heart with which they are continuous. The first functional vessels, the **right** and **left primitive aortae** arise at about 24 days (i.e. after reversal) as rostral continuations of the primitive heart tube and are formed, like the heart tube, by coalescence of islands of angioblastic tissue. The

Atrioventricular canal

The development and fusion of the endocardial cushions divide this canal into left and right orifices, and help to form the membranous part of the ventricular septum and to close the ostium primum in the atrial septum. Any defect in these cushions may, therefore, affect the valves and both septa. Complete failure of fusion will result in defects in the atrial and ventricular septa and a single abnormal atrioventricular orifice ringed by abnormal valve components. In less extreme cases the cushions may fuse partially to complete the ventricular septum but leaving an ostium primum defect in the atrial septum.

Early obliteration of the right atrioventricular aperture leads to tricuspid atresia. The foramen ovale remains patent, allowing blood to pass from the right to the left atrium, the right ventricle is small and receives blood from the hypertrophied left ventricle via a ventricular septal defect.

primitive aortae run forwards from the heart tube at first ventral to the developing foregut, then curve dorsally either side of the gut, embedded in the mesoderm of what is to become the first pair of pharyngeal arches (see p. 46), to run caudally as the paired **dorsal aortae**. Each dorsal aorta gives off branches, the **intersegmental arteries,** to the body wall, lateral branches to the intermediate mesoderm, a **vitelline artery** to the yolk sac and an **umbilical artery** to the placenta. Further fusion of the anterior part of the heart tube extends to the ventral parts of the aortae which become united from behind forwards as a common **aortic sac** (the most rostral part of the truncus arteriosus). The caudal parts of the dorsal aortae also fuse to give rise to a single midline vessel, but this fusion does not extend as far rostrally as the pharyngeal arch region.

The next stage of arterial development is closely bound up with the formation of the pharyngeal arches which is dealt with in detail in the account of head and neck development. For the present it is necessary only to appreciate that the first pair of pharyngeal arches, in which the primitive aortae curve dorsally, is joined during development by five more, each caudal to its predecessor. The six pairs of arches are not all present at the same time, and the fifth is so transitory as to give doubts as to its existence, but the concept of six pairs of arches is a useful one, allowing much more of the embryology of the area to be understood.

The aortic arches

As each pharyngeal arch develops behind its predecessor, it is supplied with an aortic arch, a vessel arising from the primitive ventral aorta, or later from the aortic sac, which curves through the developing mesoderm to join the dorsal aorta above (Fig. 2.15). The set of vessels so formed, which allows blood to percolate through the gills of lower vertebrates, is modified in gill-less mammals to serve other functions.

The **first** (or **mandibular**) **aortic arch** artery persists only in part as the maxillary artery of the upper jaw.

The **second** (or **hyoid**) **aortic** arch artery persists only as the small stapedial and hyoid arteries.

The **third aortic arch** is the first to make a major contribution to the adult arterial system. It forms the **common carotid artery** and the first part of the **internal carotid artery**, a cephalic prolongation of the primitive dorsal aorta which supplies the developing brain. The origin of the external carotid is uncertain: it may be a prolongation of the primitive ventral aorta, or a new vessel sprouting from the third arch which links up with the remains of the vessels of the first and second arches.

The **fourth aortic arch** is the only one to show major asymmetry. On the right it forms the stem of the **subclavian artery,** reaching the arm via the seventh intersegmental artery. The right side of the aortic sac becomes the brachiocephalic artery leading to the right subclavian and right common carotid arteries. There is no equivalent vessel on the left. The fourth aortic arch on the left becomes enlarged to form the **arch of the aorta,** continuous with the left dorsal aorta which persists.

The **fifth aortic arch** is transitory and leaves no memorial.

The **sixth** (or **pulmonary**) **aortic arch** gives off on each side a branch, the **pulmonary artery,** to the developing lung. On the right the connection to the dorsal aorta is lost, but on the left it persists as the **ductus arteriosus** which does not close until birth.

Whilst the above changes are taking place in the aortic arches, modifications of other great vessels are seen:

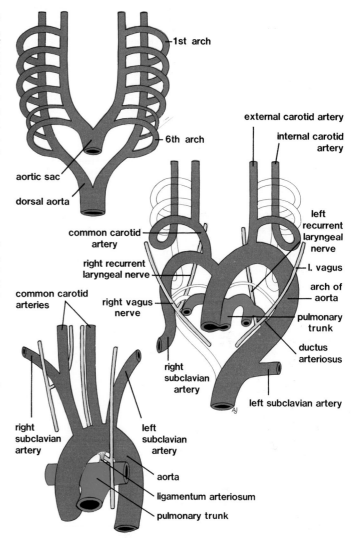

Fig. 2.15. The development of the aortic arches in ventral view.

1. The dorsal aorta, between third and fourth arches, regresses on both sides;

2. the right dorsal aorta regresses between the seventh intersegmental artery and its junction with the left dorsal aorta;

3 the **aorticopulmonary septum,** forming in the truncus arteriosus, divides the aortic sac in half, so that blood from the left ventricle is directed into the third and fourth arches and that from the right into the sixth (pulmonary) arch;

4. the formation of pharyngeal arches causes considerable elongation of the future neck region as a result of which the heart moves from its original cervical position to the chest. This is accompanied by elongation of the carotid and brachiocephalic arteries and relocation of the origin of the left subclavian artery (like the right subclavian originally the seventh intersegmental artery). The sixth arch moves down with the heart, taking with it the associated recurrent laryngeal

nerve (a branch of the vagus, p. 101). On the left side this nerve passes around the ductus arteriosus, but on the right, where the connection of the sixth arch with the dorsal aorta is lost, it passes around the subclavian artery.

Clinical aspects

It is easy to appreciate that the complex changes involved in the formation of the great vessels are liable to variation and susceptible to abnormality (Fig. 2.14).

Patent ductus arteriosus

The ductus arteriosus normally closes by muscular contraction of its walls shortly after birth. Final closure by growth of the tunica intima follows during the next 1–3 months and the ductus degenerates into a fibrous remnant, the **ligamentum arteriosum.** Persistent patency of the ductus commonly occurs, either by itself or in conjunction with other congenital heart abnormalities. This leads to a shunt of blood from the systemic to the pulmonary circulation with consequent pulmonary hypertension. If untreated this may lead to the same changes in the lung vessels as those described in the section on ventricular septal defect with eventual reversal of the shunt and cyanosis.

Coarctation of the aorta

The aorta may be narrowed just above or just below the ductus arteriosus (pre- or postductal coarctation). In the preductal form the ductus remains patent; in the postductal variety the role of the aorta is taken on by collateral circulation including the internal thoracic and intercostal arteries which may become so large as to notch the ribs, a condition easily seen on X-ray.

Double aortic arch

The right dorsal aorta between the seventh intersegmental artery and its junction with the left dorsal aorta may survive to form a symmetrical double aortic arch surrounding the oesophagus and trachea, and occasionally impeding breathing and swallowing.

Venous system

Primitively three pairs of veins drain into the heart, the vitelline, umbilical, and common cardinal; of these the cardinal veins concern us most.

Cardinal veins

The initial embryonic venous system is symmetrical and arranged in an H-shape (Fig. 2.16). The ascending and descending limbs of the H are formed by the **anterior** and **posterior cardinal veins** respectively, while the cross-piece is formed by the **left** and **right common cardinal veins.** In the centre of the cross-piece the system drains into the sinus venosus of the heart. Subsequently the pattern is complicated by additional vessels and the demise of much of the left side of the system.

Posterior cardinal veins

The posterior cardinal veins are reinforced at four weeks of development by paired **subcardinal veins** medial to and draining the intermediate mesoderm. These gradually supersede the posterior cardinal veins, anastomoses form between left and right subcardinals and the right subcardinal develops a connection with the vitelline vein. The left subcardinal regresses rostral to its anastomosis with the

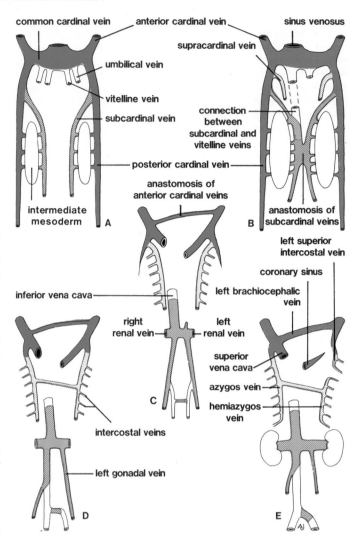

Fig. 2.16. Development of the venous system.

right; caudally it is retained as the left gonadal (testicular or ovarian) vein. The region of anastomosis becomes the renal veins. The right subcardinal vein becomes inferiorly the right gonadal vein, and superiorly, together with its connection to the vitelline vein, the **inferior vena cava.**

Azygos veins

As the posterior cardinal veins are gradually obliterated they are replaced by a third pair of cardinal veins, the **supracardinals,** which sprout medially just below the cross-piece of the H. Again a left-right anastomosis is formed and the left vein loses contact with its origin. The right supracardinal forms the **azygos vein** draining right intercostal spaces and the left supracardinal the **hemiazygos vein** draining lower left intercostal spaces into the azygos vein. The stump of the left supracardinal vein becomes the **superior intercostal vein** draining the upper left two or three intercostal spaces.

Superior vena cava

During the period under consideration the anterior part of the system has also been modified. A cross-anastomosis between the anterior cardinal veins is formed which eventually becomes the **left brachiocephalic vein.** The left common cardinal is obliterated; the right, together with the base of the right anterior cardinal, forms the **superior vena cava.** The right anterior cardinal vein cranial to the anastomosis becomes the **right brachiocephalic** and **internal jugular veins.** On the left, the anterior cranial vein cranial to the anastomosis becomes the **left internal jugular vein;** caudal to the anastomosis it becomes the **left superior intercostal vein.**

Pulmonary veins

The **common pulmonary vein** arises as an evagination of the posterior wall of the future left atrium at about 28 days. The bud grows towards the part of the primitive foregut which will produce the lungs (see below). As the atrium enlarges the common pulmonary vein is incorporated, forming the smooth part of the atrial wall. This incorporation continues as far as the first division of the left and right tributaries of the common pulmonary vein, hence the eventual entry into the atrium of four pulmonary veins, two on the right and two on the left.

Developmental abnormalities of the venous system are common. The inferior vena cava may be totally absent, blood draining instead via the azygos vein and superior vena cava; there may be a left or double superior vena cava; and finally, one or more of the pulmonary veins may drain into the right atrium instead of the left or into the superior vena cava.

RESPIRATORY SYSTEM

The trachea, bronchi, and lungs develop from a pouch, the **respiratory diverticulum,** which appears in the ventral wall of the foregut caudal to the last pharyngeal arch at about four weeks of development.

The diverticulum enlarges caudally to form the trachea. As it continues to enlarge it branches into right and left lung buds which form the right and left bronchi. With continued growth each lung bud gives rise to branches (two on the left and three on the right) which become the main bronchi to the lobes of the lung. These main bronchi undergo repeated dichotomous branching until by the time of birth approximately 17 generations of subdivisions exist. During postnatal growth of the lungs further divisions take place. The bronchi are closed tubes: when the first breaths are taken the thin-walled terminal subdivisions (the respiratory bronchioles) are inflated to form the **alveoli.** The epithelial lining of the respiratory tree is thus endodermal in origin. The associated smooth muscle and cartilage are derived from the mesoderm surrounding the developing respiratory tree. As the lungs enlarge they push into the part of the intraembryonic coelom ventral to the foregut. The mesoderm adjacent to the lungs becomes the visceral pleura, that adjacent to the body wall becomes the parietal pleura. The space between the two layers of pleura becomes the pleural cavity.

Clinical aspects

Most of the described congenital abnormalities of the lungs and bronchial tree are functionally trivial, the presence of supernumerary lobules, etc., making little difference to the efficiency of breathing, although they may make difficulties for anyone wielding a broncho-scope. Major abnormalities, such as the complete absence of lungs or agenesis of one lung, are rare. Sequestrations are areas of lung tissue which are incapable of helping to oxygenate blood. They may have a blood supply from the aorta rather than the pulmonary artery or their alveoli may not be in communication with the trachea. Sequestrations may have the appearance of normal, though uninflated, lung tissue or display prominent fluid-filled cysts.

One group of abnormalities is related to the origin of the trachea from the foregut. It includes: (i) the formation of an oesophagus which is a blind sac; (ii) the formation of an oesophagus opening into the trachea, so that food is transferred to the lungs; or (iii) the formation of a trachea opening into the oesophagus, so that air enters the stomach.

PERICARDIAL AND PLEURAL CAVITIES

We have already noted that at the end of the third week of development the lateral plate mesoderm splits to produce somatic and visceral layers, and that the space appearing between the two is termed the intraembryonic coelom. We have followed this space during embryonic folding and noted that it becomes closed off ventrally to form right and left coelomic cavities, separated in the midline by the dorsal and ventral mesenteries of the gut which persist in some areas and regress in others.

After embryonic folding the coelomic cavity is partly divided by the **septum transversum,** a thick plate of mesoderm which extends from the newly formed ventral body wall, on the rostral side of the stalk of the yolk sac, to reach and then surround the sinus venosus. Laterally there are two wide canals, the **pleuroperitoneal canals,** between the edge of the septum and the dorsal body wall. These have considerable length because of the thickness of the septum transversum in which the liver is developing.

Rostral to the septum transversum the lateral walls of the coelom are pushed inwards by the common cardinal veins and phrenic nerves, the course of which can be traced up the thoracic wall as a ridge later forming the base of the **pleuropericardial fold.**

The respiratory system develops in the part of the thorax immediately rostral to the septum transversum. When the trachea bifurcates the lung buds lie in the part of the coelom behind the pleuropericardial folds and extend downwards on each side into the pleuroperitoneal canal. With further growth of the lungs this space becomes inadequate and the developing pleural cavities (Fig. 2.17) become extended forwards around the coelom until they almost meet at the anterior midline. The pleuropericardial folds also grow, fusing in the midline with the transitory dorsal mesocardium, thus isolating the heart in the **pericardial cavity.**

The **diaphragm** is formed from the septum transversum (which gives rise to the central tendon), the two **pleuroperitoneal membranes** (folds formed caudal to the lungs by the enlargement of the pleural cavities), the mesentery of the foregut and musculature contributed by cervical myotomes. This explains the innervation of the diaphragmatic musculature by the phrenic nerve (which is a branch of the third, fourth and fifth cervical spinal nerves).

CHANGES IN THE CIRCULATORY SYSTEM AT BIRTH: THE LUNGS ARE COMMISSIONED

Before birth oxygen and nutrients are supplied to the fetus via the placenta which is incorporated in the major systemic circulation (Fig.

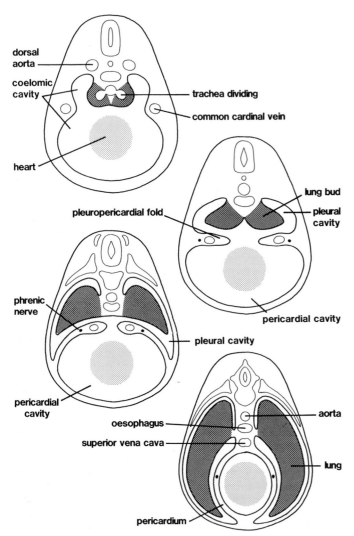

Fig. 2.17 Cross-sections through the developing embryo, rostral to the septum transversum, to show the formation of the pericardial and pleural cavities.

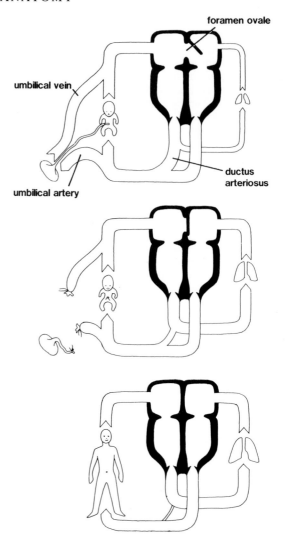

Fig. 2.18. Changes in the circulatory system at birth.

2.18). Blood is delivered to the right atrium through the vena cava from both the body tissues (deoxygenated) and the umiblical vein (oxygenated). Most of the blood arriving at the right side of the heart bypasses the lungs through two channels. Much of it is diverted (due to the hydrodynamics of the right atrium) through the foramen ovale into the left atrium and so into the systemic circulation. The remainder passes into the right ventricle whence it is diverted into the aorta via the ductus arteriosus. The two sides of the heart are, in effect, working in parallel, with a common inlet and a common outlet (the aorta). The pulmonary circulatory system of the lungs is intact from six months but is fed by only a trickle of blood, sufficient to keep the vessels patent. The substance of the lung is assured of a supply of oxygen and nutrients via the **bronchial arteries**, branches of the aorta.

At birth the placental circulation is interrupted. The lungs are emptied of amniotic fluid either by the pressure exerted on the chest during birth or by the midwife in attendance, and the lungs fill with air. The resistance to the passage of blood in the expanded lung is much diminished and blood flow through the pulmonary arteries much increased. This causes a momentary drop in the blood flow through the ductus arteriosus, the walls of which contract narrowing the lumen. The ductus is functionally closed within the next few days. The walls of the umbilical vessels connecting the newborn child to the placenta contract similarly. The foramen ovale is closed by the raised pressure in the left atrium due to the increase in blood returning from the lungs. This is a physiological closure at first. In 75 per cent of the population the closure eventually becomes anatomically complete.

Development of the head and neck

INTRODUCTION

The development of the anterior part of the embryo into the head, neck, face, and brain is one of the most fascinating parts of embryology. We have to concern ourselves with the further development of the following structures:

1. the neural tube situated dorsally;
2. below this the rod-like notochord;
3. further ventrally still the hollow gut tube;
4. the mesoderm surrounding these structures;
5. the investing layer of ectoderm.

Although these tissues develop together and interrelate, it is simpler to tackle them one at a time. We shall, therefore, look first at the somites formed from the head mesoderm.

HEAD SOMITES

We have already noted that the paraxial mesoderm undergoes metameric segmentation and that the resulting somites each becomes divided into dermotome, sclerotome, and myotome. In the head region the development of somites is atypical. Recent studies in a wide variety of non-human embryos indicate that a number (in several studies this has been reported as seven but it may well vary between species) of somitomeres are formed within the paraxial mesoderm alongside the caudal end of the forebrain, the midbrain, and the cranial half of the hindbrain but do not go on to form somites. It seems likely that mesoderm from these somitomeres gives rise to much of the striated muscles of the face, jaws, and throat. The most cephalic fully formed somites to appear are in the paraxial mesoderm adjacent to the caudal part of the hindbrain. These are four in number and are called **occipital** (or **metotic**, i.e. behind the otic capsule) **somites**. It should be emphasized that the study of head segmentation is a rapidly advancing field and that much of the modern research work is based on non-human embryos.

An older, what might be termed classical, interpretation of head segmentation exists which has yet to be fully correlated with the new research findings. A brief summary of this interpretation is necessary because it still forms much of the basis of the terminology of the cranial nerves. According to this view there were originally three pairs of **prootic** (i.e. anterior to the otic capsule) **somites** in the paraxial mesoderm of mammals but these never form separately identifiable structures in modern species. Nonetheless their myotomes are deemed to give rise to the extraocular muscles. The nerves (oculomotor, trochlear, and abducent) supplying these muscles are, therefore, judged to be equivalent to the ventral roots of the spinal nerves through which the myotomic muscles of the trunk are supplied. The dermotomes of the prootic somites are supplied by cranial nerves thought to be equivalent to the dorsal roots of the spinal nerves. These cranial nerves are the ophthalmic division of the trigeminal, the combined maxillary and mandibular divisions of the trigeminal (the trigeminal having been formed by fusion of the two originally separate dorsal cranial nerves), and the facial. The dermatomes of the postulated first and second prootic somites have enlarged enormously and the trigeminal divisions are correspondingly much enlarged and carry many cutaneous fibres. The dermatome of the postulated third prootic somite is very small and the cutaneous content of the facial correspondingly reduced. There are clearly discrepancies between this classical interpretation of anterior head segmentation and the modern findings but, presumably, the three prootic somites of the older view are equivalent to some or all of the somitomeres which have recently been shown to appear in the paraxial mesoderm of this region.

Segmentation in the occipital region is better understood, but even here there has been controversy regarding the number of somites formed. According to the classical view there were originally six (on each side) but the first has disappeared completely and the second is a transient structure only. Hence the usual description of four occipital somites (equivalent to three to six of the original series).

The mesoderm derived from the myotomes of the four occipital somites is believed to migrate to the floor of the mouth where it differentiates into the musculature of the tongue, although in extant mammals this mesoderm appears to form *in situ* in the developing tongue. The nerves supplying these myotomes are again judged to be equivalent to ventral roots of spinal nerves. In higher vertebrates they have fused to form the hypoglossal nerve. The corresponding dorsal nerves have also fused, in this case to form the vagus. The glossopharyngeal nerve, according to the classical view, is the dorsal nerve of the missing first occipital somite. The cutaneous fibres in the vagus and glossopharyngeal are few in number and most of the cutaneous innervation of the head behind the otic capsules is by the cervical spinal nerves. The relationships between the cranial nerves and head segmentation are discussed more fully on pp. 254–5.

The sclerotomes of the occipital somites are believed to become incorporated in the posterior (parachordal) part of the skull base. The number of segments which contributes in this way is still disputed.

The dorsal nerves of the head region differ from the spinal dorsal roots in that they fail to fuse with the corresponding ventral nerves, that they contain visceral motor as well as sensory fibres, and that they contain motor fibres which supply the striated muscles associated with the pharyngeal or branchial arches (hence the dorsal cranial nerves are often called **branchial nerves** although this term tends to be used more in zoology than in human anatomy).

FOREGUT AND PHARYNGEAL ARCHES

After folding is completed, the foregut is separated from the amniotic cavity by only the buccopharyngeal membrane. At the end of the third week of development this membrane ruptures, establishing a primitive mouth or **stomodeum** at the cephalic end of the foregut.

During the fourth and fifth weeks of development the walls of the anterior part of the foregut, the future **pharynx**, develop a series of pouches from before backwards (Fig. 2.19). These **pharyngeal pouches** extend outwards until the endoderm of the pharynx meets the surface ectoderm to form a **closing membrane**. As the pouches develop one behind the other, they divide the mesoderm lying between the pharynx and the ectoderm in to a series of bars, the **pharyngeal, visceral,** or **branchial arches**. The arches appear in a cephalo-caudal sequence and are not all present at the same time. Six arches are usually described as developing on each side, but the fifth is at most a transitory structure. On the outer surface of the embryo the divisions between the arches, floored by the closing membranes, are seen as depressions, the **pharyngeal clefts.** The first pouch and cleft thus lie between the first and second arch, and so on.

The mesoderm contained within each arch develops: (i) an aortic arch artery, linking ventral aortic sac and dorsal aorta (p. 41); (ii) a skeletal element (probably formed from ectomesenchyme, of neural crest origin, which has migrated into the arch); (iii) a branchial muscle mass supplied by a dorsal (branchial) cranial nerve. It was originally believed that the mesoderm from which the branchial muscles are derived was of lateral plate (i.e. visceral) origin despite the muscles being of a striated, voluntary nature. The nerve fibres supplying these muscles were, therefore, classified as visceral and given the added appelation 'special' to denote the fact that the muscles had a different structure and function from visceral muscles elsewhere in the body. From recent research, however, it appears that the mesoderm which gives rise to the branchial muscle fibres is derived initially from the somitomeres of the anterior cephalic region while that forming the connective wrappings of the muscles is ectomesenchyme of neural crest origin. If this modern view is correct then the term 'special visceral' applied to the nerve fibres supplying the branchial muscles is inaccurate and the alternative name of 'branchiomotor' is preferable. However, the former term is so deeply entrenched in human anatomy that it has been retained in the present text.

This arrangement of pouches, clefts, arches, and contents can only be understood in an evolutionary context. In ancestral aquatic vertebrates, as in modern fishes, water was drawn in through an anterior mouth and expelled through a series of gill slits in the sides of the pharynx. Oxygen was extracted as the water was passed over a gill apparatus supported by a branchial arch skeleton and moved by branchial muscle controlled by branchial nerves. In land vertebrates the function of respiration has been taken over by the lungs but the branchial or pharyngeal arches have persisted and have been modified to serve other purposes. The gill slits are represented by the closing membranes (which never quite rupture to form actual slits) and the arch elements have become incorporated into other structures of the head and neck.

We have already noted the 'descent' of the heart. In the 24-day embryo the septum transversum lies opposite the cervical somites while in a seven-week embryo it lies at the level of the first lumbar somite. This descent is actually a passive process, the heart being left

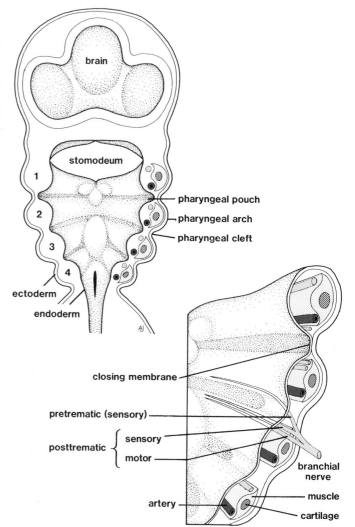

Fig. 2.19. The pharyngeal arches. Above, the dorsal part of a human embryo has been removed to give a view into the ventral floor of the pharynx — at this stage only four arches have formed. Below, the right pharyngeal wall enlarged to show fundamental vertebrate arrangement of nerves.

behind by the growth of the cranial part of the embryo. As a result of this growth the head and floor of the mouth are lifted clear of the pericardium as the neck comes into existence. Structures which grow at the same rate as the dorsal part of the embryo, such as the third aortic arch, the oesophagus, and the trachea, will maintain their relative positions. Structures growing less quickly (such as the ventral part of the third pouch which will form the thymus gland) are left behind in the root of the neck or the upper thorax.

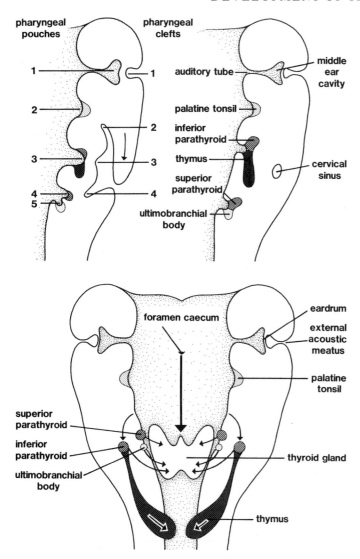

Fig. 2.20. Fate of the pharyngeal pouches. View as in Fig. 2.19.

The part nearest the closing membrane widens to form the **middle-ear cavity**, the closing membrane becomes the **tympanic membrane** or **ear drum** and the remains of the first pharyngeal cleft form the **external acoustic** or **auditory meatus**.

Second pharyngeal pouch

The second pouch is also practically obliterated by the developing tongue. The surviving dorsal portion is eventually infiltrated by lymphoid tissue to form the **palatine tonsil**.

Third pharyngeal pouch

At about five weeks parathyroid tissue begins to differentiate in the endoderm lining the dorsal part of the pouch. The ventral part differentiates into the forerunner of the **thymus**. This proliferation of the walls of the pouch leads to the eventual obliteration of the dorsal part of the lumen. As the neck grows the thymic precursor elongates into a cord of cells with a relatively massive head and a narrow tail still attached to the developing parathyroid. The eventual location of the thymus in the thorax corresponds to the head of this mass: the tail eventually breaks up into small nests of cells which disappear, or may persist as **thymic rests**. The parathyroid tissue, because it is attached to the thymus, is also held back as the neck grows, and eventually forms the **inferior parathyroid gland**.

Fourth pharyngeal pouch

The dorsal part of the fourth pouch forms the **superior parathyroid gland** which becomes associated with the developing thyroid. The ventral part of the pouch may give rise to a little thymus tissue, but this does not contribute to the gland.

Fifth pharyngeal pouch

This is the last pouch to develop and is often considered part of the fourth. If the pouch is judged to exist, then its product is the **ultimobranchial body**, later incorporated into the thyroid gland. If the pouch is judged not to exist as a separate entity, then the ultimobranchial body and the developing superior parathyroid gland are referred to together as the **caudal pharyngeal complex**.

Pharyngeal clefts

In contrast to the important structures derived from the internal pharyngeal pouches, the external clefts are of little importance apart from the first which, as already described, forms the external acoustic meatus. The second, third, and fourth clefts are overgrown by the second arch to form the transient ectodermally lined **cervical sinus**.

Pharyngeal floor

Tongue (Fig. 2.21)

The tongue appears in the floor of the pharynx at four weeks. It is seen first as two **lateral lingual swellings** and a median swelling, the **tuberculum impar**, which are derived from the ventral part of the first pharyngeal arch. Two further swellings develop in the midline behind the tuberculum impar, the **copula** or **hypobranchial eminence** derived from the second, third and the cranial part of the fourth arch, and the **epiglottis** formed from the remainder of the fourth arch. Immediately behind the epiglottal swelling lies the opening of

Pharyngeal pouches (Fig. 2.20)

Since the embryo has six pharyngeal arches, it must have five pouches between them. In practice the fifth pouch is small and atypical, and is often considered part of the fourth.

First pharyngeal pouch (or tubotympanic recess)

The ventral part of the first pharyngeal pouch is obliterated by the developing tongue (see below). The remaining dorsal part, more of a tube than a slit, retains its relationship with the first closing membrane and the first pharyngeal cleft. The part of the pouch nearest the pharynx remains narrow and forms the **auditory tube**.

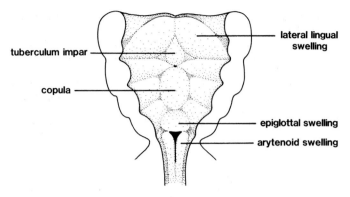

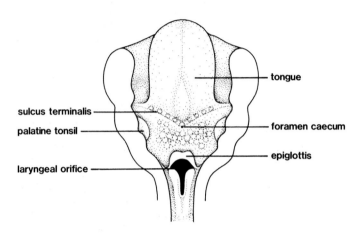

Fig. 2.21. Development of the tongue.

the respiratory system, the **laryngeal orifice,** flanked by the **arytenoid swellings.**

The lateral lingual swellings and the copula unite to form the anterior part (two-thirds) of the tongue which receives its general sensory innervation from the mandibular division of the fifth cranial nerve (the nerve of the first arch) and its taste fibres from the seventh cranial nerve (the nerve of the second arch). The posterior part (one-third) of the tongue is formed from the third arch with minor contributions from the second and fourth arches. Its mucosa is innervated (general sensory and taste) by the glossopharyngeal nerve (the nerve of the third arch). A V-shaped groove, the **sulcus terminalis,** separates the anterior two-thirds from the posterior one-third of the tongue, but during development a certain amount of tissue migrates forwards from the posterior one-third to lie just anterior to the sulcus terminalis where it gives rise to the **vallate papillae** which, hence, are innervated by the glossopharyngeal nerve. The extreme posterior part of the tongue and the epiglottis are innervated by the superior laryngeal nerve, the nerve of the fourth arch which is a branch of the vagus.

As already described the tongue muscles are traditionally described as being derived from the myotomes of the occipital somites, and are supplied by the hypoglossal nerve.

Thyroid gland

The thyroid gland can be seen as early as the 17th day of development as a proliferation of epithelium between the future tuberculum impar and copula. This point is marked in later life by the **foramen caecum** on the dorsum of the tongue. Differential growth of surrounding tissue produces relative movement of the thyroid primordium so that it appears to descend in front of the pharyngeal gut, still connected to the foramen caecum by the thyroglossal duct which subsequently disappears. By the seventh week the thyroid has passed down in front of the developing hyoid bone and laryngeal cartilages to lie in front of the trachea.

Derivatives of the pharyngeal arches

The fate of the skeletal, muscular, and nervous components of each pharyngeal arch can be determined in nearly all cases. The skeletal structures may vanish or persist as cartilage, bone, or ligament; the muscles tend to migrate but can be identified by their nerve supply which is immutable.

Skeletal elements

First arch
The main cartilaginous element of the first arch, **Meckel's cartilage,** is closely related to the part of the first pharyngeal pouch which is to become the middle-ear cavity. The dorsal end of Meckel's cartilage later ossifies to form the malleus (one of the ossicles of the developing middle ear). The middle part of the cartilage regresses, leaving only its perichondrium as the **anterior ligament of the malleus** and the **sphenomandibular ligament.** The ventral part extends towards the ventral midline where it meets its fellow. The **mandible** develops in close association with, but not from, Meckel's cartilage (see p. 57). A second, smaller first arch cartilage, the **pterygoquadrate bar,** develops close to the dorsal end of Meckel's cartilage and ossifies to form the **incus** (another of the middle-ear ossicles).

Second arch
The cartilage of the second arch (**Reichert's cartilage**) is also related at its dorsal end to the middle-ear cavity, to which it contributes the **stapes** (the third ossicle). The remainder of the cartilaginous bar gives rise to the **styloid process** of the temporal bone, the **stylohyoid ligament** and the **lesser cornu** and upper part of the **body of the hyoid bone.**

Third arch
This leaves no trace dorsally, but its ventral part completes the body of the hyoid and supplies its **greater cornu.**

Fourth arch–sixth arch
The cartilaginous elements of these arches fuse to form the **thyroid, cricoid,** and **arytenoid cartilages** of the larynx but just what represents which is not known.

Evolutionary history
The gill bars of the pharyngeal arches are very ancient and have undergone many modifications during their long history.

Our knowledge of the early jawless vertebrates is incomplete and the modern survivors of these evolutionary stages are likely to be very different from their ancestors of 400 million years ago. We must, therefore, look to the early jawed fishes for ancestral gill-arch morphology. In these fossils we find that the branchial skeletal elements are arranged as a series of hinged rods, each with a major dorsal and ventral component. The segmentation seems not to be related in any way to the segmentation of the somites, although many attempts have been made to prove it so. The upper and lower jaws appear to be derived from the transformed skeletal elements of an anterior gill arch, with the primitive jaw joint developing from the joint between the dorsal and ventral components. The mouth has expanded and the jaws have been furnished with many sets of teeth (derived from the skin). Both the upper and lower jaw elements have persisted in all vertebrates. In mammals the upper element, or pterygoquadrate bar, is much reduced while the lower element, Meckel's cartilage, is prominent in the embryo but contributes little to the adult lower jaw. Mammalian jaws are composed almost entirely of dermal bones which develop independently of the cartilaginous skeleton.

With the emergence of the land vertebrates the gills were abandoned in favour of lungs. In amphibians (after metamorphosis), reptiles, birds, and mammals new structures, the hyoid apparatus (supporting the tongue) and the laryngeal cartilages (guarding the entrance to the lungs) have been formed from the skeletal elements of the arches behind the first. Even more recently the mammals have developed a new jaw joint between the mandible and the squamous, both dermal bones, and the bones which ossify in Meckel's cartilage and the pterygoquadrate bar, which form the jaw joint in all other vertebrates, have become incorporated into the middle ear as the malleus and incus. As Romer* says, 'Breathing aids have become feeding aids and finally hearing aids'.

Pharyngeal arch nerves and muscles

Evolutionary history

The pharyngeal arches are supplied with sensory and motor fibres by the dorsal (branchial) cranial nerves. The naming (or numbering) of the cranial nerves we use today is based on their function and position in mammals. According to the classical scheme of head segmentation just described the ten 'true' cranial nerves (i.e. the third to twelfth inclusive) are each equivalent to either a ventral or a dorsal root of a spinal nerve. The ventral nerves are the oculomotor, trochlear, and abducent, which supply the extraocular muscles, and the hypoglossal which supplies the tongue muscles. The cranial nerves (trigeminal, facial, glossopharyngeal, and vagus + cranial accessory) thought to be equivalent to dorsal spinal roots contain, like their spinal equivalents, sensory fibres but they differ from their spinal counterparts in that they also convey visceral motor fibres (to glands and visceral muscle) and motor fibres to the pharyngeal arch musculature (as described on p. 46 these latter fibres are often, and probably inappropriately, called special visceral motor fibres). Each of the dorsal cranial nerves is associated with one of the pharyngeal arches and supplies exclusively the muscles derived therefrom. The trigeminal supplies muscles from the first arch, the facial muscles from the second arch, the glossopharyngeal the single muscle from the third arch, and the vagus (composed of several fused dorsal nerves) the muscles of the remaining arches. The cranial accessory is, in reality, merely a detached portion of the vagus and is included with it from a functional point of view. The vestibulocochlear nerve probably represents components of the facial, glossopharyngeal, and

*Romer, A.S. (1949). *The vertebrate body.* Saunders, Philadelphia.

vagus nerves which supplied the area of skin which has evolved into the internal ear.

Perhaps the most typical (i.e. least modified) dorsal cranial nerve encountered in modern vertebrates is the glossopharyngeal nerve of fishes. Running from the medulla oblongata of the brain this reaches the branchial region as a trunk which splits into a **posttrematic branch** (mixed) and a **pretrematic branch** (visceral sensory only). The posttrematic branch passes behind and the pretrematic branch in front of the gill slit between the second and third arches (see Fig. 2.19). The glossopharyngeal nerve also gives off a pharyngeal branch (visceral sensory only) which runs forwards beneath the pharyngeal lining. A dorsal branch, conveying somatic sensation from the skin, may be present but is commonly absent.

Behind the glossopharyngeal (which supplies the first unmodified gill slit in fish) the pattern in essence is repeated, but all the nerves connect to the brain by a common trunk, the compound vagus nerve. In front of the glossopharyngeal, the facial nerve has lost its sensory component in large measure while the trigeminal is much modified, serving a region where the arrangement of the gills has been disrupted by the development of the mouth and jaws.

The situation in man

This is discussed in detail in Chapter 5.6. The following briefly summarizes the situation. Although distinctions become a little blurred due to the migration and overlapping of dermatomes, in general the skin or mucous membrane of a particular branchial area is supplied by the sensory component of the nerve appropriate to that arch. The musculature derived from each arch, however widely it migrates, retains its innervation from the nerve of that arch. All the nerves supplying the arches, except the trigeminal, also contain parasympathetic motor fibres. To distinguish them from the neurons supplying the branchial muscles these are often termed **general visceral motor** rather than simply visceral motor.

Clinical aspects

If the second pharyngeal arch fails to grow sufficiently to bury the second, third, and fourth clefts, the clefts may retain contact with the surface by means of a branchial fistula often draining a cervical cyst, the remains of the cervical sinus. These may be found anywhere along the anterior border of the sternocleidomastoid muscle. Rarely an internal branchial fistula may open into the pharynx. A preauricular fistula (ear pit), found just in front of the external ear, may be a remnant of the dorsal end of the first pharyngeal cleft.

The tongue is occasionally large at birth (macroglossia). In most cases this is due to undergrowth of the rest of the mouth and is gradually corrected during postnatal growth. In Down's syndrome and cretinism true macroglossia occurs and persists. The tongue may be bifid if the lateral lingual swellings fail to fuse. This is often associated with a cleft lower lip.

Thyroglossal cysts may occur at any point on the path of migration of the thyroid gland where part of the thyroglossal duct persists. They are commonest close to the hyoid bone, but also occur regularly at the base of the tongue, beneath it and at either side of the thyroid cartilage. Ectopic thyroid tissue may also be found along the migratory path but occurs most commonly in the base of the tongue close to the foramen caecum (a lingual thyroid).

FACE, PALATE, AND NOSE

Face

The face develops around a shallow ectodermal depression, the stomodeum (Fig. 2.22). At first the stomodeum is closed by the buccopharyngeal membrane but about the end of the third week this ruptures to produce continuity between the outside world (represented at this stage by the amniotic cavity) and the foregut.

The stomodeum is surrounded on all sides by mesodermal swellings. One of these, the **frontal prominence**, is cranial and unpaired. The other swellings are bilaterally paired. They are derived from the ventral ends of the first pharyngeal arches. These each split into two portions to produce the **maxillary swellings (or processes)**, which lie on each side of the stomodeum abutting against the frontal prominence, and the **mandibular swellings (processes)**, which pass

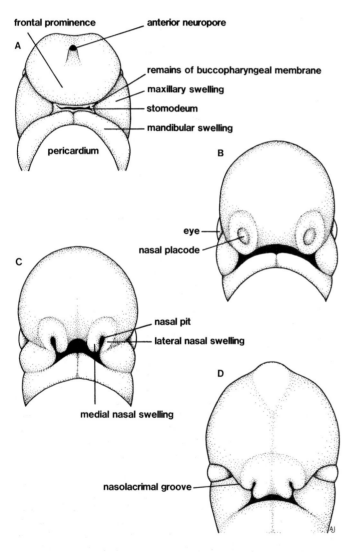

Fig. 2.22. Development of the face.

below the stomodeum and above the pericardium to unite in the ventral midline.

Bilateral **nasal placodes** develop in the ectoderm covering the frontal process just above the stomodeum. During the fifth week each of these becomes flanked by a **medial** and a **lateral nasal swelling**. The swellings unite above and below the placode so that it comes to lie in the floor of a shallow depression, the **nasal pit**. The medial nasal swellings meet each other and fuse. The unit so formed, the **intermaxillary segment,** contributes to the middle portion of the nose, the philtrum of the upper lip, and the part of the upper jaw bearing the four maxillary incisors and forming the primary palate. The lateral swellings will form the **alae** of the nose.

The nasal pits are temporarily continuous ventrally with the stomodeum but are then closed off again as the medial nasal swellings and maxillary processes unite beneath them. The furrow between the lateral nasal swelling and the maxillary process is continuous laterally with that between maxillary and frontal processes, and so runs from the upper lip to the region of the developing eye. This is the **nasolacrimal groove** and is eventually bridged by the processes on each side to form part of the **nasolacrimal (tear) duct.**

Palate

The palate is composed of two major parts, the **primary palate** and the **secondary palate**.

Primary palate

As already noted, the intermaxillary segment has an upper jaw component which is associated with the four upper incisor teeth and forms the **primary palate.** The latter is a horizontal triangular shelf with its apex directed posteriorly, separating the nasal pits above from the stomodeum below (Fig. 2.23). Along the midline of its upper surface it is continuous with the deeper part of the frontal process which separates the nasal pits and becomes relatively thinned to form the primitive **nasal septum**.

Secondary palate

The secondary palate originates as shelf-like outgrowths which appear at about six weeks from the deep surface of each maxillary process. When first formed these palatine processes are directed medially and downwards on either side of the developing tongue. Starting at the posterior extremity, the processes re-orientate themselves horizontally so that they approach each other above the tongue. The mechanism of this manoeuvre and the next stage, the fusion of the free margins of the palatine processes, has been, and is, the subject of a great deal of research but is still uncertain. Eventually fusion occurs (i) between the free edges of the palatine processes; (ii) between each process and the free edge of the primary palate anteriorly; and (iii) between the newly formed secondary palate and the inferior margin of the **nasal septum** which has become elongated by posterior growth of the primitive nasal septum. The point of union of the apex of the primary palate and the two processes of the secondary palate is marked by the **incisive foramen.** The posterior extremities of the palatine shelves unite to form the **uvula**, the posterior border of the soft palate. The palate is usually completed by 60 days.

Nasal chambers

The nasal pits are originally separated from the primitive oral cavity

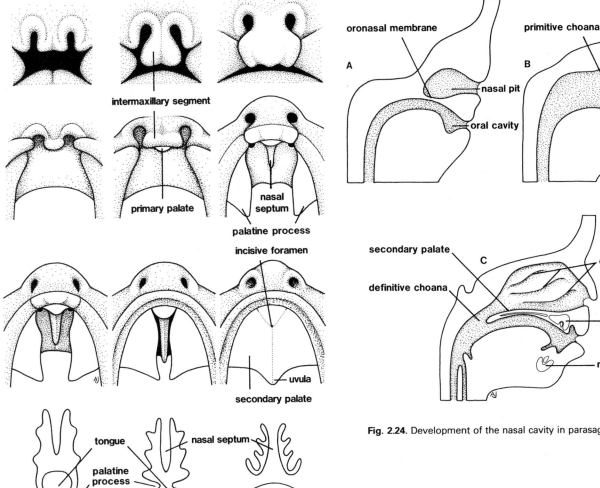

Fig. 2.23. Development of the palate. Top row — development of intermaxillary segment from in front; second and third rows — development of primary and secondary palate from below; bottom row — development of palatine processes in cross-section.

Fig. 2.24. Development of the nasal cavity in parasagittal section.

by the **oronasal membrane**. This ruptures during the sixth week of development allowing the pits or **primitive nasal chambers** to open into the oral cavity via the **primitive choanae** (Fig. 2.24) located either side of the midline behind the forming palate. With the formation of the secondary palate, the nasal cavity is greatly elongated in a posterior direction. Intercommunication between nose and mouth is then via the **definitive choanae** at the junction of nasal cavity and pharynx (i.e. behind the secondary palate). The initial smooth-walled nasal chamber develops folds in its lateral walls, the future conchae, which considerably increase its area.

Clinical aspects

Congenital abnormalities of the face, nose, and palate are of interest to dentists because there is frequently an associated disorder of the jaws and teeth which may require dental treatment.

Early defects in the formation of facial swellings (3rd–4th week) can lead to cyclopia in which there is a single median eye (due to agenesis of the frontal process and incompatible with life) or agenesis of the nasal septum with median fissure of the nose and median cleft lip (caused by incomplete fusion of the medial nasal swellings). In the first arch syndrome there is abnormal development of the first pharyngeal arch with consequent anomalies of the jaws and middle ear. Unilateral hypoplasia of the first arch leads to facial aplasia with malformation of the ear on the affected side. The Pierre Robin syndrome is also produced by abnormal development of the first arch and consists of micrognathia (small jaws) with the tongue permanently placed between the palatal shelves and a consequent cleft palate. Maxillary process defect is a recognized but rather variable condition with cleft lips and other facial fissures.

An important group of defects occurring later in development involves the palate. One scheme of classification uses the incisive foramen as a landmark. Defects anterior to the foramen are considered to be due to anomalies in the melding process of the intermaxillary segment with its neighbours. Posterior defects are due to the failure of secondary palatal union. These two types of defect are probably best regarded as separate conditions, perhaps with separate causes and operating at different times during development.

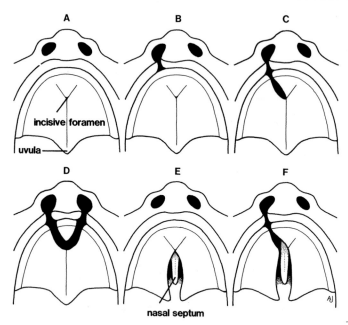

Fig. 2.25. Cleft palate and cleft lip. A = normal; B = unilateral cleft lip; C = unilateral cleft lip and anterior cleft palate; D = bilateral cleft lip and anterior cleft palate; E = posterior cleft palate; F = unilateral cleft lip and anterior cleft palate and posterior cleft palate.

Anterior palate defects

These are concentrated around the junction of the intermaxillary unit and the structures lateral to it (Fig. 2.25). A unilateral anterior lesion will often involve the palate anterior to the incisive foramen, the upper lip and the nose. Its severity may range from division of the maxilla through various degrees of lateral cleft lip to no more than a white line in the red border of the lip. A severe bilateral defect frees the central part of the lip and upper jaw from the structures on each side. The freed segment may then swing forward in a very disfiguring manner.

Defects belonging to this group are often referred to as 'hare-lips'.

Posterior palate defects

These are the result of failure of fusion of the palatine processes of the secondary palate. They tend to run from behind forwards. The least severe cases will merely have a bifid uvula. Progressively more severe cases will have a larger midline defect extending as far as the incisive foramen. The two conditions, hare-lip and cleft palate, can occur in one individual, producing a cleft which runs from the posterior border of the palate to the lip.

The causes of palatal defects are complex and uncertain. Anterior palate defects are commoner in males than females, vary somewhat in prevalence in different population groups and increase with increasing maternal age. The condition is certainly familial and genetic factors are probably involved. The chances of a second child born to parents who already have a child with an anterior palatal defect being similarly affected are about 40 per 1000, compared to 1 per 1000 in the general population, while the chances of a third child being affected are 90 per 1000. There is a persistent but unfounded belief that the cause of a hare-lip is a confrontation beween a pregnant woman and a hare or rabbit.

Posterior palatal defects (cleft palate) have a different basis. They are less common than the anterior type of defect (1 in 2500), are more common in females than males, and are unrelated to maternal age. Again, the probability of recurrence is higher in families with one affected individual than in the general population.

4

Development of the skeletal system

INTRODUCTION

The skeleton is derived from mesoderm, with important contributions in the head from the neural crest. The skeletogenic tissue first associates as a **blastema** in the region where the element is to be formed. This **mesodermal** or **mesenchymal condensation** may be transformed into cartilage which, in turn, may be replaced by bone. Alternatively the cartilaginous stage may be omitted, bone being formed directly in the mesodermal condensation. Some cartilages (such as those of the larynx) never ossify, others (such as the costal cartilages) may ossify partially or pathologically.

AXIAL SKELETON

Vertebral column and ribs

The vertebral column forms in relation to the unsegmented **notochord** and the **neural tube**. The skeletogenic mesoderm is provided by the sclerotomic subdivisions of the somites which form on each side of the neural tube. In the fourth week of development cells of the sclerotomes migrate around the notochord. The rod of tissue so formed betrays its segmental origin, being denser at levels corresponding to somites than between them. In the traditional view of vertebral development, the vertebrae are believed to be formed by a process of resegmentation in which the cranial half of each sclerotome segment unites with the caudal half of the segment in front to produce a new unit, the **vertebral body** (Fig. 3.7, p. 80), which is, therefore, intersegmental. A layer of sclerotomic tissue located between the cranial and caudal segments goes on to form the **intervertebral disc**. The notochord regresses at the level of each vertebral body but persists and even enlarges at the level of the disc to form the **nucleus pulposus** of the disc. Sclerotome cells also migrate dorsally on either side of the neural tube between the successive spinal ganglia (formed from neural crest tissue) to outline the future **neural arches** and **transverse processes** of the vertebrae.

An alternative view of vertebral development, based on extensive work in sheep, suggests that resegmentation does not, in fact, occur. In this species at least it appears that the vertebral bodies are derived from **perichordal mesenchyme**, which is unsegmented, and only the vertebral processes are somitic in origin.

Within the vertebral body or **centrum** a pair of lateral areas begins to chondrify and soon fuses to form a single centre of chondrification. Chondrification centres appear in each neural arch and spread ventrally towards the centrum as the **pedicles** and dorsally as the

laminae, the latter not meeting in the midline until the fourth month. Transverse and articular processes also chondrify from these centres.

The **costal processes** chondrify separately and in the thorax are large, curving round the body wall towards the developing **sternal plates**, so forming the **ribs**. Outside the thorax the costal processes become incorporated into the transverse processes of the adult vertebrae.

Towards the end of the second month the vertebrae start to ossify. Each vertebra typically ossifies from three centres, one in each half of the arch and one in the body.

Clinical aspects

Failure of fusion of the vertebral laminae can result in spina bifida, which may be purely skeletal, but often involves the spinal cord as well (p. 59). Occasionally the process of resegmentation is imperfect, resulting in the formation of a wedge-shaped half vertebra or in the fusion of two adjacent vertebrae. A half vertebra can cause disabling lateral angulation of the spine (scoliosis) and trapped nerve roots may cause pain.

Skull

On developmental grounds the skull can be divided into (i) the chondrocranium in which the skeletal elements develop first as cartilage which is then replaced by bone and (ii) a dermal component in which the bones ossify directly in mesenchyme without an intervening cartilaginous stage. In early vertebrates the chondrocranium was a well-developed structure forming protective boxes around the brain and special sense organs as well as contributing, through the pterygoquadrate and Meckel's cartilages and their replacing bones, to the upper and lower jaws. Dermal bones were added to the skull to provide further protection for the braincase and sense organs and to complete the jaws.

In most modern vertebrates the chondrocranium is reduced although still forming major skull components. This reduction is particularly evident in the mammalian skull where the chondrocranium and its replacing bones are restricted to the cranial base and the capsules around the inner ears and nasal cavity. The chondrocranial element of the lower jaw, Meckel's cartilage, is a transient structure over most of its extent, the mandible being a dermal bone which ossifies in the mesenchyme lateral to the cartilage. The only part of the cartilage to ossify is its dorsal extremity which forms the malleus. The chondrocranial element of the upper jaw, the palatoquadrate or pterygoquadrate cartilage, is even more reduced appearing as just a small piece of cartilage, adjacent to the dorsal extremity of Meckel's cartilage, which ossifies to form the incus. The more anterior part of the pterygoquadrate cartilage is believed to have been incorporated into the cranial base (as part of the greater wing of the sphenoid). The cranial vault, the upper facial skeleton, apart from some of the bones around the nose, and the lower jaw are made up of dermal bones.

Before going on to describe the formation of the various parts of the skull, a few words of explanation are needed about the terms applied to developing bones. Bones that ossify in cartilage are referred to variously as cartilage bones, endochondral bones or cartilage replacing bones. The latter term is the most accurate and is used here. Bones that ossify directly in mesenchyme are referred to as membrane bones, intramembranous bones or dermal bones. Since the first two terms sometimes carry other connotations, the name dermal bone is to be preferred. This name has the further advantage of reflecting the evolutionary origin of this type of skeletal element from the bony plates which developed in the dermis of early vertebrates and provided a protective armour plating.

Braincase and sense capsules

It is apparent from the foregoing that the braincase, the box of bone around the brain, can be divided into the cranial base, which is developed from part of the chondrocranium and is composed of cartilage-replacing bones, and the cranial vault composed of dermal bones ossifying in mesenchyme.

Cranial base

This region extends from the front of the head to the cervical flexure of the brain. Early in development it contains the following landmarks (Fig. 2.26): (i) the front part of the notochord, which runs in the midline; (ii) the infundibulum, a pouch pushing down from the floor of the brain which forms part of the pituitary gland. The infundibulum lies just anterior to the termination of the notochord.

In the mesoderm separating the brain above from the foregut below cartilages begin to appear at about seven weeks of development. These may be considered as a **central stem** and paired **lateral structures.** Between the central stem and the lateral structures pass the various cranial nerves and blood vessels.

The first element of the central stem to appear is parachordal (i.e. near the notochord). It is in the form of two plates, one each side of the notochord, which soon fuse across the midline enclosing the front end of the notochord as they do so. The cartilage spreads backwards to include the sclerotomes of the metotic somites (except the first which disappears). In the process it surrounds the roots of the hypoglossal nerve, then spreads around the neural tube to unite dorsal to the brain as the **occipital tectum** and so marginate the foramen magnum.

Anterior to the parachordal plate are the paired **hypophysial cartilages,** one each side of the developing pituitary stalk. These soon unite in front of and beneath the pituitary gland, so flooring the pituitary fossa, and fuse posteriorly with the parachordal cartilage. This unit will form the body of the **sphenoid bone.**

Anterior to the hypophysial cartilages is a median rod of cartilage which extends forwards between the nasal capsules and is involved in the formation of the nasal septum. The median rod and the hypophysial cartilages are believed to represent the paired trabeculae

cranii which form the anterior part of the central stem in non-mammalian vertebrates.

Lateral to the three pairs of cartilages making up the central stem of the neurocranium were originally three **sense capsules,** i.e. the cartilages surrounding the **nasal, optic,** and **otic** sense organs. In mammals the optic capsule is not seen as cartilage (in fact, it forms the **sclera** of the eye) but in reptiles and birds ossifies as a series of bony plates protecting the eye.

The otic (or auditory) capsule condenses around the developing inner ear. The growing capsule meets the parachordal plate ahead of and behind the glossopharyngeal, vagus, and accessory nerves thus defining the jugular foramen. The vestibulocochlear nerve enters the capsule and the facial nerve runs on its superior aspect between the parts enclosing semicircular canals and cochlea.

The medial walls of the two nasal capsules unite in the midline to form, with the median rod, the **nasal septum.** The lateral walls unite with the medial walls superiorly, leaving a large central aperture which later becomes the **cribriform plate** which gives passage to the olfactory nerves.

Two bilaterally paired cartilages develop in the region between the otic and nasal capsules: anteriorly the **alae orbitalis** and posteriorly the **alae temporalis.** The ala orbitalis, which ossifies as the lesser wing of the sphenoid, unites with the central stem at its anterior and posterior boundaries, leaving a foramen for the passage of the optic nerve. Ossification in the ala temporalis, together with adjacent intramembranous ossification, gives rise to the greater wing of the sphenoid. This grows posteriorly to enclose the maxillary and mandibular divisions of the trigeminal nerve in the foramen rotundum and foramen ovale respectively. Between orbitalis and temporalis is the superior orbital fissure through which pass the oculomotor, trochlear and abducent nerves and the ophthalmic division of the trigeminal nerve. Between the ala temporalis and the otic capsule runs the **internal carotid artery.**

By the end of the second month the chondrocranium is fully differentiated. The nasal capsules grow enormously around this time, doubling in length between 10 and 14 weeks and increasing six-fold by 36 weeks. The parachordal region grows less quickly, increasing four-fold between 10 and 32 weeks. This rapid growth of the nasal capsules is responsible for the change in the shape of the head in the late fetal period.

Centres of ossification later appear in the cartilages of the braincase and sense capsules. These include:

1. centres for the basioccipital and lateral parts of the occipital bone in the parachordal region, and for the supraoccipital part of the occipital bone in the region of the tectum; the latter forms the more ventral area of the squamous part of the adult occipital bone;

2. centres for the lesser wings and base of the greater wings of the sphenoid in the alae orbitalis and temporalis respectively; centres for the body appear in the adjacent part of the central stem;

3. centres for the petrous part of the temporal bone in the otic capsule; the dermal tympanic bone ossifies lateral to the petrous and supports the ear drum. The region between the petrous and tympanic becomes surrounded by bony processes from the petrous enclosing the ear ossicles and forming the middle-ear cavity;

4. centres for the ethmoid and inferior conchae in the nasal capsule. The ethmoid centres include one (the mesethmoid) for the perpendicular plate and crista galli and one for each labyrinth. The ossification centres for the labyrinths and inferior conchae appear in the fifth month in the lateral walls of the nasal capsules. The meseth-

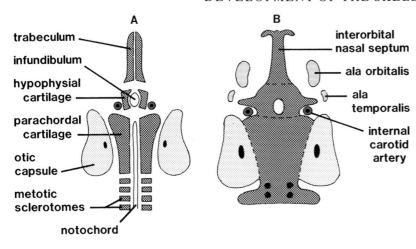

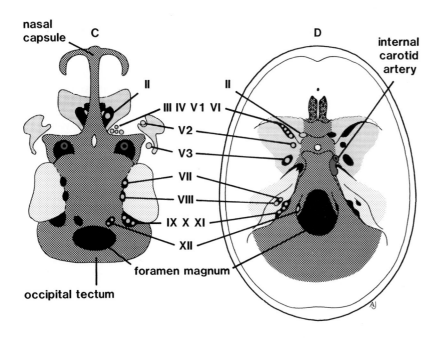

Fig. 2.26. Development of the cranial base showing the main structural elements and their approximate contribution to the adult skull. Roman numerals refer to cranial nerves. The evolutionary and developmental history of the region of the greater wing of the sphenoid is complex and still disputed (see for example, *The Mammalian Skull* by W J Moore, Cambridge University Press, 1981).

moid ossification appears in the upper part of the nasal septum shortly after birth. The anteroinferior part of the nasal septum remains cartilaginous and is called the **septal cartilage**. Elsewhere the cartilage of the lateral walls regresses and is replaced by the dermal maxillary, palatine and lacrimal bones. The mesethmoid and labyrinth components of the ethmoid unite by ossification of the cribriform plate by the third year.

Cranial vault

The vault of the skull (Fig. 2.27) is formed by dermal bones. Centres of ossification appear in the mesenchyme surrounding the dorsal aspect of the developing brain. These extend and eventually form the frontal and parietal bones and the more dorsal part of the squamous component of the occipital bone. At a later stage the squamous part of the temporal bone, which develops initially in the maxillary pro-

cess, becomes added to the lateral wall of the vault. With continued growth the vault bones meet each other at joints, the **sutures,** representing remnants of the original mesenchyme.

Facial skeleton and the contribution of the pharyngeal arches to the skull

The adult facial skeleton, except for that part of the nasal region developing from the nasal capsule, is made up of dermal bones. Nevertheless the cartilages of the first or mandibular pharyngeal arch provide a major component of this part of the skull for a brief period of fetal life. The cartilage of the second or hyoid arch is also involved to a small degree in skull development. The first and second arch cartilages and their contribution to skull development are described on page 48. The remaining arches chondrify at only their ventral ends where they become incorporated into the larynx.

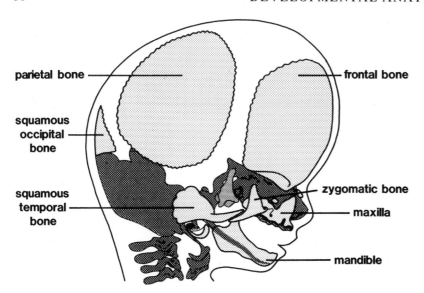

Fig. 2.27. Development of the cranial vault. Fetus aged approximately 4 months. Dermal bone in light stipple; cartilage and cartilage replacing bone in dark stipple; ala temporalis in intermediate stipple.

Dermal bones of the facial skeleton

An arcade of dermal bone is laid down in the mesoderm of the maxillary process consisting of four bones, the **premaxilla, maxilla, zygoma,** and **squamous part of the temporal bone.** The last named becomes incorporated into the braincase, where it fuses with the outer aspect of the otic capsule (the petrous bone). On the deep aspect of the maxillary process are laid down the **palatine bone** and **vomer** and on its superior aspect the **lacrimal** and **nasal** bones.

Further development of the facial skeleton

Maxilla

The human maxilla is usually described as being formed by fusion of two initially independent ossifications – the **maxilla proper** and the **premaxilla.** In other mammals these two ossification centres give rise to separate maxillary and premaxillary bones. There is some recent evidence that the traditional view of the development of the human maxilla is incorrect and that the bone, in reality, ossifies from a single centre which extends into the incisor region in such a manner as to give the appearance of a separate premaxillary ossification in serial sections of the developing jaws. However, this newer view is inconsistent with the situation in most other mammals and with the observation of what appear to be sutures between the maxillary and premaxillary ossifications in the fetal and infant skull (see below).

According to the traditional view, the maxilla proper first appears as a membranous ossification in the maxillary process at about 40 days. Ossification begins adjacent to the lateral wall of the nasal capsule just below the infraorbital nerve at the point where it gives off its anterior superior alveolar branch. This is the position eventually occupied by the upper canine teeth. Ossification spreads backwards below the orbit and forwards towards the premaxillary ossification to produce a curved strip of bone. A trough containing the infraorbital nerve crosses the superior surface of the developing bone (Fig. 2.28). Several extensions develop from the main mass of bone to form the various maxillary processes. An upwardly directed extension develops from the anterior part of the bone mass which, together with a similarly directed extension from the premaxilla, forms the **frontal**

process. Posteriorly ossification extends into the zygomatic arch where it forms the **zygomatic process,** medially it extends into the palate forming the **palatine process** and inferiorly it extends either side of the developing tooth germs as the **medial** and **lateral alveolar plates.** Later the tooth germs are separated by transverse septa to produce a series of **alveoli** or **tooth sockets.**

A mass of cartilage (the malar cartilage) is temporarily present on the zygomatic process of the maxilla. This is a piece of secondary cartilage (p. 57) which soon undergoes endochondral ossification and disappears.

The premaxilla forms at the junction of frontonasal and maxillary processes. It ossifies a little later than the maxilla from two centres. The major centre is close to the nasal capsule and in front of the anterior superior alveolar nerve (i.e. above the germ of the second incisor). From here ossification spreads above and behind the incisor tooth germs to form the posterior alveolar walls and the **palatal premaxilla,** upwards to form the premaxillary component of the

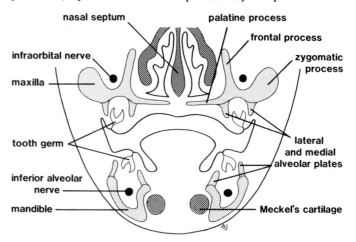

Fig. 2.28. Development of the maxillae and mandible in cross section. Dermal bone in light stipple; cartilage in dark stipple.

frontal process and backwards to unite with the maxilla. The minor (paraseptal) centre develops near the midline.

Bone from the maxillary ossification centre spreads anterior to the premaxilla to form the anterior alveolar walls. As a result the suture between the maxilla and premaxilla on the anterior aspect of the upper jaw has disappeared by the third month of prenatal life. On the palatal aspect the suture, running from the incisive fossa to the region of the canine tooth, usually remains visible until after birth.

By the time of birth the maxilla has all the constituents of the adult bone although the alveolar process is relatively small and the body of the bone is shallow due to the small size of the contained **maxillary air sinus**.

Palatine bone

The palatine is a dermal bone which develops adjacent to the cartilaginous nasal capsule. In the seventh or eighth week ossification extends upwards to form the **perpendicular plate** and horizontally to form the **horizontal plate**. As the nasal capsule regresses locally the palatine bone meets the medial surface of the maxilla to form a major part of the lateral nasal wall.

Other upper facial bones

The **vomer** develops from two centres which appear in membrane close to the inferior margin of the septal cartilage during the ninth week. These unite beneath the cartilage and extend backwards to form a bony trough whose posterior margin eventually meets the body of the sphenoid. A vertical stem which develops on the underside of this trough descends towards the hard palate.

The **lacrimal** bone develops in the third month from an intramembranous centre adjacent to the nasal capsule. With regression of the nasal capsule it forms a small part of the lateral wall of the nose and of the medial wall of the orbit.

The **nasal** bone develops in the second month as an intramembranous ossification on the anterior roof of the nasal capsule.

The **zygomatic** bone ossifies in the second month from an intramembranous centre lateral to the eyeball. With development it soon contacts the temporal bone and maxilla and later the frontal bone.

The development of the ethmoid and inferior conchae is described on page 71.

Mandible

The mandible is a dermal bone which develops in close association with Meckel's cartilage. By six weeks the latter element is an unbroken rod of cartilage stretching from the otic capsule to the midline. The ventral end is united with its fellow of the opposite side by a bridge of mesenchyme.

Closely related to the cartilage is the mandibular division of the trigeminal nerve and its branches. The mandibular nerve issues from the braincase and reaches the cartilage at the junction of dorsal and middle thirds (Fig. 2.29). Here it divides into lingual and inferior alveolar nerves. The lingual nerve runs medial to the cartilage, the inferior alveolar nerve lateral to it to a point where it divides again into mental and incisive branches. Ossification of the mandible commences at seven weeks at a centre cradled in the V of the mental and incisive nerves, close to the future mental foramen. Ossification spreads posteriorly beneath the inferior alveolar nerve and anteriorly beneath the incisive nerve, leaving the nerves in a groove on the upper surface of the bony rudiment. The mental nerve is surrounded by this mass of bone running at first in a groove which is later roofed over from before backwards to form the **mental canal**. In a similar

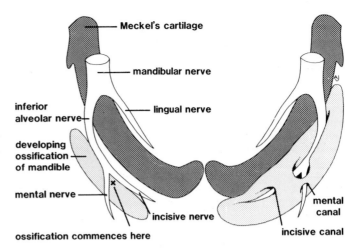

Fig. 2.29. Development of the mandible as seen from above. Left — ossification has just begun; right — slightly later stage. Dermal bone in light stipple; cartilage in dark stipple.

fashion the incisive nerve becomes immured in the **incisive canal**. Ossification proceeding backwards has the same effect on the inferior alveolar nerve, although at a later stage. From this single centre of ossification is thus produced the **body of the mandible**, running from the symphysis in the anterior midline, to the area which will become the mandibular foramen.

At this stage the tooth germs still lie above the mandible and are not connected to it. As the germs develop, however, they come to lie in a gutter formed by **medial** and **lateral alveolar plates** which grow upwards from the body of the mandible. Later in development the gutter is divided into individual alveoli for the roots of the teeth by the formation of transverse septa.

The ventral part of Meckel's cartilage becomes surrounded by the intramembranously ossifying bone of the mandibular body and is resorbed apart from one or two small remnants close to the midline.

The **ramus** is produced by further backward spread of ossification which occurs so rapidly that the coronoid and condylar processes are visible by the tenth week. The part of Meckel's cartilage lying medial to the ramus regresses apart from its perichondrium which becomes the sphenomandibular ligament.

Two cartilages appear in the ramus, one in the condylar and the other in the coronoid process, which, since they are not related to Meckel's (i.e. the primary) cartilage, are called **secondary cartilages**. Secondary cartilage is unusual in several respects. First, it is derived not from primitive mesenchymal cells but from cell lines which are already producing dermal bone. Secondly, although secondary cartilage undergoes endochondral ossification, it does so by a mechanism different in several ways from that seen in primary cartilage. These differences are described on page 71.

The **condylar cartilage** is the largest and most important secondary cartilage. It first appears at about 11 weeks as a fringe to the superior and lateral aspects of the condylar process. During subsequent growth it undergoes relative enlargement and within a few weeks has formed a conical mass occupying the condylar process as far inferiorly as the mandibular foramen.

The cartilage is replaced inferiorly by trabecular bone, easily distinguished from the membrane bone of the body. By five months much of the original cartilage has ossified, only a narrow zone of cartilage persisting beneath the articular surface of the head of the mandible. Nevertheless, this zone is an important site of mandibular growth (p. 71).

The **coronoid cartilage** is first seen at about 14 weeks as a cartilaginous strip on the anterior border of the summit of the coronoid process. By birth it has been completely replaced by bone. The development of the coronoid process and also of the angle of the mandible is intimately related to the development of the major muscles of mastication. The **temporalis** muscle is attached to the coronoid process, the **masseter** and the **medial pterygoid** to the angle.

The mandible at birth is still separated into right and left halves by a midline joint (the **mental symphysis**). The ramus is small relative to the body and the alveolar process is incompletely developed. The mandibular angle (i.e. the angle formed between the inferior border of the body and the posterior border of the ramus) is more obtuse than in the adult. The mental symphysis fuses at about the end of the first postnatal year, being aided by the appearance of a number of ossicles. Some of these ossicles may ossify in the ventral end of Meckel's cartilage but others are believed to ossify in small nodules of secondary cartilage which have been described as developing in the symphysis.

5

Development of the central nervous system

INTRODUCTION

We have already noted (p. 33) the specialization of the ectoderm into **neurectoderm** with the formation of the **neural plate** during the third week of development. We have also described the **neural folds** and the way they come together in the midline to produce the **neural tube** and pinch off the **neural crest**. Final closure of the **anterior neuropore** and **posterior neuropore** defines the developing nervous system as a closed tube with a cylindrical caudal portion, the future **spinal cord,** and a much larger diameter cephalic portion, the future **brain.**

The development and histological differentiation of the spinal cord and brain are similar in essence. The brain is much more complex in terms of size, folding and numbers of cells, so it is convenient to consider the spinal cord first.

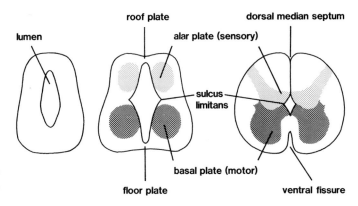

Fig. 2.30. Development of the spinal cord.

Differentiation of the spinal cord

The neurectoderm which will give rise to the neural tube is originally a single layer of cells. By the time the neural tube has formed, this original single layer has become separated into three concentric layers of cells, each with a different function. (i) Surrounding the central lumen is a layer of **ependymal** cells, an actively dividing pseudostratified epithelium. The cells of this layer are closely packed, and cells about to divide seem to retract and round up adjacent to the lumen; mitotic figures are most frequently seen in this location. (ii) The middle or **mantle layer** is made up of primitive neuroblasts provided by the proliferating ependymal cells. This layer will go on to become the **grey matter** of the spinal cord. (iii) The outer or **marginal layer** has relatively few cells, being composed mainly of **nerve fibres** emerging from the neuroblasts of the middle layer. It will ultimately form the **white matter** of the spinal cord.

The brain and spinal cord, as well as being enclosed within the braincase and vertebral canal, are further protected by a series of wrappings, the **meninges**. In fish there is a single meninx but in land vertebrates this has become divided into the outer fibrous **dura mater** and an inner layer applied to the surface of the nervous tissue. In mammals this delicate inner layer is further divided into the outer **arachnoid mater** and the inner, vascular **pia mater.**

Proliferation of cells within the neural tube causes it to change its shape (Fig. 2.30). A pair of dorsolateral and a pair of ventrolateral cell masses form the **alar** and **basal plates,** respectively. The basal plates develop into parts of the spinal cord and brainstem which are essentially motor in function; the derivatives of the alar plates are mainly sensory and coordinative in function. The lumen of the neural tube is transformed from a vertical slit to a lozenge shape by the formation of these thickenings. The furrow on the lateral wall of the lumen between alar and basal plates is known as the **sulcus limitans**. The roof and floor of the tube in the midline are known as the **roof** and **floor plate** respectively. They are thin and contain nerve fibres crossing from one side of the cord to the other. Further growth of the basal plates is in a ventral direction and results in the formation of the **ventral fissure** of the spinal cord. The alar plates expand medially, compressing the dorsal part of the lumen or **central canal** until it is obliterated and so forming the **dorsal median septum**.

During neural tube formation, cells immediately lateral to the forming tube become cut off as a dorsal mass, the **neural crest**. This zone extends from midbrain to caudal segments. The neural crest of the head is discussed on page 33; in the trunk the neural crest migrates to form the spinal ganglia, one per somite, and the autonomic ganglia of the trunk, as well as contributing to non-nervous tissue.

Clinical aspects

Occasionally the neural tube fails to close, either along its whole length, including the future brain, or in a localized area (complete or localized rachischisis). More commonly the tube closes but the protective vertebral arches which surround it are defective dorsally. Both types (tube open and closed) are referred to as spina bifida if they occur at any point along the spinal cord. Spina bifida may thus involve only the non-closure of the neural arches of the vertebrae (usually in the sacrolumbar region) and thus be seen only on X-ray (spina bifida occulta) or be a more serious defect in which the meninges bulge through the opening in the vertebral column and appear on the body surface as a fluid-filled sac (meningocele) or one containing a portion of the closed spinal cord (meningomyelocele). Failure of the neural tube to close results in a plate of nervous tissue being exposed on the dorsal surface of the body (myelocele).

BRAIN

Divisions of the brain

In all vertebrates there is a concentration of nervous tissue, the brain, at the anterior end of the body. In an active bilaterally symmetrical animal this is the part that contacts the environment first. Primitively, no doubt, the brain was simply a centre for the receipt of sensory impulses from organs which were naturally placed at the anterior end of the body. In vertebrates there has been an elaboration of this system with the involvement of extra neurons. This has led to a greatly increased number of possible responses to a given stimulus and to the development of functionally specialized groups of neurons. In these **brain centres** afferent impulses are correlated and integrated for appropriate response and motor mechanisms are co-ordinated. They are also the areas where such complex neural functions as consciousness, memory, emotional response, and intellect reside.

The topography of the adult human brain is most easily under-stood through a study of its development, both in the individual and during the evolution of the vertebrates. In the early embryo, the anterior end of the developing neural tube tends to fold ventrally (Fig. 2.31), probably because the neural tube is growing faster than the more ventral tissues. This is the **cephalic flexure** marked by the **ventral sulcus.** Anterior to the ventral sulcus a central sac-like en-largement, the **prosencephalon** or **forebrain,** is delineated. A little later a second, more **caudal (pontine) flexure** occurs in the opposite direction, separating the **mesencephalon** or **midbrain** anteriorly from the **rhombencephalon** or **hindbrain** posteriorly. The hindbrain merges posteriorly with the spinal cord.

The three primary divisions of the brain are represented in the adult by the **brainstem** (= hindbrain + midbrain) and its upward continuation, the **diencephalon** (= primitive forebrain). These are evolutionarily the oldest part of the brain and the seat of many primitive but literally vital neural mechanisms.

In primitive vertebrates, these divisions of this ancient part of the brain are associated with the sensory inputs from the nose (to the forebrain), eye (to the midbrain), and ear (plus the lateral line organs found in fishes) (to the hindbrain). To deal with the number of neurons needed to cope with these very large inputs each division of the brain developed, during the course of evolution, a dorsal extension: the **cerebral hemispheres** from the forebrain, the **tectum** of the midbrain, and the **cerebellum** from the hindbrain.

In man, as in other mammals, this simple picture has become blurred by the appearance of many new features. Nevertheless, the basic vertebrate structure of the brain is maintained as is readily apparent from its further embryonic development. From the front part of the hindbrain, now called the **metencephalon,** a dorsal out-growth, the **cerebellum,** appears. The metencephalon ventral to the cerebellum forms the **pons.** The remainder of the hindbrain, or **myelencephalon,** gives rise to the **medulla oblongata.** Meanwhile, the forebrain is changing even more dramatically. Paired outgrowths

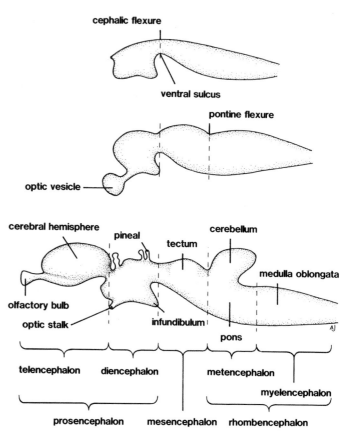

Fig. 2.31. Development of the brain.

grow outwards and forwards towards the nasal region. From these develop the **cerebral hemispheres** and more anteriorly the **olfactory bulbs.** These structures together make up the **telencephalon.** The unpaired remainder of the forebrain is the **diencephalon** (Table 2.1).

At the three-vesicle stage of embryonic development **optic vesicles** push out on either side from the forebrain to which they remain attached by **optic stalks** which later develop into **optic nerves.** The distal end of each optic vesicle comes into contact with surface ectoderm to form the eye. More posteriorly a median projection, the **infundibulum,** pushes downwards towards **Rathke's pouch,** a pocket of epithelium growing up from the roof of the stomodeum. These will later meet to form the **pituitary gland.** Dorsally the **pineal organs** grow from the roof of the forebrain.

Ventricles

The original cavity of the neural tube persists within the brain as a series of spaces filled with cerebrospinal fluid. As the cerebral hemi-spheres grow outwards, the cavity expands into them to form the **lateral ventricles.** Each of these connects via an **interventricular foramen** with the cavity of the diencephalon, or **third ventricle.** The cavity of the midbrain is reduced to a narrow canal, the **aqueduct of the midbrain,** communicating rostrally with the third ventricle and caudally with the **fourth ventricle** in the pons and upper part of the medulla oblongata. The latter is continuous with the central canal of the lower part of the medulla which, in turn, is continuous with the

Table 2.1. *Divisions of the developing brain and their adult derivations*

Prosencephalon	Telencephalon	Cerebral hemispheres, olfactory pathway
	Diencephalon	Epithalamus, thalamus, hypothalamus, subthalamus
Mesencephalon		Midbrain
Rhombencephalon	Metencephalon	Pons, cerebellum
	Myelencephalon	Medulla oblongata

canal of the spinal cord. The walls of the ventricles are in most regions made up of thick layers of neural tissue. In two areas, one at the junction of the hemispheres with the diencephalon and the other in the roof of the fourth ventricle, the walls are very thin, being composed of no more than a layer of ependyma. In these areas develop **choroid plexuses,** folds of vascular tissue which invaginate the ependyma and through which selective exchange of materials between blood and cerebrospinal fluid can take place.

Cranial nerve nuclei

Several cranial nerves emerge from the brainstem and are associated with nuclei which make up much of the grey matter of this part of the brain. It has already been noted that in the spinal cord the motor neurons develop ventrally and the sensory neurons dorsally. Since the brain is a development of the rostral end of the spinal cord, a similar arrangement might be expected there. If we consider the part of the brain which is directly continuous with the spinal cord (the caudal part of the medulla oblongata), the similarity is immediately apparent, the motor nuclei tending to lie ventral to, and the sensory nuclei dorsal to, the central canal. In the rostral part of the medulla and in the pons the expansion of the central canal to form the fourth ventricle has resulted in the originally dorsal areas being pushed laterally but the arrangement of the grey matter in the floor of the fourth ventricle is essentially unchanged (Fig. 2.32).

The sensory region is separated by the sulcus limitans from the motor region. Motor and sensory regions are each divided further into somatic and visceral portions. Most ventrally is the somatic motor column for the supply of muscles derived from myotomes,

then the special visceral motor column for the supply of pharyngeal arch muscles and, next to the sulcus limitans, the general visceral motor column, the source of autonomic efferents. Dorsal to the sulcus limitans is the general visceral sensory column, then the special visceral sensory (taste) column, and finally the somatic sensory (cutaneous and proprioceptive) column.

In higher vertebrates the columns tend to be interrupted, so that in a longitudinal section through the human brainstem (Fig. 2.33) we see discrete **nuclei,** each a collection of cells of similar function, rather than continuous columns. The somatic motor column is fragmented into several small nuclei in the midbrain and pons which supply neurons to the oculomotor, trochlear, and abducent nerves for the extraocular muscles and a single nucleus in the medulla which supplies the tongue muscles through the hypoglossal nerve. The special visceral motor column for branchial musculature is broken up into separate nuclei located in the pons for the trigeminal and facial nerves (to muscles of the first and second arches) and the nucleus ambiguus in the medulla for the glossopharyngeal, vagus, and cranial accessory nerves (to the muscles of the remaining arches). Autonomic (parasympathetic) nuclei of the third column are present in the midbrain for autonomic eye reflexes (oculomotor nerve) and in the medulla for the salivary glands (facial and glossopharyngeal nerves) and for most of the viscera of the trunk (vagus nerve).

The sensory columns are less disrupted. The nuclei associated with general visceral sensation (glossopharyngeal and vagus nerves) and taste (facial, glossopharyngeal, and vagus nerves) remain together in the medulla as the nucleus of the tractus solitarius. The somatic sensory column remains intact as a single elongated nucleus, associated principally with the trigeminal nerve, which traverses the

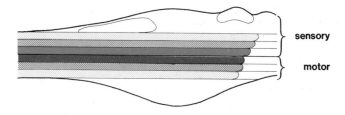

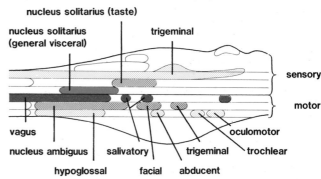

Fig. 2.33. The position of the cranial nerve nuclei in the human brainstem, longitudinal section. Above, the idealised arrangement of the sensory and motor columns; below, the position of the nuclei shown in diagrammatic form—during development some of these nuclei migrate (see Fig. 5.36). The most rostral nucleus (unlabelled) in the general visceral motor column is the Edinger–Westphal.

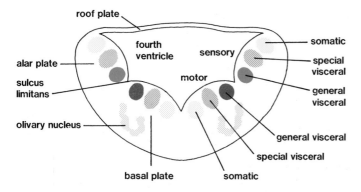

Fig. 2.32. The position of the cranial nerve nuclei in the open medulla, transverse section.

brainstem and extends into the cervical part of the spinal cord. Although anatomically continuous it is divided on functional grounds into the spinal nucleus (in medulla and cord), the chief sensory nucleus (in the pons) and the mesencephalic nucleus (in the midbrain).

The motor and sensory nuclei are sheathed thickly by tracts of fibres running to and from the higher brain centres. The motor and sensory neurons of the cord and brainstem have the necessary connections to make up relatively simple reflex arcs between the sensory receptors and the responding effector organs. However, the brain works at a more complex level and behaviour above the reflex level requires that information is passed to higher centres for processing. The main processing centres are located outside the brainstem, comprising the three specialized dorsal additions to the ancient brain, viz. the cerebellum, the midbrain tectum, and the cerebral hemispheres.

Cerebellum

The roof of the metencephalon (i.e. the roof of the anterior part of the fourth ventricle) is wide posteriorly and very narrow anteriorly. Because of this, the alar plates in this region lie almost at right-angles to the midline and are termed the **rhombic lips**. The rostral parts of the rhombic lips become thickened to form the **cerebellar plate**. By the 12th week of development the cerebellar plate shows a small midline part, the **vermis** and paired **lateral cerebellar hemispheres.** The cerebellum is functionally part of the motor system, playing a major role in the maintenance of balance and the co-ordination of muscle activity.

Specializations of midbrain and diencephalon

The cranial nerve nuclei reach as far rostrally as the midbrain. The region ahead of this (i.e. the diencephalon and most rostral part of the midbrain) contains nuclei which, in those vertebrates where the cerebral hemispheres are not well developed, are important centres for correlation and co-ordination. In mammals, these roles have been taken over to a considerable extent by the cerebral hemispheres. The centres in the midbrain and diencephalon now act as relay stations between lower centres and the hemispheres, as well as retaining some of their original correlative function.

In a bisected human brain (Fig. 5.21), the diencephalon can be seen to surround the third ventricle, being buried below and between the cerebral hemispheres. It contains, each side of the ventricle, a large collection of nuclei, called collectively the **thalamus,** which are concerned, amongst other things, with the relay of visual, auditory, and somatic sensory information. Above the thalamus is the **epithalamus;** below is the **hypothalamus** and **subthalamus**. The epithalamus includes the **pineal organ(s)** and a number of small nuclei concerned with responses to olfaction. The hypothalamus is an important autonomic centre to which passes information from olfactory and taste organs as well as from viscera. From the centre, fibres pass to visceral motor nuclei. Amongst other functions the hypothalamus controls the secretions of the pituitary gland and plays a part in temperature regulation and sleep. The subthalamus is a small collection of grey matter which is associated functionally with the basal nuclei of the cerebral hemispheres (p. 63).

In the floor of the diencephalon the **optic chiasma** is a prominent anterior feature. The optic nerves enter the chiasma ventrolaterally.

In all vertebrates except mammals the visual fibres run upwards and backwards to the roof of the midbrain to reach the primary visual centre in the tectum. In mammals the roof of the midbrain loses this function which is transferred to the cortex of the occipital lobes of the cerebral hemispheres.

As already noted, the pituitary gland develops from a midline evagination from the floor of the diencephalon, the **infundibulum,** and an upgrowth from the ectodermal roof of the stomodeum, **Rathke's pouch**. The greater part of the gland, the **adenohypophysis,** is derived from Rathke's pouch. The **neurohypophysis** is a product of the infundibulum.

The roof of the third ventricle is thin and mostly non-nervous. It develops a whole series of outgrowths, of varying importance in different vertebrate groups. Among the most prominent structures in this region are the pineal organs. In some groups (e.g. lizards), the pineal organs form functional eyes. Although this visual function is absent in mammals the pineal persists as an endocrine glandular structure (and hence is often termed the **pineal gland**).

The midbrain is continuous above with the diencephalon and below with the pons. Much of its ventral and lateral part is made up of ascending and descending fibres, the latter being congregated on the front of midbrain to form a swelling, the basis pedunculi, on each side of the midline. Deep to these swellings is the **tegmentum** which is essentially a forward continuation of the motor areas of the caudal part of the brainstem, co-ordinating stimuli from the diencephalon, tectum, and cerebellum and transmitting to motor nuclei in the brainstem and spinal cord. Although rather diffuse in lower vertebrates, well defined nuclei, such as the **red nucleus,** are found in the tegmentum of the midbrain in mammals.

The grey matter dorsal to the aqueduct of the midbrain is thickened to form the **tectum.** In man the tectum has lost its function as the primary visual cortex, but its superior part (the **superior colliculi**) still functions as a relay station for fibres concerned with reflexes to visual stimuli. The inferior part of the tectum (the **inferior colliculi**) provides relays for the auditory pathway from the cochlear nuclei to the thalami.

Cerebral hemispheres

Evolutionary history

It is perhaps ironic that man, whose sense of smell is so poor, should have developed his highest mental faculties in a region of the brain originally devoted to olfaction.

The paired outgrowths at the anterior end of the brain began as centres of olfaction. In the primitive living vertebrates, the jawless fishes, each half of the telencephalon is subdivided into two, the **olfactory bulb** and the **hemisphere**. The bulb is a terminal swelling in which fibres from the olfactory organ relay. The hemisphere is merely an **olfactory lobe** for the assembly and relay of olfactory sensation.

During the course of evolution, much of the grey matter of the cerebral hemispheres has tended to move outwards to the surface to become the **cerebral cortex** (Fig. 2.34). In amphibia there is a band of lateral grey matter, the **paleopallium,** which retains its olfactory connections. Dorsally and medially is the **archipallium,** a correlation centre receiving ascending fibres from the diencephalon as well as olfactory input. Ventrally, the grey matter is concerned with the correlation of sensory information received from the nuclei of the

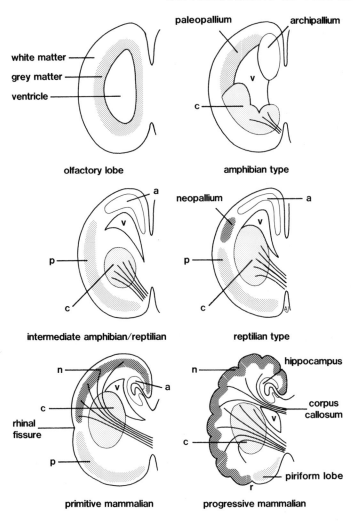

Fig. 2.34. Stages in the evolution of the cerebral hemispheres; a = archipallium, c = corpus striatum and its precursor in non-mammalian vertebrates (see text), n = neopallium, p = palleopallium, r = rhinal fissure, v = ventricle.

diencephalon with olfactory sensation. This area will become the **corpus striatum** of mammals. The term corpus striatum refers to the striated appearance of this area of grey matter in mammals caused by the passage through it of numerous fibre bundles on their way to and from the neopallium (see below and on next page). In the more primitive vertebrates this area is often called the **basal nuclei,** but in human anatomy the latter term is used to include structures in addition to the corpus striatum (p. 242).

Reptilian hemispheres have progressed further with the exteriorization of grey matter, apart from that which becomes the corpus striatum which has moved inwards to occupy most of the centre of the hemisphere and developed numerous connections with the thalamus and brainstem. Certain reptiles show a new development, the **neopallium,** a small area of grey matter between paleopallium and archipallium. This is again a correlative centre with fibres relaying sensory information from the brainstem.

The neopallium of mammals, even in the less advanced types, has

expanded over the roof and side walls of the hemispheres to form most of the cerebral cortex and crowd the archipallium and paleopallium to the medial surface. With further enlargement of the neopallium the archipallium becomes restricted to a small area on the medial side of each hemisphere, called the **hippocampus** (a major part of the limbic system and so called because it is alleged to look like a seahorse), while the paleopallium is represented by the small ventral **piriform lobe.**

With the increase in size of the neopallium came new functions, this structure taking over duties formerly assigned to the brainstem and basal nuclei. The tectum of the midbrain remains as a reflex centre for responses to visual stimuli and a relay station in the auditory pathway (although it retains important correlative functions as well). The optic and somatic sensory pathways are relayed to the neopallium through the thalamus, where a further relay also occurs in the auditory pathways to the neopallium.

Acting on all these sensory data motor decisions are despatched from the neopallium to the cerebellum via the pons, to the basal nuclei and through the pyramidal tract directly to the voluntary motor nuclei of the brainstem and cord.

The expansion of the hemispheres requires physical space. In primitive mammals the cerebrum leaves much of the midbrain exposed. But in most living mammals the midbrain and part of the cerebellum are overlaid dorsally by the enlarged hemispheres. The piriform lobe, the hippocampus and associated nuclei have been moved relative to each other and to the rest of the brain.

There is a limit to the increase in volume of the cerebral cortex which can be achieved by simple expansion of the hemispheres. Further increase is most simply achieved by folding. Although the cerebral surface is smooth in small primitive mammals, it is convoluted in more advanced types into **gyri** separated by **sulci.** These folds serve to increase the surface area and do not accurately delimit functional areas.

Development of the cerebral hemispheres in man

Because of the importance and complexity of the cerebral hemispheres in man, it is worthwhile considering their development in a little more detail. The cerebral vesicles which evaginate from the median part of the forebrain, and which will form the cerebral hemispheres, take with them the lateral parts of the thin roof plate of the forebrain. Each vesicle is hollow, containing a primitive lateral ventricle continuous with the cavity of the diencephalon over a wide area which will eventually be narrowed to form the **interventricular foramen (of Monro).** The caudal wall of this foramen connects the lateral wall of the diencephalon with the medial wall of the hemisphere; the anterior wall, the **lamina terminalis,** represents the original rostral end of the neural tube and forms a bridge connecting the hemispheres.

The cerebral hemispheres grow rapidly, especially in the rostro-caudal plane, so that they come to project ahead of and behind the interventricular foramen. This elongation of the hemisphere is accompanied by elongation of the contained lateral ventricle and of the roof plate. The caudal prolongation of each hemisphere lies lateral to the diencephalon, from which it is separated by only a narrow cleft containing mesoderm.

Both diencephalon and hemisphere now become more than simple hollow vesicles (Fig. 2.35). Thickenings of the walls of the diencephalon give rise laterally to bilaterally paired **thalami** and ventrally to the **hypothalamus.** The division between the thalamic and hypothalamic

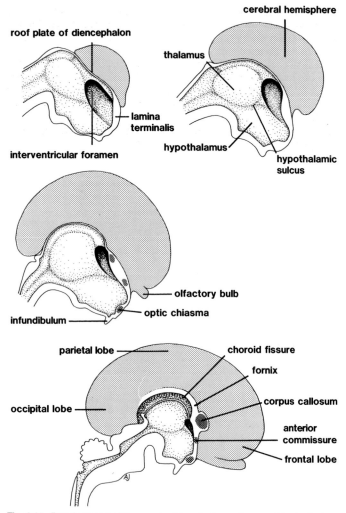

Fig. 2.35. Development of the cerebral hemispheres in man. The brain has been bisected to give a medial view of the left cerebral hemisphere.

obstruction of the foramen most of this expansion takes place in a posterior direction.

The fibres running through the corpus striatum form a thick tract called the **internal capsule** which divides the corpus striatum into two parts. Superomedial to the internal capsule, and bulging into the lateral ventricle, is the head and body of the **caudate nucleus;** infero-lateral to the capsule is the **lentiform nucleus.**

The thickening of the posterior wall of the interventricular foramen, and the consequent abolition of the cleft between diencephalon and hemisphere, incorporates the thalamus into the hemisphere. Because of the great expansion of the hemisphere, the ependymal roof plate comes to form part of the medial wall of the lateral ventricle rather than its roof. Together with its covering of vascular pia mater, the ependymal layer is invaginated into the ventricle to produce its choroid plexus. The line of the invagination can be seen on the medial surface of the hemisphere as the **choroid fissure.**

Perhaps because of its intimate association with the diencephalon, or perhaps because of limited space in the developing skull, the caudal extension of the cerebral hemisphere begins to turn ventrally, then rostroventrally so that the final shape of the hemisphere as seen in lateral view is that of a letter C. The hemisphere now has, in anteroposterior and then ventral sequence, a frontal, parietal, and temporal lobe. This curvature is, or course, reflected in the final shape of the lateral ventricle and choroid fissure, the caudate nucleus and the fornix (see below). An occipital lobe is added posteriorly at a late stage, so modifying somewhat the essentially simple shape of the hemisphere. The choroid plexus is confined to the area of the original roof plate; the projections of the lateral ventricle into the frontal lobe (the frontal horn) and into the occipital lobe (the occipital horn) were never adjacent to the roof plate and so lack a choroid plexus.

On the medial aspect of each hemisphere a curved strip of cortex abutting the outer edge of the choroid plexus at the **choroid fissure** is termed the **limbic lobe.** This area, much of it derived from the archipallium, is concerned with emotional behaviour in man and has connections with the hypothalamus which enable the cortex to influence the autonomic nervous system and endocrine glands. The most important of these connections is the **fornix** which runs along the edge of the choroid fissure to the anterior wall of the interventricular foramen whence neurons pass ventromedially into the hypothalamus. Further development of the limbic lobe is complex; those parts of the lobe which lie inferior to the ventral part of the curved choroid fissure become folded into the temporal horn of the ventricle which projects into the temporal lobe of the hemisphere.

The right and left hemispheres are connected by numerous fibres which cross the midline in the **commissures.** The major commissure is the **corpus callosum** which, in the adult, carries many millions of fibres. It first appears as a small bundle of fibres passing transversely across the upper part of the lamina terminalis and cutting through the fornix. As the number of fibres increases, the corpus callosum spreads backwards and upwards, following the line of the fornix which it splits into a small upper part, which becomes attenuated and virtually disappears, and a larger lower one adjacent to the choroid fissure, the definitive fornix. Further enlargement is brought about by bending and thickening of the corpus callosum which becomes markedly concave inferiorly and pulls away from the fornix. The vertical space so produced is occupied by the **septum pellucidum,** a very thin sheet of nervous tissue lying in the medial wall of each lateral ventricle above the fornix. In practice the left and right septa are very close and usually fuse in the midline.

parts of the diencephalon is marked by a groove, the **hypothalamic sulcus,** on the lateral wall of the third ventricle. The floor of the diencephalon becomes specialized to form the neurohypophysis of the pituitary gland and its roof becomes invaginated by pia to produce the choroid plexus of the third ventricle. In the hemispheres the major change is a thickening of the floor, the future corpus striatum, which bulges up into the cavity of the lateral ventricle.

The only possible route for nerve fibres passing to and from the cerebral hemispheres is via the walls of the interventricular foramen, which at this stage are quite thin. The most convenient route for fibres passing from the lateral walls of the hemispheres to the rest of the brain is across the thickened floor of the hemisphere (and so through the developing corpus striatum) to the caudal or posterior wall of the interventricular foramen and hence to the diencephalon. Large numbers of fibres following this route lead to thickening of the tissue forming the posterior wall of the foramen. In order to prevent

Clinical aspects

Anencephalus is the result of failure of closure of the anterior part of the neural tube. Little normal brain tissue develops. There is an associated failure of development of the cranial vault. The condition is fatal before, or shortly after birth.

Hydrocephalus (water on the brain) is an accumulation of excess cerebrospinal fluid in the brain ventricles or in the subarachnoid space. As a congenital defect, it is usually attributable to obstruction of the aqueduct of the midbrain which prevents fluid secreted by the choroid plexuses of the lateral and third ventricles draining into the fourth ventricle and so into the subarachnoid space whence it is normally reabsorbed into the blood stream. Accumulation of fluid, if not treated, may result in a greatly enlarged brain enclosed in a large, thin-walled skull.

There is often surprisingly little correlation between morphological deficiencies of the brain and its function. Absence of the corpus callosum may be associated with few symptoms and absence of the cerebellum may lead to only a slight impairment of co-ordination. Similarly, there appears to be little relationship, within wide limits, between the size of the cerebral hemispheres and intelligence or intellectual capacity.

Postnatal growth and the growth of the skull

GENERAL CONSIDERATIONS

Human beings increase in both complexity and size during the **growth period** which lasts from conception until about 20 years of age. Much of the increase in complexity occurs during the early stages of this period, especially in the prenatal phase. Increase in size is also rapid prenatally but continues with changes in rate throughout the remainder of the growth period. Some increase in overall size may occur in mature individuals due to obesity or pathological conditions but this is not usually counted as growth.

Localized proliferation continues in many tissues after the growth period has ended to make good the losses from wear and tear. This is most marked in epithelial tissues. In some parts of the alimentary tract, for example, epithelial cells are replaced every two to three days.

Growth in overall proportions

Growth in overall size can be conveniently studied by examining the changes which take place with age in the easily measured parameters of height and weight. There are two ways in which such data can be presented (Fig. 2.36). The simplest method is to plot a graph of the

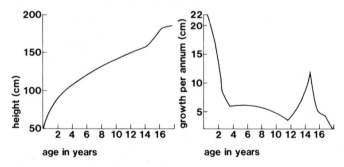

Fig. 2.36. Distance curve (left) and velocity curve (right) for the growth of an individual human being.

measurement against age. This is called a **distance curve**. Changes in the rate of growth are demonstrated more clearly by plotting the increment in the measurement per unit of time (e.g. the increase in height per year) against age. This is a **velocity curve**.

Both height and weight follow the **somatic growth pattern** (Fig. 2.37). Growth is rapid in the prenatal and early postnatal period but begins to slow down after about four years of age. During the early teens (at about 11 years in girls and 13 years in boys) the gonads

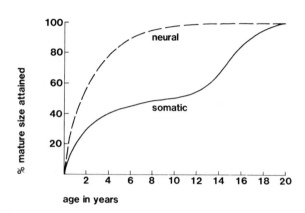

Fig. 2.37. Somatic and neural growth patterns.

undergo maturation, a period known as **puberty**, and this is followed almost immediately by the **adolescent growth spurt** (**adolescence** is the period between puberty and completion of the growth period). During the adolescent growth spurt, height and weight increase rapidly for a time and then slow down again as maturity is approached.

Many other features of the body besides total height and weight follow the somatic growth pattern. These include the size of many of the internal viscera, the length of the limbs and limb segments and, of particular significance for dental students, many of the dimensions of the face and jaws.

Relative growth

Although many of the major bodily components grow according to the somatic pattern, this does not imply that their rates of growth are identical. The increase in both lower limb length and trunk length, for example, follow the somatic pattern yet during the growth period the increase in limb length is consistently greater than that of trunk length so that the limbs become progressively longer in relative as well as absolute terms. In some cases the relationship between the growth rates in two dimensions is more or less constant over the growth period (a **linear** relationship) but in other cases one growth rate increases or decreases relative to the other (an **allometric** relationship).

Adolescent growth spurt

In the period before puberty one of the principal factors governing the rate of somatic growth is the **growth hormone** secreted by the pars distalis of the pituitary gland. Amongst the specific target organs upon which this hormone acts are the epiphysial cartilages and other growth sites in the skeleton. As the gonads mature during puberty their secretion of sex hormones, **testosterone** and **oestrogen**, increases greatly. These hormones, as well as influencing the development and growth of the primary and secondary sex organs, are powerful stimulators of general body growth. Their sudden increase in the bloodstream at puberty is responsible for the adolescent growth spurt. In addition to stimulating growth the sex hormones bring about the maturation of the growth centres and eventually the cessation of growth. A eunuch is tall, despite the lack of the growth stimulating effect of sex hormones, because the growth centres do not mature and growth is, therefore, greatly prolonged.

Until puberty there is little difference in body size or shape between the two sexes. In fact, girls are usually a little bigger than boys during this period since they are, age for age, physically more mature. During adolescence this trend is reversed because the adolescent growth spurt is more pronounced and prolonged in boys than in girls owing to the greater growth stimulating effect of testosterone as compared to oestrogen. The different growth effects of the two sex hormones are also responsible for the development of sexual dimorphism in body shape which becomes increasingly marked during adolescence. The sex hormones also have differential effects upon many other features including hair growth, disposition of body fat, muscular strength, and behavioural characteristics.

A pronounced adolescent growth spurt appears to be a characteristic of our own species. A slight increase in growth rate has been reported in certain body dimensions of adolescent great apes but in other extant mammals growth declines progressively throughout the postnatal growth period with no evidence of an acceleration equivalent to the human growth spurt. The significance of the growth spurt in human beings is not understood. One suggestion is that during the course of human evolution there was a selective advantage in keeping offspring small, and therefore easily contained within the protective family group, while the function of the enlarged brain matured but that once this had been achieved the advantage lay with the individual who reached full physical maturity as quickly as possible and who therefore stood a better chance of survival outside the family group. The adolescent growth acceleration may have evolved to provide the means whereby this rapid maturation was achieved.

Growth of the nervous system

The brain and spinal cord, together with such associated structures as the eyeballs and organs of hearing, follow a separate growth course, often referred to as the **neural growth pattern** (Fig. 2.37). In this case growth is rapid in prenatal and early postnatal life but then declines smoothly and progressively and is virtually complete before puberty. The brain, for example, has reached some 90 per cent of its final size by the age of 10 years. Those parts of the skull that surround the brain, eyeballs, and organs of hearing follow the neural growth pattern.

Maturation

Individuals of the same chronological age may differ from each other in their degree of maturity as well as in their rate of growth and size attained. In general more mature children tend to be taller than those who are less mature because they have progressed further along their distance growth curve. Clearly chronological age is not always the best guide in comparing the relative growth between individuals. This is particularly true in the early teens where one individual may be well into the adolescent growth spurt whereas another, of the same age but less mature, may not yet have entered the phase of accelerated growth. As already noted, this difference in maturity is responsible for the somewhat greater size of girls in the preadolescent period, a difference which becomes more marked in the early teens as girls enter the adolescent growth spurt earlier than boys.

Discrepancies between chronological age and maturity are of practical significance when assessing growth abnormalities. Growth may be retarded by a disorder of the growth mechanisms or may be the result of delayed maturation. It is obviously desirable therefore to be able to assess maturity separately from growth. This can be done by using one of the **indices of maturity** such as the development of centres of ossification (those in the wrist bones are frequently used). The degree of development and eruption of the teeth is also a measure of maturity although not so reliable on its own as the appearance of ossification centres.

SKULL GROWTH

It will be apparent from the preceding section that the growth of a particular organ or part of the body will have its own rate and timing. It may also proceed more rapidly in some directions than in others. These three attributes of growth – **rate, timing,** and **direction** – can be referred to collectively as the **pattern** of growth. In some organs growth is achieved by cell division and matrix proliferation throughout its structure. This is not so in bones where the mineralized nature of the matrix precludes interstitial growth. Instead bones grow by apposition at pre-existing surfaces. As illustrated in Fig. 1.3 (p. 6) it is impossible for a bone of adult size and proportions to be achieved from the corresponding immature bone by surface deposition alone. There must also be surface resorption. During the growth period virtually all bone surfaces, both internal and external, undergo deposition or resorption, the two processes being known collectively as **remodelling.** Surfaces at which particularly large amounts of growth take place are often referred to as **sites** of bone growth.

In the following account the pattern of skull growth is described first. This is followed by a description of the sites of growth and the remodelling processes which produce the pattern of growth.

Pattern of skull growth

There are numerous ways of measuring the pattern of skull growth. One widely used method has been to take measurements of dried skulls of different ages. The two main problems with this approach are that the skulls of children are, fortunately, not easy to obtain and that it is obviously impossible to follow the progress of an individual child since each skull can appear only once in the analysis (such growth data are termed **cross-sectional**). Following the growth of individual children requires that the measurements be taken at successive intervals on the same child (data of this type are called **longitudinal**) using methods appropriate for living subjects. Longitudinal data are greatly preferable to cross-sectional data for several reasons including the fact that the latter tend to blur growth patterns because of the individual differences which exist in rates of maturation. In the past longitudinal data have been collected either by taking measurements directly on the heads of children or on radiographs of heads. Both have disadvantages. Direct measurements are limited to those which can be made from externally locatable landmarks while radiographs are subject to distortion of the image, are limited to two-dimensional representation, and often produce overlapping, and hence obscuring, of the structures to be measured. Despite the inherent problems these methods have been widely used especially that based on X-rays where special procedures have been developed for standardizing the orientation of the head and X-ray machine for different views of the skull and for taking the measurements and correcting them for distortion (the resulting techniques are called **cephalometric radiography** or, in the USA, **roentgenographic cephalometry**). More recently a number of studies based on **computed tomography** have been published. This uses a special computerized radiographic technique to reconstruct a transaxial image (i.e. a visualization of structures in a single plane) of the head in which there is virtually no distortion and no overlap of structures. By using multiple transaxial images a three-dimensional representation of the skull can be built up. The following account is based mainly on findings from cephalometric radiography. In general these are supported by such studies as have been published using the potentially much more powerful technique of computed tomography.

For the purpose of describing the pattern of skull growth it is convenient to divide the skull into cranial vault, cranial base, and facial skeleton. Of these three components the cranial base and facial skeleton are of particular importance for the dental student.

Cranial vault

The growth of the cranial vault follows closely that of the enclosed brain. The vault enlarges rapidly in prenatal life and in the first few years of postnatal life so that by the age of puberty the cranial cavity has attained virtually adult size. Subsequent growth is restricted to some thickening of the cranial bones and enlargement of the superciliary arches and of the various muscle markings on the vault. There is no adolescent growth spurt in the major dimensions of the braincase. The overall shape of the cranial vault is usually established early in infancy. If the outlines of an individual skull at progressive growth stages are superimposed on the anterior cranial base, enlargement of the vault appears to take place in a largely concentric manner.

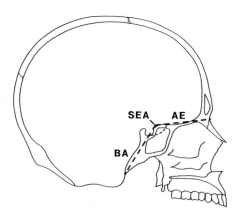

Fig. 2.38. The basicranial axis (BA), anterior extension (AE), and sphenoethmoidal angle (SEA).

Cranial base

The cranial base is a key region in understanding the growth changes which take place in the skull for it not only forms a junctional zone between the braincase and facial skeleton but also gives separate attachment to the upper and lower parts of the facial skeleton. For the purposes of growth studies the cranial base is often divided into two zones (Fig. 2.38). These are represented in the midline by the **basicranial axis**, stretching from the anterior border of the foramen magnum (the **endobasion**) to the region of the pituitary fossa, and an **anterior extension**, stretching from the pituitary fossa to the junction of the internasal and frontonasal sutures (the **nasion**) on the bridge of the nose. The growth changes in the cranial base are then represented by the changes that take place in the anteroposterior dimensions of the basicranial axis and the anterior extension and in the angle (the **sphenoethmoidal angle**) between them. Although this scheme of measurement is obviously unsatisfactory, in that no account is taken of the lateral regions, practically all the growth data collected for the cranial base relate to these (or similar) midline dimensions. One of the main reasons for this is the ease with which midline structures can be seen in lateral head radiographs.

Many studies have been made of the growth changes in the anteroposterior dimensions of the basicranial axis from which it is apparent that this part of the cranial base continues to elongate throughout the growth period with a well-marked acceleration during adolescence. It follows, therefore, the somatic growth pattern. When measured to the nasion, the anterior extension also follows the somatic growth pattern. If the anterior extension is measured to the anterior edge of the cribriform plate, however, it is found to follow the neural pattern more closely and to cease growing early in the postnatal growth period. This discrepancy is attributable to the growth changes in the thickness of the frontal bone, between the cribriform plate and the nasion, following the somatic pattern and so obscuring the neural growth pattern of the anterior part of the cranial base.

During prenatal life the sphenoethmoidal angle increases from about 130°, at the time the various components of the cranial base first become established, to some 150° at birth. Postnatally the angle decreases again by an amount almost equalling the prenatal increase, with most of the decrease occurring in the first two years of life. Postnatal decrease in the sphenoethmoidal angle is an entirely human characteristic; in all other mammals the angle increases progressively throughout the growth period. This contrast reflects the differing orientation of the facial skeleton, relative to the braincase, between man and other mammals. In most adult non-primates the facial skeleton lies completely anterior to the braincase and the sphenoethmoidal angle increases from a value well below 180° in the prenatal period to about 270° at maturity. In monkeys and apes, where the facial skeleton lies below as well as in front of the braincase, the angle increases to about 170°. The human facial skeleton remains tucked well under the anterior part of the braincase throughout life and correspondingly the sphenoethmoidal angle shows little or no overall change during growth, the prenatal increase being almost completely offset by the postnatal decrease.

Since the upper facial skeleton is attached principally to the anterior part of the cranial base while the mandible articulates with the more posterior part, it is often suggested that growth changes in the angulation of the cranial base affect the relationship between the upper and lower jaws. As described in the following section,

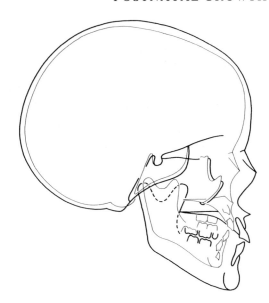

Fig. 2.39. Growth of the facial skeleton illustrated by superimposition of radiographic outlines of the heads of a six-year-old (thin lines) and a 16-year-old (thick lines). Outlines superimposed on anterior extension of cranial base. Note that anterior points on the facial skeleton move downwards and forwards whereas posterior points move more directly downwards.

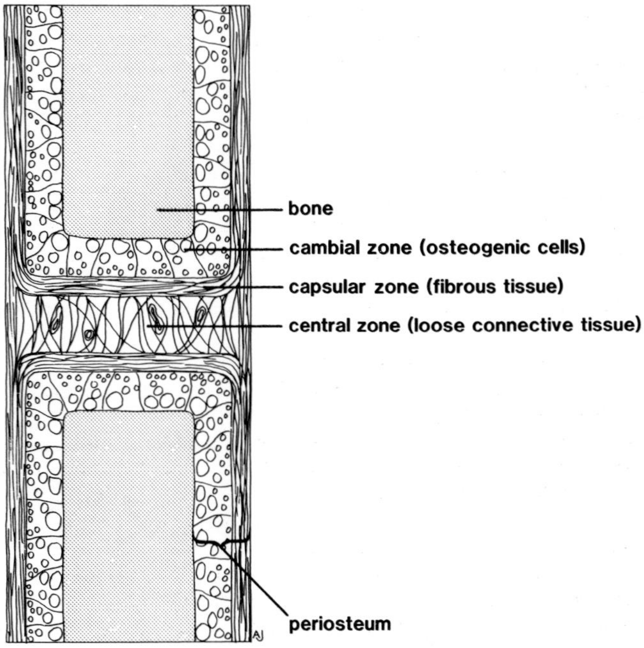

- bone
- cambial zone (osteogenic cells)
- capsular zone (fibrous tissue)
- central zone (loose connective tissue)
- periosteum

Fig. 2.40. Cross-section through a suture.

however, there is now evidence, at least so far as the postnatal period is concerned, that these changes in the human skull may reflect localized growth movements of the landmarks used to define the basicranial axis and anterior extension rather than any fundamental realignment of the two segments of the cranial base.

Facial skeleton

In non-primates the facial skeleton grows much more rapidly in anteroposterior length than in height or width. In monkeys and apes this predominance of growth in length is less pronounced and results, together with the relatively modest increase in the sphenoethmoidal angle, in the face being much less protrusive than in other mammals. This primate trend is even more marked in man where growth in length is, on average, rather less than in height although still exceeding growth in width. Coupled with the tendency for the sphenoethmoidal angle to undergo little overall growth change, this results in a face which protrudes hardly at all beyond the forehead region of the braincase.

The orbital region completes its growth earlier than the lower face following, like the contained eyeballs, the neural growth pattern. Most of the increase in facial height taking place after infancy is in the suborbital compartment. Whether or not there are regional variations in height increments within this compartment is uncertain, studies of this aspect of facial growth having produced conflicting results.

Growth in length exhibits a gradient within the facial skeleton, being least in the orbital region, somewhat greater in the suborbital part of the upper face and greatest in the mandible. As a result there is a tendency for the lower parts of the face to become progressively more prominent as growth proceeds.

The combined effect of growth in height and length is that the lower part of the facial skeleton is transposed downwards and somewhat forwards relative to the braincase (Fig. 2.39). Anterior points on the facial skeleton (such as the anterior nasal spine, interdental spines between the central incisors, and point of chin) tend to move along fairly constant pathways which are directed antero-inferiorly with respect to the cranial base whereas posterior points (such as the posterior edge of the hard palate and angle of the mandible) pursue a more directly downward path.

Growth sites and remodelling in the skull

Cranial vault

The bones of the cranial vault are covered on both their ectocranial and endocranial surfaces by periosteum, although the potentially confusing names of pericranium, for the ectocranial periosteum, and endosteal layer of the dura mater, for the endocranial periosteum, are often used. All internal surfaces of the bones (i.e. the surfaces facing into the marrow cavity) are lined by endosteum. As elsewhere in the skeleton these periosteal and endosteal membranes contain unspecialized cells whch can differentiate into osteoblasts for the deposition of bone. Osteoclasts for bone resorption are also present.

In the immature skull the bones of the vault are separated from each other by fibrous joints or **sutures,** remnants of the fibrous membrane in which these dermal bones ossify. A typical suture has five distinct layers (Fig. 2.40) comprising a **cambial zone,** containing osteogenic cells, covering each of the bone surfaces entering into the suture, a fibrous **capsular zone** next to each cambial layer, and a **central zone** of loose cellular tissue, between the two capsular zones. The cambial and capsular zones are continuous with the correspond-

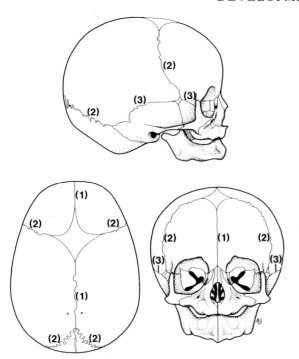

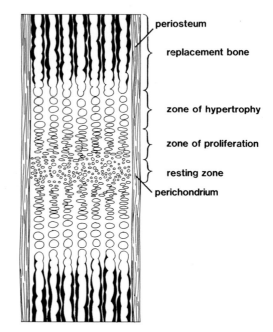

Fig. 2.43. Cross-section through a synchrondrosis of the cranial base.

Fig. 2.41. Sutures of the cranial vault of the newborn: (1) = sutures of sagittal group; (2) = sutures of coronal group; (3) = sutures of horizontal group.

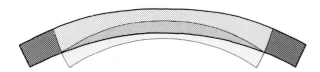

Fig. 2.42. Remodelling of the bones of the cranial vault. Sections of a vault bone at younger and older growth stages superimposed to show areas where bone is added and areas where it is resorbed. Bone added at sutures shown in dark shading.

ing layers of the periosteum on the ectocranial and endocranial surfaces of the bones. Increments of new bone are added to the sutural margins of the bones by the activity of the osteoblasts of the cambial zones which form the essential growth sites. The presence of two growth zones separated by the relatively inactive tissue of the capsular and central zones allows growth at each bone margin to be independent in rate and timing. Much tissue is deposited at the sutural margins as a result of which the area of the bones is progressively increased.

As can be seen from Fig. 2.41 the sutures in the cranial vault can be divided into three main groups: (i) sagittal (comprising the sagittal and frontal sutures); (ii) coronal (coronal and lambdoid sutures); and (iii) horizontal (squamoparietal suture). Growth at the sutures of the sagittal group results in the braincase enlarging in width, at those of the coronal group in enlargement in anteroposterior length and at those of the horizontal group in increase in height.

Sutural growth proceeds actively during the first years of the growth period, during which most of the enlargement of the cranial

vault is completed. Subsequently the sutures develop a serrated interlocking form which increases their resistance to deformity but renders any major amount of further growth impossible. Later still, the bones begin to unite across the sutures which are obliterated. Fusion usually begins in the coronal suture at about 30 years and all the sutures are obliterated by middle age.

As the cranial vault enlarges, the curvature of its individual bones must decrease. This is achieved by remodelling on the ectocranial and endocranial surfaces. The traditional view of these remodelling activities is illustrated in Fig. 2.42 but recent evidence suggests that this type of differential activity is not as widespread in the cranial vault as was once assumed.

Cranial base

As described in Chapter 2.4 the bones of the cranial base ossify in the cartilage of the chondrocranium. The joints between these bones are formed by remnants of this cartilage and are called **synchondroses.**

As in the study of the pattern of growth in the cranial base, attention has tended to concentrate upon events occurring in the midline and especially at the **sphenoccipital** and **sphenoethmoidal joints.** The sphenoccipital joint is a typical cranial base synchondrosis (Fig. 2.43). Its structure is rather like two epiphysial cartilages placed back-to-back. There is a central zone containing resting cells flanked, on either side, by zones in which the chondrocytes proliferate, hypertrophy, and then degenerate and are replaced by bone. The sphenoethmoidal joint (Fig. 2.47) is also at first a typical cranial base synchondrosis but shortly after birth the cartilage is replaced by fibrous tissue. A third cartilaginous joint, the **midsphenoidal synchondrosis,** is present in the midline of the prenatal skull, located between the presphenoid and basisphenoid ossifications (Fig. 2.47). These ossifications fuse in man at about the time of birth to form the

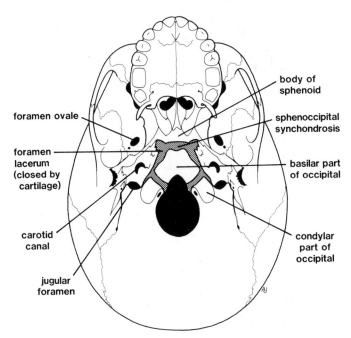

Fig. 2.44. Principal synchrondroses of the cranial base of a skull bearing a full deciduous dentition and with the first permanent molar about to erupt (i.e. 5–6 years old).

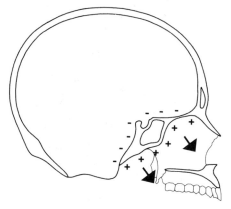

Fig. 2.45. Cortical drift in the cranial base. + = bone deposition; − = bone resorption; arrows indicate direction of growth. (Based on Enlow.)

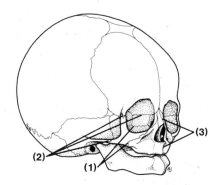

Fig. 2.46. Sutures in the facial skeleton of the newborn. Some of the sutures belonging to the (1) circummaxillary, (2) craniofacial, and (3) sagittal groups are shown. In the interests of clarity not all the facial sutures are labelled.

body of the sphenoid bone and the midsphenoidal synchondrosis is obliterated.

Considerable quantities of bone are formed at the sphenoccipital and sphenoethmoidal joints, growth at the latter continuing after its conversion to a suture. Growth continues in the sphenoccipital synchondrosis until the early teens and during this time it is believed to be the principal site of elongation of the basicranial axis. Ossification at the sphenoethmoidal joint contributes to the enlargement of the anterior extension. The midsphenoidal synchondrosis is believed to be an active growth site during the prenatal period.

It has become apparent in recent years that remodelling at the periosteal surface of the bones of the cranial base plays a major part in the growth of this part of the skull. Bone deposition takes place over much of the ectocranial surface of the base and resorption over most of the endocranial surface. As a result the whole cranial base is relocated downwards and forwards relative to the centre of the braincase. This method of growth is termed **cortical drift** (Fig. 2.45). The superior surfaces of the petrous temporal bones and the sella turcica are isolated areas of bone deposition in the generally resorbing floor of the cranial cavity and consequently become increasingly prominent as growth proceeds.

The mechanism by which the growth changes in the angulation of the cranial base are produced is less well understood. At least part of the postcranial growth change has recently been shown to be brought about by asymmetric growth at the sphenoccipital synchondrosis. Growth and bone deposition proceed more rapidly towards the endocranial surface of this synchondrosis than they do in its lower part with the result that the endobasion is relocated downwards and the sphenoethmoidal angle decreased. It also seems probable

that part of the postnatal decrease in this angle is the result of the increasing prominence of the region of the pituitary fossa brought about by bone deposition in this area in contrast to the resorption occurring over the most of the remainder of the endocranial surface of the cranial base. If true, this would mean that this part of the postnatal decrease in the sphenoethmoidal angle is merely a reflection of the local remodelling around the pituitary fossa and does not represent any real change in angulation between the basicranial axis and anterior extension.

Facial skeleton

There are numerous growth sites in the facial skeleton, including the sutures of the upper facial skeleton, the primary cartilage of the nasal capsule, and the secondary cartilages of the mandible. There is also extensive remodelling on the periosteal and endosteal surfaces.

The sutures of the upper facial skeleton are similar in structure and mode of growth to those of the cranial vault. They can be grouped into three major systems: (i) **circummaxillary** – the sutures separating the maxillae from the neighbouring bones; (ii) **craniofacial** – the sutures separating the facial bones from the bones of the braincase; (iii) **sagittal** – the internasal, intermaxillary and median palatal

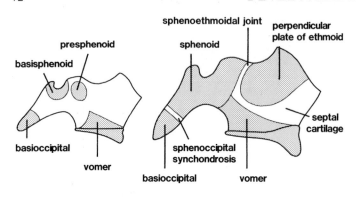

Fig. 2.47. Development of the nasal septum. Ossifications shaded. Left, before birth; right, during the first few years of life.

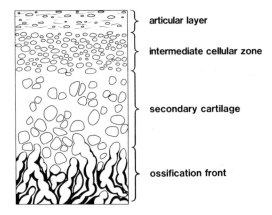

Fig. 2.48. Tissues of the mandibular head during growth.

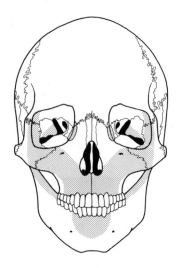

Fig. 2.49. Remodelling in the facial skeleton. Shaded areas undergo resorption during much of the growth period; unshaded areas undergo deposition. (Based on Enlow.)

One of the main sites of bone deposition in the mandible is the condylar cartilage. As described on page 57 secondary cartilages appear in the coronoid and condylar processes of the developing mandible. By birth the coronoid cartilage has been entirely replaced by bone but the condylar secondary cartilage persists throughout the growth period and into adult life.

The arrangement of the tissues in the mandibular head is unusual (Fig. 2.48). The upper surface is covered by a fibrocartilaginous layer which provides the articular covering. Beneath this is an intermediate zone of connective tissue cells. Below the intermediate zone is the condylar cartilage. During the growth period the intermediate zone is a site of rapid cell division. The cells produced function as chondrocytes, secreting matrix about themselves so adding new layers to the upper surface of the condylar cartilage. As successive layers are added, previously formed chondrocytes are passively relocated into ever deeper zones of the cartilage. As they do so, they hypertrophy but undergo no further division so that the cell columns typical of the hypertrophic zones in epiphysial and synchondrotic cartilages are not formed. At the deep border of the condylar cartilage the matrix is eroded and replaced by bone and the chondrocytes emerge, still living, into the marrow spaces below the cartilage. There are thus two major differences between growth at the condylar cartilage and at a primary cartilaginous growth site: (i) primary cartilages grow interstitially whereas the condylar cartilage grows mainly by apposition of cells produced in the intermediate layer, and (ii) the chondrocytes in a primary cartilage eventually degenerate and die but the cells in the condylar cartilage emerge still living at the ossification front.

Growth at the condylar cartilages moves the head of the mandible, relative to the remainder of the bone, in a predominantly superior direction. Since the head abuts against the under surface of the cranial base at the temporomandibular joint, this intrinsic growth results in the body of the mandible being moved inferiorly so adding to the height of the facial skeleton.

Growth at the various sites just described must clearly be accom-

sutures (Fig. 2.46; see also Fig. 2.41). The generally oblique orientation of the circummaxillary and craniofacial systems ensures that their growth contributes to increase in both the length and height of the upper face. Growth of the sagittal system leads to increase in facial width.

The nasal capsules are preformed in cartilage. The principal bone to ossify in this cartilage is the ethmoid. The labyrinths ossify in the lateral walls of the nasal capsules from centres which appear about the middle of prenatal life. The perpendicular plate is formed from the mesethmoid ossification centre which appears in the cartilage of the nasal septum in the first postnatal year (Fig. 2.47). The vomer ossifies from centres which develop close to the lower edge of the septal cartilage. For the first few years of life the perpendicular plate of the ethmoid and the vomer remain separated by septal cartilage. A zone of endochondral ossification is established at the junction of the perpendicular plate and septal cartilage. This, together with interstitial growth of the septal cartilage, produces a growth mechanism resembling that seen in an epiphysial cartilage and which results in the hard palate being moved downwards relative to the cranial base. According to some authorities this septal growth mechanism is a principal determinator of the rate and direction of upper facial growth.

INTRINSIC

EXTRINSIC

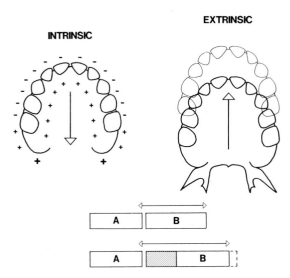

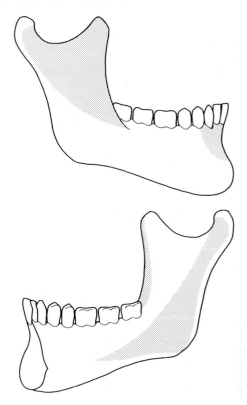

Fig. 2.50. Growth of the maxillary alveolar arch in occlusal view. Upper left: intrinsic remodelling (+ = bone deposition; − = bone resorption; arrow indicates direction of intrinsic growth); upper right: the direction of the extrinsic growth movement; below: diagrammatic representation of the growth movement – bone is added to the posterior surface of the maxilla (B) at its suture with the pterygoid buttress (A) and removed, in lesser amount from the anterior surface of the maxilla. (Based on Enlow.)

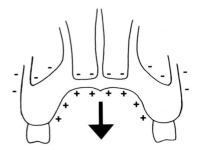

Fig. 2.51. Growth of the maxillary alveolar arch in coronal section through the premolar region. Symbols as in preceding Figure. (Based on Enlow.)

Fig. 2.52. Remodelling in the mandible. Areas undergoing resorption shaded; areas undergoing deposition not shaded. (Based on Enlow.)

panied by extensive surface remodelling to maintain the proportions of the facial skeleton and the spatial relationships of its various components.

The frontal region of the braincase is depository in nature. This area of deposition continues downwards to include the superior orbital borders and the external surfaces of the frontal processes of the maxillae. In the prenatal period the remaining external periosteal surfaces of the upper facial skeleton are also depository but during the first year or so after birth deposition is replaced by resorption over a progressively enlarging area which eventually includes the premaxillary region below the nasal cavity, the maxillary bodies as far posteriorly as the roots of the zygomatic processes, and the anterior surfaces of the zygomatic bones (Fig. 2.49). The external surface of the maxillary alveolar arch thus becomes resorptive in nature, apart from the small areas which lie posterior to the roots of

the zygomatic processes. The inner surface of the arch, the posteriorly facing tuberosities and the oral surface of the palate all remain depository.

If the maxillary alveolar arch is viewed from below it has a rounded V-shape with the open end of the V facing posteriorly (Fig. 2.50). The combination of deposition on the inner aspect and free ends (i.e. the tuberosities) of the V and resorption from its outer aspect results in the whole region growing **intrinsically** in a posterior direction. The posterior surfaces of the tuberosities are sites of especially rapid bone deposition. Since these surfaces abut onto the pterygoid processes of the sphenoid, which act as fixed buttresses, deposition here results in the maxillary complex being translocated in a forwards direction. In other words the posteriorly directed **intrinsic** growth results in an **extrinsic** growth movement in an anterior direction. It appears that the resorption of bone from the front of the maxillary alveolar arch is insufficient in amount to result in a wholesale posterior movement of the dental arcade but is related to the smaller scale remodelling of the periosteal surfaces of the maxillary complex.

In coronal section (Fig. 2.51) the maxillary alveolar arch and palate form a second V-shape with, in this case, the open end of the V facing inferiorly. Again, the outer aspect of the V (i.e. the floor of the nasal cavity and maxillary sinuses and the buccal surfaces of the alveolar processes) is resorptive and the inner aspect (the oral surface of the palate) is depository. The **intrinsic** growth movement of the maxillary arch in the vertical plane is, therefore, in a downward direction and adds a further component of downward growth to that produced extrinsically by bone deposition at the circummaxillary and craniofacial groups of sutures.

The internal surfaces of the nasal cavity are predominantly resorptive, as a result of which the cavity increases in size. The outer sides of the bones forming the lateral walls and floor of the cavity (i.e. the medial walls of the orbits and maxillary sinuses and the oral surfaces of the palate) are depository. Most of the internally facing surfaces of the orbits are sites of deposition. As in other V- or cone-shaped regions this results in the orbit growing towards its open end and increasing in overall size.

One of the principal sites of periosteal bone deposition in the mandible is along the posterior border of the ramus (Figs 1.3 and 2.52). As a result the mandible undergoes a posteriorly directed intrinsic growth movement. Because the mandible is anchored to the cranial base at the temporomandibular joints this intrinsic growth movement results in the mandible being transposed forwards. The anterior border of the ramus undergoes resorption at a somewhat lesser rate than deposition takes place posteriorly so that the length of the ramus, as well as that of the body, is increased.

In the anterior part of the ramus, the lateral surface and anterior border of the coronoid process are resorptive and the medial surface, posterior to the temporal crest, is depository. In the posterior part of the ramus, on the other hand, the lateral surface is depository and the medial surface resorptive. A line of reversal runs obliquely across each surface of the ramus separating these regions of differential remodelling.

The medial surfaces of the coronoid processes face superiorly and posteriorly, as well as medially, so that the combination of medial deposition and lateral resorption results in the processes growing upwards and backwards and in their apices moving apart. At one and the same time the coronoid process enlarges in height, the body of the mandible is elongated and the separation between the processes of the two sides is increased. The coronoid process merges at its base into the more medially located inferior part of the ramus which itself merges anteriorly into the still more medially located body. The combination of medial deposition and lateral resorption results in the medial relocation of the base of each coronoid process into the ramus and of the ramus into the body as the overall proportions of the mandible increase.

In horizontal section the ramus is somewhat curved with the convexity facing laterally. As the ramus grows intrinsically in a posterior direction areas originally at the posterior border of the ramus must be relocated first laterally and subsequently medially in order to preserve this convexity. The distribution of remodelling in the ramus enables this relocation to be achieved. The lateral deposition and medial resorption over the posterior part of the ramus is responsible for the initial lateral movement and the reverse changes in the region of the coronoid process bring about the subsequent medial relocation.

Increase in length of the mandibular body is an inevitable consequence of the remodelling changes in the ramus. Increasing separation of the two sides of the body is likewise an inevitable consequence of the mode of increase in length. The body grows in height principally by deposition along its inferior border and in thickness by deposition on its buccal surface. After the eruption of the primary dentition an area of resorption becomes established on the labial surface of the body below the incisor teeth. Its presence results in an increasing prominence of the mental protuberance, itself an area of deposition, and the appearance of the characteristic human chin.

FURTHER READING

Enlow, D.H. (1975). *Handbook of facial growth.* Saunders, Philadelphia.

Moore, W.J. and Lavelle, C.L.B. (1974). *Growth of the facial skeleton in the Hominoidea.* Academic Press, London.

Sinclair, D. (1978). *Human growth after birth,* 3rd edn. Oxford University Press, London.

Slavkin, H.C. (1979). *Developmental craniofacial biology.* Lea and Febiger, Philadelphia.

Tanner, J.M. (1962). *Growth at adolescence,* 2nd edn. Blackwell Scientific, Oxford.

Waitzman, A.A., Posnick, J.C., Armstrong, D.C., and Pron, G.E. (1993). Craniofacial measurements based on computed tomography. *Cleft Palate Craniofac. J.*, **29**, 118–28.

Section 3

Thorax

1

Surface anatomy and thoracic cage

SURFACE ANATOMY

Anatomy is learned mainly from cadavers which have certain disadvantages as anatomical subjects. They are the mortal remains of usually old (often senile) people and are often emaciated or obese. In addition the texture of the tissues is greatly changed from that in the living body by the preservatives used to avert decay and by the fact that dissection is carried out at room temperature which is many degrees lower than body temperature.

Fortunately each anatomy student has access to a living body, his or her own. Much of the surface of this can be seen or felt while the more inaccessible parts can be examined in a fellow student. This process allows you to determine the disposition of internal thoracic organs in relation to surface landmarks and palpable bony features in the young, fit, living body.

Anterior thoracic surface (Fig. 3.1)

Reference landmarks

In the clinical examination of the living subject the position of the internal thoracic organs is defined with reference to a set of vertical and horizontal lines running through surface or bony landmarks. The vertical lines are (Figs 3.1 and 3.6):

1. midsternal line – in the median plane anteriorly;
2. midclavicular line – through the midpoint of the clavicle;
3. anterior axillary line – through the anterior axillary fold;
4. posterior axillary line – through the posterior axillary fold;
5. midaxillary line – midway between 3 and 4;
6. scapular line – through the inferior angle of the scapula (with the arms alongside the body);
7. median posterior line.

The horizontal lines can be defined either with reference to the vertebrae or, more usefully in the living subject, the ribs. The first rib lies deep below the clavicle and is difficult and painful to palpate. It is customary, therefore, to start counting the ribs from the second. This is found by first locating the **suprasternal notch** on the superior margin of the manubrium sterni. It lies in the midline between the medial ends of the clavicles and is opposite the body of the second thoracic vertebra (T2 – Fig. 3.2). About an 2½ cm below the notch you will be able to feel a ridge made by the joint between the manubrium and the body of the sternum. This is the **sternal angle** (of Louis) and lies opposite the intervertebral disc between T4 and T5. If you now slide your finger laterally, it will pass on to the skin over the second costal cartilage and, further laterally still, over the second rib. Below this rib and costal cartilage is the second intercostal space. Having identified the second rib and space, it is an easy matter to

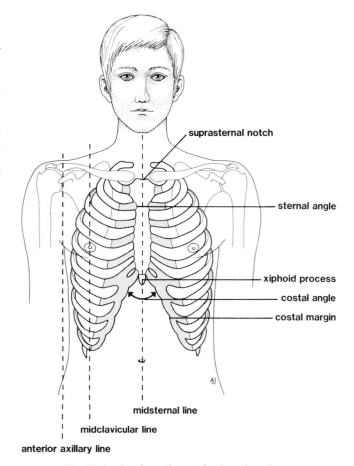

Fig. 3.1. Landmarks on the anterior thoracic surface.

count down (moving laterally as you reach the lower part of the thoracic cage).

There are usually twelve pairs of ribs in all but you will probably not be able to feel the lowermost unless you are thin.

Xiphoid process and costal margin

Feel downwards from the sternal angle in the midline until you reach an indentation, the inferior end of the body of the sternum. Just below this and a little deeper the **xiphoid process** may be felt. A horizontal line through here would pass through the body of T9. If

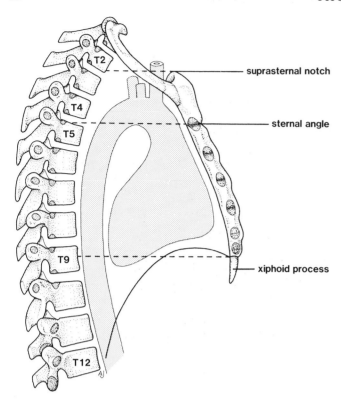

Fig. 3.2. Thoracic landmarks in lateral view.

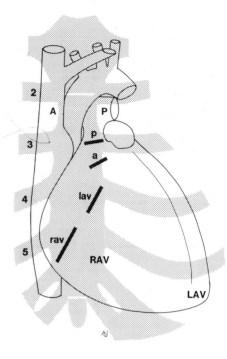

Fig. 3.3. Surface markings of the heart in anterior view. The actual position of the aortic, pulmonary, left and right atrioventricular valves is shown by the relevant lower case letters. The site of maximum propagation (i.e. where heard loudest with a stethoscope) of the valve sound is shown in upper case.

you move your fingers laterally from the xiphisternal joint, you will be able to feel the **costal margin**, the lower boundary of the thorax formed by the cartilages of the seventh, eighth, ninth, and tenth ribs, and perhaps the cartilaginous free ends of the eleventh and twelfth ribs. The angle between the costal margins in the midline is known as the **costal angle.**

Nipple and breast

The male **nipple** usually lies in the fourth intercostal space (below the fourth rib) just lateral to the midclavicular line. In women its position is inconstant due to the development of the breast, and it is a poor landmark. The **breast**, or **mammary gland**, is rudimentary in children and men, and variably developed in women. Lying in the superficial fascia of the chest wall, this fatty organ is hemispherical in young women, overlying the second to sixth ribs, and extending from the lateral margin of the sternum to the midaxillary line.

Apex beat of heart (Fig. 3.3)

The **apex beat** of the heart can be found as follows. If the flat of the hand is placed on the chest wall over the heart, the beat of the latter should be felt. The apex beat is the lowest and outermost point of definite cardiac pulsation. It is produced by the left ventricle and is usually located in the left fifth intercostal space in the midclavicular line in the seated healthy subject. Its position varies to some degree with posture, build, and height, and in pathological conditions where the heart is enlarged or displaced. It must be emphasized that this is a

point located on the chest, not from a textbook. If you cannot feel the apex beat try leaning forwards a little. From the apex beat the location of the rest of the heart can be visualized or marked out on the chest wall.

Trachea

This runs in the midline from the level of C6 in the neck to the level of the sternal angle. Its rings can be felt by placing a finger in the suprasternal notch. If you say 'Aah', you will feel the air in the trachea vibrating.

Lungs and pleura

The surface markings of the lungs and pleura (that is the projection of these structures on to the anterior and posterior chest walls) are shown in Figs 3.4 and 3.5. The position of the lower border of the lung varies as you breathe in and out. The projection usually given is a compromise, the position in mid-inspiration. Between the lower border of the lungs and that of the pleura is a space, the costodiaphragmatic recess (see p. 86) which is roughly two ribs wide at its greatest extent.

Note that the lungs are lobed, and that the fissures between lobes may be mapped as follows: both lungs have **oblique fissures** running along a line from the spine of T3 to the sixth rib at the costochondral junction; the right lung has a second, **horizontal fissure** which corresponds to a line drawn horizontally along the fourth costal cartilage to meet the oblique fissure at the midaxillary line.

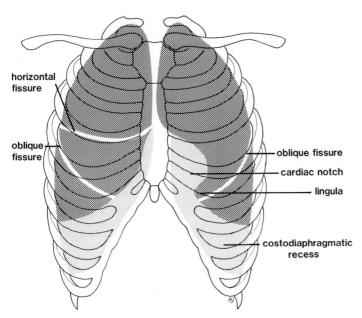

Fig. 3.4. Surface markings of the lungs (dark stipple) and pleura (light stipple) in anterior view.

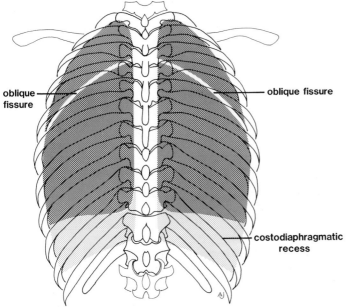

Fig. 3.5. Surface markings of the lungs (dark stipple) and pleura (light stipple) in posterior view.

Great vessels

The **arch of the aorta** and the roots of the **brachiocephalic** and **left common carotid artery** lie behind the manubrium, as do the **superior vena cava,** and right and left **brachiocephalic veins.** The **internal thoracic (mammary)** arteries and veins lie about 1 cm lateral to the margins of the sternum.

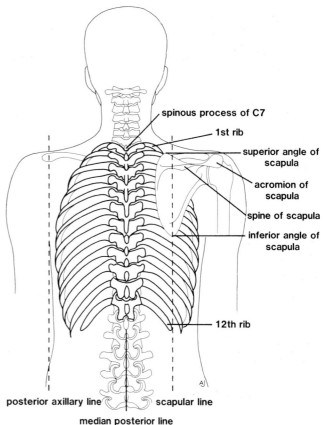

Fig. 3.6. Landmarks on the posterior thoracic surface.

Posterior thoracic surface (Fig. 3.6)

On your own back (or on that of another student) you should be able to feel, in the midline, the spinous processes of vertebrae from the **seventh cervical** (C7, the most inferior vertebra in the neck, also called the **vertebra prominens** because of its prominent spine) downwards. The tip of each vertebral spine lies over the body of the vertebra below (Fig. 3.2). The angles and borders of the **scapulae** (shoulder blades) may also be felt. The **superior angle** lies opposite the spine of T2, the **inferior angle** opposite the spine of T7. The acromion and spine of each scapula should also be identified.

THORACIC CAGE

The thoracic cage is made up posteriorly by the thoracic part of the vertebral column, laterally by the ribs and anteriorly by the sternum and costal cartilages.

Thoracic vertebral column

Vertebrae

The thoracic vertebral column is concave anteriorly and made up of twelve thoracic vertebrae and their intervertebral discs. Thoracic vertebrae (Fig. 3.7) have the following components:

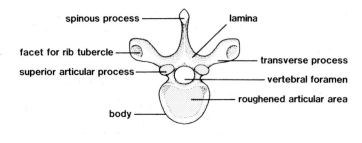

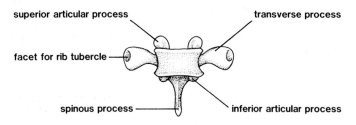

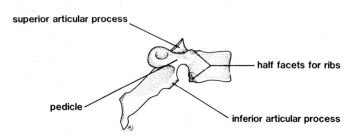

Fig. 3.7. Superior, anterior, and lateral views of a typical thoracic vertebra.

1. a heart-shaped **body** carrying, on each side, two **half facets** for the **heads** of two ribs in the case of T2–T9 or a single complete facet for the head of one rib in the case of T1 and T10–T12;

2. stout **transverse processes** running laterally and slightly posteriorly and becoming progressively shorter from first to twelfth rib; each transverse process carries near its tip a facet for the **tubercle** of a rib (except T11 and T12);

3. a long **spinous process** directed inferiorly in the middle four vertebrate (T5–8) but becoming progressively more horizontal above and below these levels;

4. **articular processes** set vertically with the facets on the superior processes facing posterolaterally and those on the inferior processes anteromedially; the relative movement of the vertebrae is thus mainly rotary;

5. the **vertebral foramen** (containing the spinal cord and its coverings) is about the diameter of a fingertip and is round; the walls of the vertebral foramen are made up anteriorly by the vertebral body, laterally by the **pedicles** grooved above and below to allow ample space for the passage of spinal nerves and posteriorly by the **laminae** which meet behind in the median plane;

6. the central area of the superior and inferior face of each vertebral body is roughened for attachment of the thin layer of hyaline cartilage which separates bone from **intervertebral disc**.

The intervertebral disc has an outer ring of fibrocartilage (the annulus fibrosus) and an inner **nucleus pulposus,** an ovoid gelatinous mass containing a few collagen fibres and cartilage cells. The annulus (which runs from vertebra above to vertebra below) and the nucleus together form a shock-absorbing mechanism. Sudden downward forces will tend to compress the nucleus vertically, but the concomitant lateral expansion (because the nucleus has a fixed volume) will be restrained by the fibres of the annulus. Sometimes the force generated is so great that the nucleus herniates through the annulus (slipped disc—usually confined to the lumbar region). The slight degree of movement possible between adjacent vertebral bodies occurs by a rolling movement on the relatively incompressible nucleus with the annulus being stretched on one side and compressed on the other. With increasing age the nucleus becomes thinner, less aqueous and is eventually converted to fibrocartilage.

Sternum (Fig. 3.8)

This may be divided into three parts.

Manubrium

You have already felt the concave upper border in the suprasternal notch, deepened by the sternal ends of the clavicles articulating with the manubrium at the sternoclavicular synovial joints each containing a fibrous articular disc. Immediately below the clavicle is the synchondrosis (cartilaginous joint) between manubrium and first rib.

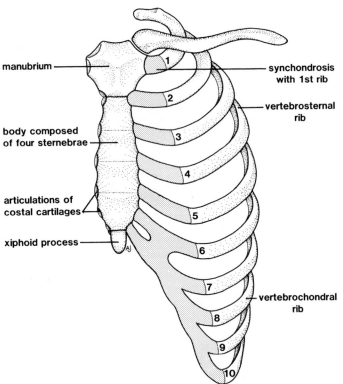

Fig. 3.8. To show the articulations of the sternum.

Body

This is composed of four **sternebrae** which are sometimes incompletely fused leaving a deficiency often mistaken for a bullet hole. The second costal cartilage articulates with the sternum at a notch at the sternal angle, the third, fourth, and fifth costal cartilages at the junctions between sternebrae and the seventh costal cartilage at the lower margin of the fourth sternebra. Only the sixth costal cartilage articulates close to the centre of a sternebra.

Xiphoid process

This extends downwards and slightly backwards from the body for a variable distance. It is half as thick as the body, and arranged so that the inner surfaces of sternum and xiphoid are flush. The anterior surface of the xiphoid is thus inset.

Ribs and their cartilages (Figs 3.8, 3.9)

Each rib articulates posteriorly with the vertebral column. The costal cartilages of the first seven ribs articulate directly with the sternum (true or vertebrosternal ribs). The remaining five pairs may be subdivided further. The cartilages of ribs 8, 9, and 10 articulate with the cartilages immediately above them (false or vertebrochondral ribs). The cartilages of ribs 11 and 12 are free (floating or vertebral ribs). Additional articulations commonly form between the cartilages of ribs 7, 6, and 5.

A typical rib has the following features. The **shaft** has an internal (concave) and an external (convex) surface, a superior (rounded) and inferior (sharp) border. The medial surface is marked along its lower border by the shallow **costal groove**. The posterior quarter of the shaft is circular in section, the anterior three-quarters compressed laterally. The shaft has a non-uniform curve of smallest radius at its **angle**.

The **head** carries two articular facets (except 1, 10, 11, and 12 which have only one). The **neck** is stout. The **tubercle** (absent in 11 and 12) has a roughened, non-articular region and a small facet which articulates with the transverse process of a vertebra.

The **first rib** (Fig. 3.10) is atypical in being flattened from above downwards. Its head carries a single facet for articulation with T1. It is shorter and more curved than any other rib and has prominent roughenings on its upper surface for the attachment of the scalene muscles. In front of the attachment of scalenus medius the rib may be grooved by the roots of the brachial plexus and the subclavian artery, while in front of the attachment of scalenus anterior a similar marking may be made by the subclavian vein.

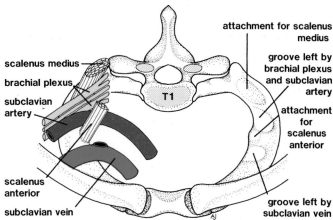

Fig. 3.10. The first rib and its relationships.

Costal joints

Ribs have several articulations (Fig. 3.9).

1. The head of a typical rib (2–9) articulates with demifacets on the body of the corresponding vertebra and of the vertebra above and with the intervertebral disc between them. The rib is attached to the disc by an **intra-articular ligament**. A **capsule**, strongest anteriorly where its fibres are arranged radially, surrounds the joint. The heads of ribs one, ten (usually), eleven and twelve articulate with a single (the corresponding) vertebra, have a rounded head and no intra-articular ligaments. These joints are all synovial.

2. The tubercles of the first ten ribs articulate with the facets of the transverse processes of the corresponding vertebrae forming synovial joints. Rib and vertebra are united by strong **costotransverse ligaments.** These are separated by the joint into **medial** and **lateral** portions. A **superior** costotransverse ligament descends from the transverse process of the vertebra above to be inserted into the neck of each rib.

3. The first costal cartilage is united with the manubrium by a synchondrosis. The cartilages of the remaining true ribs articulate with the sternum at synovial joints. The cavities of the synovial joints are often obliterated by fibrous union.

4. Interchondral joints between the lower costal cartilages may be synovial, fibrous, or completely united.

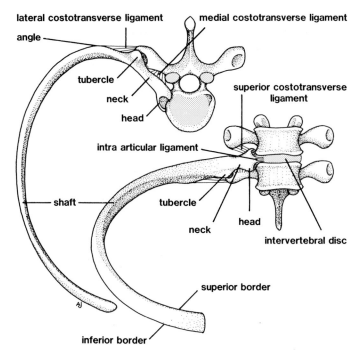

Fig. 3.9. The articulations between a rib and vertebrae; superior (left of figure) and anterior (right of figure) views.

Thoracic cage

The following features of the thoracic cage should be confirmed on a mounted skeleton.

1. The typical rib runs anteriorly and downwards; its cartilage runs anteriorly and upwards. The first rib and costal cartilage run downwards throughout.

2. The sternal end of each costal arch lies lower than the vertebral end.

3. The middle of each arch lies lower than either end (except again the first).

4. Ribs and cartilages increase in length from the first to the seventh.

5. The transverse diameter of the thorax increases progressively from ribs one to eight.

6. The ribs increase in obliquity from one to nine.

7. The inferior margin of the cage is formed by the twelfth thoracic vertebra posteriorly, the twelfth ribs and the tips of the eleventh ribs at the sides and by the cartilages of the tenth to seventh ribs in front. In the anterior midline the margin is formed by the xiphoid process.

Clinical aspects

Because of the large amount of cartilage present, the ribs not being fully ossified until adult life, the rib cage of children is very flexible and fractures are rare. In adults, rib fractures tend to occur near the angle. The upper two ribs (protected by the clavicle) and the lower two are least often fractured. In a severe crush injury several ribs may fracture in front and behind, freeing a whole section of chest wall. This flap is sucked in on inspiration and blown out on expiration (paradoxical respiration). A cervical rib attached to C7 (Fig. 3.11) occurs unilaterally in about one in 200 of the population, bilaterally in about one in 400. This may press on the lower trunk of the brachial plexus, causing paraesthesia (tingling) and muscle wasting, or on the subclavian artery, impairing circulation in the upper

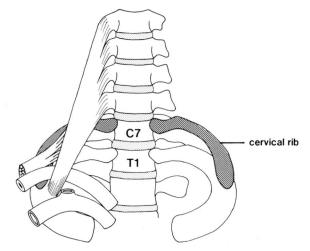

Fig. 3.11. Cervical ribs.

limb. A lumbar rib is more common, sometimes causing confusion of vertebral levels in radiographs or being misinterpreted as a fractured vertebral transverse process. Bifid, forked, and fused ribs are not uncommon.

Fractures of the sternum are infrequent and are usually caused by direct violence such as hitting the steering wheel in a motoring accident. The broken pieces are usually held in place by the fibrous layers surrounding them but if the violence is great enough they may be driven into the chest rupturing great vessels or damaging the heart. Ossification at the xiphoid may result in middle-aged people reporting to their doctors with a newly occurring hard lump in the pit of the stomach. The sternum has a readily accessible marrow cavity allowing the removal of a sample of haemopoietic marrow by sternal puncture.

2

Thoracic muscles and diaphragm

THORACIC MUSCLES AND INTERCOSTAL SPACES

Except for a small area posteriorly, the thorax is entirely clothed in muscles. Many of these are inserted into the upper limb and do not concern us here. Beneath this muscle layer are the muscles of the thoracic wall proper, uniting vertebrae, ribs, and sternum.

Intercostal muscles

The spaces between the ribs, the **intercostal spaces**, are occupied by intercostal muscles whose fibres unite the ribs above and below each space. These are in three layers (Fig. 3.12).

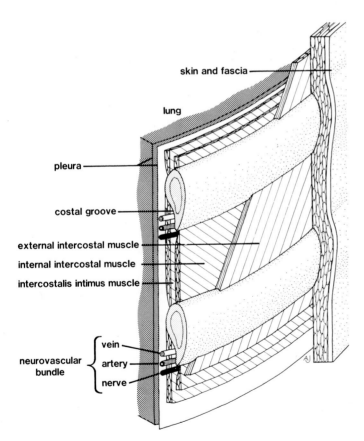

skin and fascia

lung

pleura

costal groove

external intercostal muscle

internal intercostal muscle

intercostalis intimus muscle

vein

neurovascular bundle — artery

nerve

Fig. 3.12. The intercostal muscles.

Outer layer

The fibres of the **external intercostal muscle** run forwards and downwards. The muscle sheet is complete from the tubercle of the rib posteriorly to the costochondral junction anteriorly, where it is replaced by a fibrous aponeurosis, the **external (anterior) intercostal membrane**.

Middle layer

Internal intercostal muscle fibres run backwards and downwards. The muscle is complete from the sternum anteriorly to the angles of the ribs where it is replaced by the **internal (posterior) intercostal membrane**.

Inner layer

The fibres of the incomplete **intercostalis intimi** run in the same direction as those of the internal intercostals, from which they are thought to be derived.

The action of the intercostal muscles is still disputed. One view is that both external and internal groups of fibres are elevators of the ribs; another that the external intercostals are elevators and the internal intercostals depressors of the ribs.

Neurovascular bundle

The main vascular and nervous supply to the intercostal space runs as a neurovascular bundle just below the costal groove on the rib forming the upper boundary of each space and protected by its sharp inferior margin. The bundle runs in the plane between the internal intercostals and intercostalis intimi.

Intercostal vessels

There are two sets of intercostal vessels, anterior and posterior (Fig. 3.13). The **posterior intercostal arteries** arise from the aorta (lower nine spaces) or from the costocervical trunk (upper two spaces). Each runs obliquely upwards in the corresponding intercostal space to the angle of the rib where it enters the costal groove, being located at first between pleura and internal intercostal membrane and then between intercostalis intimi and the internal intercostal muscle. It gives off a collateral branch which passes along the upper border of the rib below, a lateral branch which pierces the intercostal muscles to supply the skin and subcutaneous tissues over the side of the chest wall and numerous muscular and pleural branches. The posterior intercostal artery and its collateral branch anastomose in front with the anterior intercostal arteries.

The **anterior intercostal arteries** arise from the internal thoracic artery (upper six spaces) or its branch, the musculophrenic artery

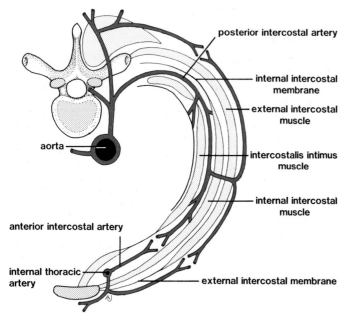

Fig. 3.13. Intercostal vessels.

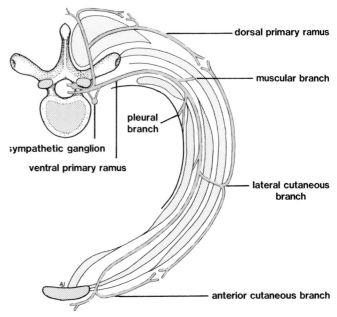

Fig. 3.14. An intercostal nerve.

(lower five spaces) as the latter runs along the lower border of the thorax. There are two arteries for each space, running immediately below and above the ribs between intercostalis intimi and internal intercostal muscles. Perforating branches pierce the chest wall to supply pectoralis major (upper five or six spaces) and the breast (spaces 2–4). In the lactating female these may be of considerable size.

Corresponding veins run with the arteries and drain into the brachiocephalic, azygos and hemiazygos veins posteriorly (p. 100) and the internal thoracic or musculophrenic veins anteriorly.

Intercostal nerves

The intercostal nerves (Fig. 3.14) are the ventral primary rami of the upper eleven thoracic spinal nerves. The spinal nerves emerge from the intervertebral foramina and immediately split into **dorsal** and **ventral primary rami**. At or close to its origin each ventral ramus in the thoracic region gives off a **white ramus communicans** to and receives a **grey ramus communicans** from the corresponding sympathetic ganglion. The intercostal nerves then pass forwards in the intercostal spaces with the intercostal vessels. The following branches are given off:

1. a collateral branch running inferior to the main nerve, on the superior border of the rib below;
2. a lateral cutaneous branch near the midaxillary line to the skin over the side of the chest;
3. an anterior cutaneous branch near the edge of the sternum to the skin on the front of the chest;
4. numerous branches to intercostal muscles;
5. pleural and peritoneal (the latter from the lower intercostal nerves) branches, conveying sensory fibres from pleural and peritoneal membranes;
6. articular branches to the joints of the ribs.

The dorsal primary rami supply the muscle and skin of the back.

The **first intercostal nerve** is atypical because it sends a large contribution to the upper limb via the brachial plexus. This contribution replaces the lateral cutaneous branch and the anterior cutaneous branch is absent. The **second intercostal nerve** also contributes to the upper limb via its lateral cutaneous branch, the intercostobrachial nerve.

The **lower six intercostal nerves** also supply the abdominal wall. The seventh turns upwards and medially on leaving the subcostal groove to run parallel to the subcostal margin (where it is vulnerable during abdominal surgery). The **tenth nerve** supplies the region of the umbilicus.

Lymphatics

The superficial lymphatics of the anterior thoracic wall drain to the **anterior axillary nodes**, the deeper ones to the **internal thoracic nodes** lying along the internal thoracic vessels. Posteriorly superficial vessels drain to the **posterior axillary nodes**, deeper ones to the **intercostal nodes** near the head of each rib. The **lymphatic drainage of the breast** is of considerable importance due to the frequent development of carcinoma in this organ and subsequent spreading (**metastasis**) via the lymphatics. The lymphatic capillaries of the breast form a network communicating with those of the contralateral breast and with the vessels draining the anterior thoracic and abdominal wall. The lymphatics (Fig. 3.15) run with the veins draining the gland, laterally to the axillary nodes and medially to nodes lying along the course of the internal thoracic artery. A few vessels follow the posterior intercostal arteries and drain to the intercostal nodes.

Clinical aspects

Blood, pus, or air may be aspirated from the pleural cavity via a needle inserted between the ribs. If the needle is kept close to the upper border of a rib, the main neurovascular bundle is safe (but the

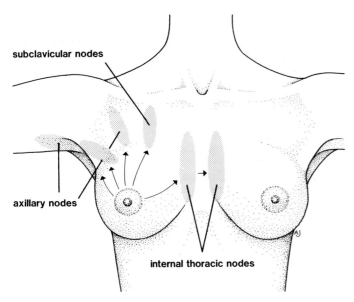

Fig. 3.15. The lymphatic drainage of the breast.

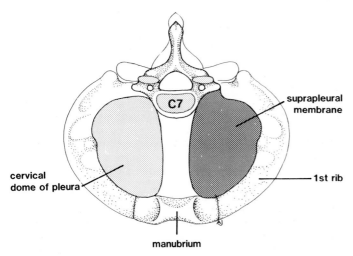

Fig. 3.16. The thoracic inlet.

THORACIC INLET AND OUTLET

Suprapleural membrane and thoracic inlet

The upper boundary of the thorax, the thoracic inlet, is the junction of thorax and neck. The inlet (Fig. 3.16) is bounded by the superior border of the manubrium sterni, the deep borders of the first ribs and by the body of T1.

The inlet transmits important structures between thorax and neck (including the trachea, oesophagus, large blood vessels, vagus and phrenic nerves, etc.). These structures all lie towards the midline (see Fig. 3.24 for details). Laterally the thoracic inlet is closed on each side by a dome of dense fascia, the **suprapleural membrane**. This is attached to the medial border of the first rib and costal cartilage, to the fascia investing the structures passing to and from the neck and posteriorly and superiorly to the tip of the transverse process of C7. Immediately below the suprapleural membrane lies the **cervical dome** of the pleura.

It should be appreciated that the pleural cavity rises above the level of the first rib arteriorly (Fig. 3.4). A local injection of anaesthetic around the site of a fractured clavicle could well penetrate the pleura, which rises to about 2½ cm above the clavicle near its midpoint.

Thoracic outlet: diaphragm (Fig. 3.17)

The lower border of the thorax, the thoracic outlet, divides thorax from abdomen. The outlet is bounded by the xiphisternal joint, the inferior costal margin and the body of T12 and closed by a musculotendinous sheet, the **diaphragm**. Numerous important structures (notably the aorta, inferior vena cava, oesophagus, nerves, and

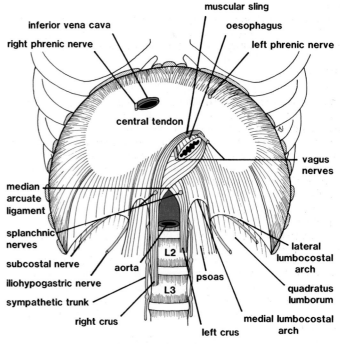

Fig. 3.17. The inferior surface of the diaphragm.

smaller collateral branches of the nerve and vessels are at risk!). Local anaesthesia may be produced by injecting anaesthetic around the origin of an intercostal nerve (intercostal nerve block). To guarantee full anaesthesia two or more roots must be anaesthetized, as the exact area supplied by each nerve is variable.

Infection of the spinal ganglia by Herpes zoster (chickenpox) virus leads to a burning pain followed by a rash over the dermatomes supplied by the affected ganglia, a condition known as shingles.

Pus originating near the vertebral column tends to work its way along neurovascular bundles to reach the surface (point) where the cutaneous branches of intercostal nerves pierce the muscles to reach the skin (midaxillary line, lateral to sternum).

thoracic duct) are transmitted through apertures in or behind the diaphragm.

Shape of the diaphragm

Seen from the front, the diaphragm is a double dome. The right dome (over the liver) is higher than the left. Both are a little higher than the **central tendon** which lies at the level of the xiphisternum, and is relatively flat. The curvature of the muscular part of the diaphragm means that it makes an acute angle where it meets ribs and sternum, forming a narrow gutter, the **costodiaphragmatic** (lateral) and **costomediastinal** (behind the sternum) **recesses.**

Morphology of the diaphragm

The diaphragm has a peripheral muscular part surrounding a central tendon. The muscle fibres (which are striated, a point often unappreciated by students) arise in three main parts:

1. small right and left slips from the posterior surface of the xiphoid process;

2. six paired slips from the lower six costal cartilages;

3. a posterior vertebral part; this is complex and made up as follows.

(a) The **lateral lumbocostal arch (lateral arcuate ligament).** Posteriorly the twelfth rib descends behind the large **quadratus lumborum muscle.** The posterolateral edge of the diaphragm is attached to the fascia covering this muscle, and is consequently arched (convexity upwards).

(b) The **medial lumbocostal arch (medial arcuate ligament).** Medial to quadratus lumborum lies **psoas,** another large muscle. The diaphragm crosses the fascia of psoas in another arch.

(c) The **right** and **left crura.** Medial to psoas the **right crus,** a substantial band of muscle fibres, arises from the vertebral bodies of L1–3. The smaller **left crus** arises from the bodies of L1 and L2. The medial borders of the two crura are joined as the **median arcuate ligament.**

Contraction of the muscle fibres (with the lower ribs fixed) pulls the central tendon downwards, so enlarging the vertical dimension of the thoracic cavity and pushing the abdominal viscera downwards. Movement of the abdominal viscera can take place only within the limits of extensibility of the abdominal wall. When these are reached, the central tendon can descend no lower and continued contraction of the diaphragm elevates the lower ribs and, because of the nature of the costovertebral joints, moves them laterally.

Apertures

The diaphragm has three major apertures:

1. the **aortic opening** (at the level of T12), behind the median arcuate ligament and in front of the twelfth thoracic vertebra, transmits the aorta, azygos vein and thoracic duct (a large lymphatic vessel). Strictly speaking, the aortic opening is behind the diaphragm;

2. the **oesophageal opening** (T10) transmits the oesophagus, the vagal trunks, oesophageal branches of the left gastric vessels supplying the lower parts of the oesophagus, and lymphatics draining the same region. The oesophageal opening is surrounded by a sling of muscles derived mainly from the right crus (although it lies to the left of the midline), the so-called 'diaphragmatic pinchcock' which plays an important part in preventing reflux of stomach contents, being in a contracted state as intra-abdominal pressure rises during descent of the diaphragm;

3. the **caval opening** (T8) transmits the inferior vena cava and terminal branches of the right phrenic nerve. It is situated in the central tendon to the right of the midline and its diameter is not, therefore, reduced by the contraction of the muscle fibres of the diaphragm (i.e. venous return to the heart is unimpeded).

In addition to the structures in these major openings, several other nerves and vessels traverse the thoracic outlet:

1. greater, lesser and least **splanchnic nerves** (autonomic to structures in the abdomen) pierce the right and left crura;

2. the left phrenic nerve pierces the muscle adjacent to the central tendon to supply the peritoneum beneath the diaphragm;

3. the sympathetic trunk passes behind the medial arcuate ligament on each side;

4. superior epigastric blood vessels pass between sternal and costal muscle origins on each side;

5. the neurovascular bundles of spaces 7–11 pass between costal muscle origins on each side.

Nerve supply

The motor nerve supply to the dome of the diaphragm is from the phrenic nerve (from the ventral rami of spinal nerves C3–5). The crura are supplied by lower intercostal nerves. The sensory supply to the parietal pleura and the peritoneum covering the upper and lower surfaces of the diaphragm respectively and of the diaphragm itself is from the phrenic nerve centrally and from the lower five intercostal nerves peripherally.

Functions of the diaphragm

1. As a muscle of respiration.

2. As an aid to micturation, defecation, and parturition. If you take a deep breath and hold it by closing the glottis, the diaphragm is unable to rise. Contraction of the muscles of the abdominal wall will now raise the intra-abdominal pressure.

3. As a lifting mechanism. If the diaphragm is used as above, the vertebral column will be discouraged from flexing, helping the muscles of the back in lifting heavy weights.

Despite the complex embryology of the diaphragm, congenital defects are uncommon, though various herniae may arise due to malunion of embryological structures. Far more common are acquired herniae, usually in patients of middle-age, when the oesophageal opening (or hiatus, hence **hiatus hernia**) has become weakened and widened. In the commonest type the abdominal part of the oesophagus and upper part of the stomach rise through the hiatus when the patient lies down or bends over. Unpleasant reflux of acid stomach contents may follow causing heartburn and, if long continued, ulceration of the oesophageal mucosa.

Before the discovery of suitable antibacterial drugs, one or other dome of the diaphragm was often paralysed (by crushing the phrenic nerve in the neck) as part of the treatment for tuberculosis. This rested the lower lobe of the lung on the same side for a variable period while the damaged nerve regenerated and was believed to retard the progress of the disease.

3

Pleural cavities and lungs

The thoracic cavity is divided into three – the right and left pleural cavities, each containing a lung, and the central **mediastinum**, containing the heart within its pericardium and the great vessels, trachea, thymus gland, and other structures in transit to the abdomen (oesophagus, vagus and phrenic nerves, and thoracic duct).

PLEURAL CAVITIES

Left and right pleural cavities are entirely separate from each other. Each (Fig. 3.18) is formed as the developing lung bud invades a space (part of the coelomic cavity, see page 43) by pushing before it a layer of the wall (just as a finger may invaginate a partially inflated balloon). The structures involved are the lung bud (finger), inner layer of pleura (nearer wall of balloon), pleural cavity (air space), outer layer of pleura (far wall of balloon).

The pleura may thus be divided into three parts:

1. **parietal layer,** lining the thoracic wall, the thoracic side of the diaphragm and the medial wall of the mediastinum;

2. **visceral layer,** closely covering all surfaces of the lungs;

3. a junctional region, the **pleural cuff** surrounding the **hilus** or root of the lung where the two layers join. The pleural cuff has some slack, leading to the formation of a fold called the **pulmonary ligament,** to allow relative movement of the lung and mediastinum.

The **pleural cavity** is located between the two layers of pleura and is normally a potential space only over most of the lung surface as the visceral and parietal pleurae are in virtual contact, being separated by only a thin layer of watery lubricating **pleural fluid**.

The parietal pleura is often arbitrarily divided into **costal, diaphragmatic,** and **mediastinal** areas; this is useful when considering their nerve supply. The costal pleura is supplied segmentally by intercostal nerves, the mediastinal pleura by the phrenic and the diaphragmatic pleura centrally by the phrenic and peripherally by the lower five intercostal nerves. The visceral pleura receives only an autonomic vasomotor supply, and is insensitive to pain and touch.

Clinical aspects

Disease states of the lung (e.g. pneumonia) are often painless until the parietal pleura becomes involved. Local infection of the pleural cavity may lead to a breakdown of lubrication between pleural layers which may then adhere due to the formation of fibrous scar tissue. Local breakdown of lubrication can give a painful and (through a stethoscope) audible pleural rub. General infection of the pleura (pleurisy) is a painful condition, the pain often being referred to the cutaneous distribution of the segmental nerves supplying the pleura. (Interestingly, pleural pain may be abolished by applying local anaesthetic to the appropriate skin area.)

Adhesions may be deliberately induced, by placing a slightly irritant powder in the pleural cavity, to cure chronic leakage of air from a diseased lung.

The pleural cavity may become infiltrated by:

1. Air (pneumothorax). This usually enters via a diseased lung, much less commonly by a stab wound through the chest wall. Spontaneous pneumothorax may occur in the healthy lung after great exertion. The most dangerous type of pneumothorax is where the ruptured lung has a valvular effect, allowing air to pass from the lung to pleural cavity but not vice versa. This is a tension pneumothorax and leads to a progressive build-up of pressure in the pleural cavity and hence collapse of the lung. The effects include breathlessness and, because the mediastinal structures are displaced towards the opposite side, pain.

2. Excess serous pleural fluid (pleural effusion). This will also affect the efficiency of the lung and displace the mediastinum. Infection of this fluid is common.

3. Pus (empyaema).

4. Blood (haemothorax).

Fluid is usually aspirated from the pleural cavity by means of a pleural tap, a wide bore needle being inserted through a lower intercostal space so as to pass into the pleural cavity beneath the lung but above the diaphragm. Pus from a lung abscess, blood, or air is usually aspirated locally after ascertaining its exact position on X-ray.

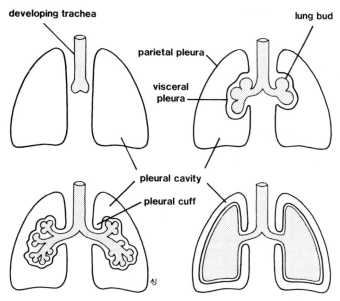

Fig. 3.18. Development of the pleural cavities.

TRACHEA

The trachea (Fig. 3.19) is a tube about 12.5 cm long and 2.5 cm in diameter running from the lower border of the cricoid cartilage in the neck to its bifurcation into left and right main bronchi at the level of the sternal angle. It is stiffened by U-shaped rings of cartilage, incomplete posteriorly to allow the passage of food boli in its posterior relation, the oesophagus. The wall between the rings is made up of fibrous tissue and the lumen lined by respiratory (ciliated columnar) epithelium. The posterior wall of the trachea contains a considerable amount of smooth muscle.

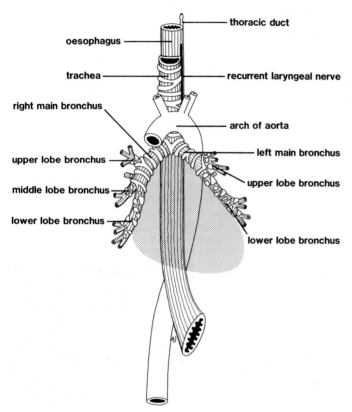

Fig. 3.19. The trachea and its relationships.

The trachea shares the upper mediastinum with the following structures – anteriorly: the thymus gland, brachiocephalic veins, arch of the aorta and origin of the brachiocephalic artery; posteriorly: the oesophagus and left recurrent laryngeal nerve; right side: the azygos vein and right vagus and phrenic nerves; left side: the left common carotid, left subclavian artery and left vagus and phrenic nerves.

The right main bronchus is shorter, wider and more vertical than the left. About 2½ cm long, it gives off a branch to the upper lobe before entering the right lung. The left main bronchus is about 5 cm long and passes to the left and downwards below the arch of the aorta, in front of the oesophagus to enter the left lung. Right and left main bronchi are subdivided further within the substance of the lung, each lobe having its own **lobar bronchus.**

The structure of the walls of the bronchi is similar to that of the trachea although the cartilages become increasingly irregular below the bifurcation.

Clinical aspects

Despite the cartilaginous rings, an enlarged thyroid gland or dilated aortic arch (aneurism) may compress the trachea with resultant difficulty in breathing.

Inflammation of the trachea (tracheitis) or bronchi (bronchitis) gives a burning sensation referred to the sternum.

Foreign bodies entering the larynx and trachea will stimulate a powerful cough reflex. None the less, small toys, peanuts, and a wide range of other objects are not uncommonly inhaled by small children. The cough reflex is in abeyance in the unconscious subject so that blood and vomit may enter the lungs in the victims of road accidents and other violence. When a patient is given a general anaesthetic for dental extraction, procedures (such as packing the throat or passing an endotracheal tube) must be adopted to ensure that tooth fragments and other foreign bodies are not inhaled. The ridge (carina) formed by the bifurcation of the trachea is the last area to contain sensory nerve endings capable of eliciting the cough reflex and may thus be considered a last line of defence. When foreign bodies do pass the carina, they usually enter the right main bronchus and thence the middle and lower bronchi of the right lung. An inhaled foreign body may block one of the bronchi leading to collapse of the lung or part of it or, if infected, may cause a lung abscess.

Carcinoma of the bronchus is the most common form of cancer, responsible for 30 per cent of malignancies. Because of the arrangement of the lymphatic drainage, it may spread to the pleura and to lymph nodes at the hilus of the lung and in the mediastinum. From these lymph nodes the tumour soon metastasizes to more distant organs (especially brain). Pressure or invasion from an enlarged hilar lymph node may involve the phrenic nerve with paralysis of the corresponding half of the diaphragm, the recurrent laryngeal nerve causing hoarseness or the adjacent sympathetic trunk producing Horner's syndrome (see p. 253).

The interior of the bronchi as far as the main branches of the lobar bronchi can be viewed by means of a bronchoscope passed through the mouth and larynx. A bronchoscope can also be used to take samples of mucosa for examination, to remove foreign bodies and to aspirate accumulations of fluid.

Tracheostomy (the provision of an opening in the anterior wall of the trachea) may be necessary to bypass laryngeal obstruction (foreign bodies, tumours) or to drain copious secretions (in a post-operative patient too weak to cough) or for long-term artificial respiration (poliomyelitis).

LUNGS

Both lungs are conical, covered by visceral pleura (which adheres tightly to their surfaces) and attached to the mediastinum by a lung root. Each has a blunt apex projecting about 2½cm above the medial third of the clavicle, a concave base over the diaphragm, an extensive costal surface and a concave mediastinal surface. In fixed *post mortem* specimens evidence of lung relations in the form of grooves moulded around the aorta, ribs, etc. can be seen. These are, of course, not

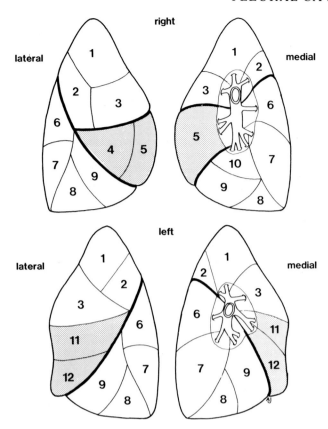

Fig. 3.20. Lobes and bronchopulmonary segments of the lungs.

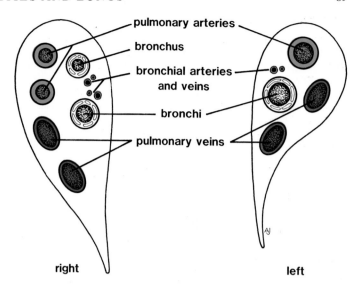

Fig. 3.21. The roots of the lungs.

present in the living, where the lung has a very light frothy texture, rather like foam rubber.

The right lung is slightly larger than the left (because of the offset of the heart which decreases the size of the left pleural cavity). Both are divided by an **oblique fissure** (Fig. 3.20). The upper part of the right lung is subdivided by a **horizontal fissure** into upper and middle lobes. The left lung has a recess, the **cardiac notch,** in its medial side which accommodates the heart. Below the notch the upper lobe may be extended into a **lingula.**

Each lung is further functionally divided into a number of pyramidal **bronchopulmonary segments** whose bases are illustrated in Fig. 3.20. These are of interest to the physician and thoracic surgeon as they form functional units supplied by segmental bronchi and blood vessels. A single segment may, therefore, be removed with minimal loss of blood or leakage of air.

Root of lung (Fig. 3.21)

Communication between the lung and the rest of the body is via the lung root which accordingly contains many important structures. Inferiorly in each lung root are two **pulmonary veins.** Above them run **pulmonary arteries** (anteriorly) and **bronchi** (posteriorly). A **bronchial artery** accompanies or is embedded in the wall of each bronchus. In the left lung root the pulmonary artery and bronchus are single: in the right lung root both have divided into superior and

inferior branches. The structures forming the root enter or leave the lung at a shallow depression called the **hilus.**

Pulmonary vessels and nerves

Blood supply

It is important to realize that there are two blood supplies to each lung. The bronchi and bronchioles, connective tissue, and visceral pleura receive oxygenated blood from the **bronchial arteries.** There are usually two left bronchial arteries, branches of the aorta, and one right, a branch of the third right posterior intercostal artery. Drainage is via the **bronchial veins** (usually two on each side) to the azygos and hemiazygos veins. The alveoli receive deoxygenated blood from the right and left **pulmonary arteries,** branches of the pulmonary trunk arising from the right ventricle of the heart, and drain via the four **pulmonary veins.** which open into the left atrium. Anastomoses between these systems become important when either is occluded by disease.

Lymphatic drainage

Lymphatic drainage follows the bronchi and pulmonary vessels to the lung root. There are many lymph nodes, often in the angles formed by branching bronchi, which may be stained black by dirt and carbon inhaled from the air, even in non-smokers. The bronchial nodes and those alongside the trachea drain through paired bronchomediastinal trunks to the brachiocephalic veins or thoracic duct.

Nerve supply

Nerve supply is again via the lung root in the shape of the autonomic pulmonary plexus (fibres from the sympathetic trunk plus vagus). Sympathetic activity produces bronchodilatation and parasympathetic bronchoconstriction. Afferent fibres from the mucous membrane of the bronchi and stretch receptors in the alveolar walls are both sympathetic and parasympathetic.

Clinical aspects

Because of the lack of pain fibres in the lung, pneumonia (inflammation of the alveoli) may be painless until the parietal pleura becomes involved. The pain then experienced may be referred to the abdomen (via the lower five intercostal nerves) or the shoulder (via the phrenic nerve).

At *post-mortem* examination a healthy lung will be found to be full of air and will make a rattling sound (crepitation) when squeezed. A diseased lung may be waterlogged and will sink when placed in water as will the lungs of a stillborn child.

Some knowledge of bronchopulmonary segments is helpful in managing the bedridden patient. A patient with infection of the left lung, for example, should be placed on the right side to allow secretions from the infected lung to gravitate towards the carina, causing coughing and removal of pus and purulent sputum. The position of very ill or unconscious patients should be changed frequently so as to drain all areas and reduce the risk of bacteria from the nose and mouth entering the lungs.

Bronchial asthma, due to spasm of the smooth muscles of the bronchi and sticky secretions causing wheezing and difficult breathing, is a major problem with multiple causes, including allergies to inhaled or ingested substances. A psychological component is not uncommon.

Pulmonary thromboembolism is due to transport of a blood clot from an often distant site (such as leg veins) to the lung through the right ventricle and pulmonary arteries. A large clot can be fatal, a small one cause damage to a bronchopulmonary segment by blocking an artery although collateral circulation may prevent this in healthy individuals.

MECHANISM OF RESPIRATION

Although respiration is the term commonly used in anatomy to cover breathing, it is more accurately called ventilation. The term respiration includes not only ventilation but also the passage of oxygen and carbon dioxide through the alveolar wall and complex biochemical events within the tissues throughout the body.

The mechanism of ventilation is still not completely understood. Many attempts at simplification, regarding the thorax as a box which can increase in size only along fixed axes and invoking pincer movements, bucket and pump handle movements of the ribs, and other such analogies, serve to confuse rather than enlighten. The increase in thoracic volume leading to inspiration of air has two main components: an increase in vertical height of the thoracic cavity and an increase in diameter in the anteroposterior, lateral and all intermediate axes.

Increase in vertical dimension is brought about principally by contraction of the diaphragm, although straightening of the normally anteriorly-concave thoracic vertebral column may be called on *in extremis*. Increase in diameter is the result of movement of the ribs. In babies and young children respiration is entirely diaphragmatic; amongst adults men are said to move the ribs less than women.

In **quiet inspiration** the muscular fibres of the diaphragm contract. Since they are firmly anchored peripherally their action is to pull the central tendon downwards, pushing the abdominal viscera before it. This decreases pressure in the thorax. Eventually a point is reached where the limited extensibility of the abdominal wall prevents further descent of the abdominal viscera and diaphragm. During this time the first rib is held fixed by the scalene muscles, and the upper inter-

costal muscles are electrically active, although little movement of the upper ribs occurs. These muscles may be contracting to prevent the tissues of the intercostal spaces from being sucked inwards, as occurs in a space in which the muscles have been paralysed by the injection of local anaesthetic solution.

Quiet expiration is mainly a passive event brought about by elastic recoil of the lungs and chest wall. The diaphragm is progressively relaxed to control the rate of outflow of air.

In **deep forced respiration** the capacity of the thorax during the inspiratory phase is increased by a much larger amount by movement of the ribs and contraction of accessory muscles.

To understand rib movement a knowledge of the movements of the joints between the ribs and vertebral column is required. It must be appreciated that movement takes place simultaneously at the joints at the heads of the ribs and at the costotransverse joints and that the degree of movement is small at both joints because of the strong ligaments uniting the ribs and vertebrae. Although the articulations between ribs and vertebral bodies are all similar, those between tubercles and transverse processes form a series, each differing a little from those above and below (Fig. 3.22). In the upper six costotransverse articulations the articular surface on the rib is convex and that on the vertebra is concave. A muscle acting on the upper margin of the shaft of one of these ribs would obviously raise it, the rib rotating about a long axis running through its neck from the joint at the head to the costotransverse joint. In the seventh to tenth joints the articulating surfaces are flat and angled, so that the surfaces on the rib tubercles face downwards and medially as well as

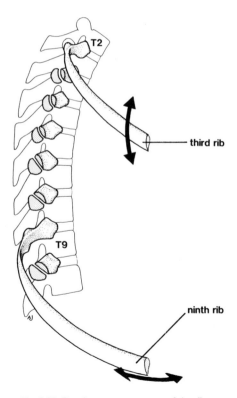

Fig. 3.22. Respiratory movements of the ribs.

backwards. Hence no rotation about the axis of the rib neck is possible. The joint surfaces can only slide over each other a little, a movement which displaces the rib principally outwards and only slightly upwards.

The sternum, attached to the upper ribs, is moved forwards and upwards during inspiration because of the obliquity of the ribs. The middle ribs are able to move laterally because of the flexibility of the long inclined cartilages which connect them to the sternum. The costal angle increases appreciably during deep inspiration.

In **deep forced inspiration** the first rib is raised a little by the contraction of scalenus anterior and medius. Contraction of the intercostal muscles moves the second rib in relation to the first, the third in relation to the second, and so on, the effect being maximal at about the seventh or eighth rib. The small triangular levatores costarum muscles, running from transverse processes of C7–T11 to the outside of the rib below, also contract although with their poor mechanical advantage their effect must be small. Continued contraction of the diaphragm after the point where it can descend no further causes the lower ribs to move upwards but, because of the constraints imposed by the shape of the costovertebral joints, principally outwards. Back muscles may contract to straighten the thoracic spine. The sternum is pulled up by sternocleidomastoid and the strap muscles (sternohyoid, sternothyrohyoid) descending from the hyoid bone, the clavicle is elevated by trapezius and sternocleidomastoid. In extreme cases the pectoral muscles, running from the upper limbs to the thorax, may be powerfully involved, the subject fixating the limbs by grasping a fixed object or placing his hands on his knees.

In **forced expiration** the normal elastic recoil of ribs and anterior abdominal wall is enhanced by contraction of the muscles of the abdominal wall forcing up the diaphragm and pulling down the lower ribs.

During inspiration the bronchial tree expands so that the lung roots move downwards, outwards and forwards; during deep inspiration the carina may descend by 5 cm. In quiet breathing the central tendon of the diaphragm moves up and down by about 1 cm; in deep forced breathing it may move through a considerably greater range. The average volume of air exchanged in quiet respiration is 500–600 ml and the normal ventilation rate is about 15 per minute for a healthy adult not taking exercise or under stress. By contrast the normal respiratory rate at birth is about 40 per minute.

The ventilatory movements of the chest wall are accompanied by expansion and contraction of the lungs. The layers of the pleura play an essential part in this, behaving like two sheets of glass separated by a thin film of water. These glass plates may be slid easily over each other but can only be pulled apart by the use of enormous force. The pleural layers similarly slide over each other wherever they are in contact, and resist the separating forces generated by the movement of the chest wall and the elasticity of the lungs.

Clinical aspects

Artificial respiration has been practised in many forms. The best is probably mouth-to-mouth, a technique with which all dentists should be familiar. The patient is laid supine, with his head fully back. This is important to ensure that the airway is patent. False teeth (patient's) should be removed and the tongue moved forwards if necessary. With one hand the reviver holds the jaw open, with the other he pinches the patient's nostrils shut. He then takes a deep breath and blows in to the patient's mouth until his chest rises. He then stops and allows passive expiration to occur. The cycle should be repeated 12–20 times a minute for as long as necessary. Note that the lungs will not work if filled with water: if the patient has inhaled a large amount of water remove this first by appropriately positioning the patient.

4

The mediastinum, pericardium, and heart

MEDIASTINUM

The mediastinum, the territory between the pleural sacs and bordered laterally by the mediastinal pleura, contains the heart, the great vessels, the trachea and bronchi, the oesophagus, the vagus and phrenic nerves, and the thoracic duct.

Divisions of mediastinum

The mediastinum is divided for convenience in description into several parts (Fig. 3.23):

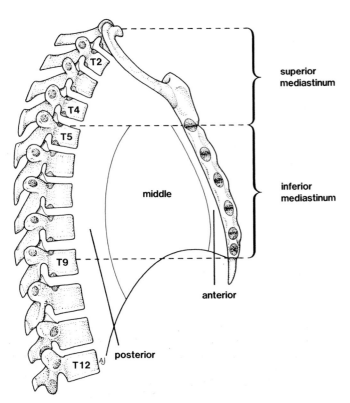

Fig. 3.23. Divisions of the mediastinum.

1. Superior mediastinum

The superior mediastinum occupies the space between the thoracic inlet above and a horizontal plane joining the sternal angle and the disc between T4 and T5 below.

2. Inferior mediastinum

The inferior mediastinum, which lies below the superior mediastinum, is further divided into three parts:

    (a) Anterior: anterior to the fibrous pericardium, and very small.

    (b) Middle: the fibrous pericardium and its contents.

    (c) Posterior: the structures posterior to the fibrous pericardium.

Contents of mediastinal divisions

Superior mediastinum (Figs 3.24 and 3.25)

    Immediately behind the sternum:

        sternohyoid and sternothyroid muscles

        thymus gland

        superior vena cava and brachiocephalic veins.

    Immediately in front of the vertebrae:

        oesophagus

        trachea

        thoracic duct

        left recurrent laryngeal nerve.

    Intermediate:

        aortic arch and its branches

        vagus and phrenic nerves.

Inferior mediastinum

    Anterior:

        no contents of importance; a little fat, fascia, and occasionally the inferior part of the thymus.

    Middle:

        the pericardium and heart and the vessels entering and leaving the heart

        trachea dividing into right and left bronchi

        phrenic nerves

    Posterior:

        the contents of the posterior mediastinum may be divided into two groups, vertical – near the heart – and horizontal – mainly posterior.

        Vertical:

            descending aorta

            oesophagus and oesophageal plexus of nerves

            azygos and hemiazygos veins

            thoracic duct.

        Horizontal:

            intercostal veins, arteries, and nerves.

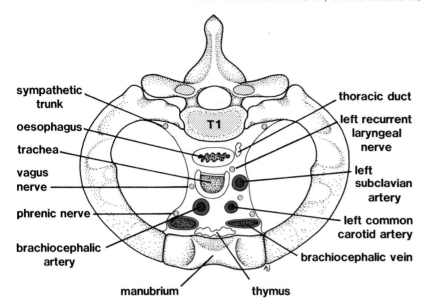

Fig. 3.24. Structures in the superior mediastinum at the level of first rib.

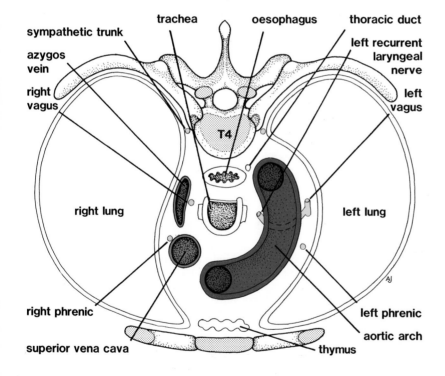

Fig. 3.25. Structures in the mediastinum at the level of T4.

From the above list it will be seen that the key to the mediastinum is the middle portion containing the heart and pericardium. Any attempt to deal with the contents of the other divisions on a strictly regional basis would lead to artificial division of the aorta, oesophagus, and vagus nerves, all of which pass through more than one mediastinal division. We shall therefore deal with the middle mediastinum as an entity, then with aorta, oesophagus, etc., under the portmanteau heading 'other mediastinal structures'.

Infection of the mediastinum may occur through pathological fluids tracking into it along the carotid sheath or following rupture of the oesophagus. The mediastinum may be pushed towards the opposite side by a space-occupying lesion in one of the pleural cavities or pulled towards the same side by a collapse of the lung.

MIDDLE MEDIASTINUM: PERICARDIUM AND HEART

Pericardium

The heart is enclosed in a tough bag, the **fibrous pericardium.** Between the fibrous pericardium and the heart is the **serous pericardium.** During development the heart has invaginated into the serous pericardium in the same way that the lung invaginates into the pleura (p. 87). Hence there are two layers of serous pericardium, an outer **parietal layer** and the inner **visceral layer** (cf. parietal and visceral pleura). Between the two layers is a potential space, the **pericardial cavity,** lubricated by a little serous fluid. The parietal and visceral layers are continuous at the roots of the great arteries and veins. The pericardial space is divided into a **general pericardial space,** a **transverse sinus** and an **oblique sinus,** a blind pocket which is open inferiorly and passes between the paired left and right pulmonary veins (Fig. 3.26).

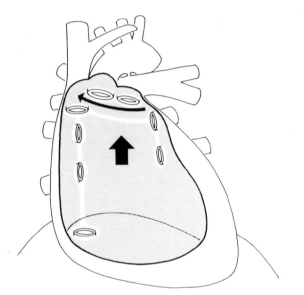

Fig. 3.26. The posterior wall of the pericardial cavity with the heart removed. Serous pericardium in stipple with reflections (i.e. where visceral and parietal layers continuous) in white. Narrow arrow in transverse sinus; broad arrow in oblique sinus.

The pericardium conforms to the external surface of the heart, although allowing free movement of the muscular walls of the ventricles and atria. The fibrous pericardium blends with the great vessels not very far from their roots and is firmly attached to the central tendon of the diaphragm and the anterior chest wall by fibrous ligaments which help to anchor the heart. The heart is also indirectly anchored by its vessels, especially by the fixation of the pulmonary veins to the lungs.

Clinical aspects

Inflammation of the pericardial sac (pericarditis) may follow bacterial or viral infection. It may also be a sequel to rheumatic fever. It is accompanied by severe substernal pain and frequently by pericardial effusion, the latter often copious enough to compress the pulmonary veins and interfere with the action of the heart. Acute pericarditis often produces a pericardial rub (cf. pleural rub). A wound penetrat-

ing the pericardium commonly injures the heart wall causing bleeding into the pericardium, again compressing and embarrassing the heart. Fluid may be drained from the pericardial sac via a wide bore needle inserted through the fifth or sixth intercostal space near the sternum, taking care to miss the internal thoracic artery.

Heart

Although the chambers of the heart are conventionally referred to as the right and left atria and ventricles, this nomenclature does not reflect the position of the heart as it lies in the chest. The right side of the heart as conventionally defined is, in fact, anterior to the left (Figs 3.27 and 3.28). The right side of the heart silhouette, as seen, for example, in a posterior/anterior radiograph, is occupied by the right atrium, with the superior and inferior venae cavae entering as their names suggest. The right atrioventricular (tricuspid) valve,

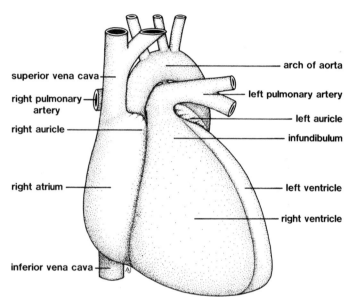

superior vena cava — right pulmonary artery — right auricle — right atrium — inferior vena cava

arch of aorta — left pulmonary artery — left auricle — infundibulum — left ventricle — right ventricle

Fig. 3.27. Anterior view of the heart.

separating right atrium from right ventricle, lies almost vertically behind the lower end of the sternum so that the right ventricle lies to the left of the atrium. Blood leaves the right ventricle superiorly through the pulmonary valve and flows into the pulmonary trunk which, after a short course, splits into right and left pulmonary arteries.

Blood returns from the lungs via the four pulmonary veins to the left atrium, situated on the posterior side of the heart and virtually symmetrical about the median plane (Fig. 3.28). It is separated from the right atrium by the atrial septum. From the left atrium blood passes through the left atrioventricular (mitral) valve to the left ventricle which lies posterior to the right ventricle and separated from it by the fibromuscular ventricular septum. Blood leaves the left ventricle via the aortic valve to enter the aorta which runs at first upwards and then curves backwards over the bifurcation of the pulmonary trunk. Note that the origin of the aorta lies to the right of the pulmonary trunk. The cusps of the valves guarding the atrioven-

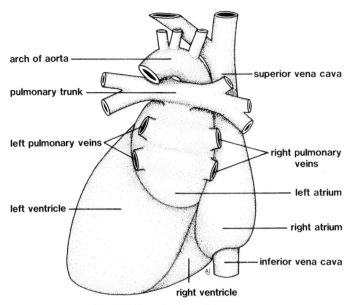

arch of aorta

pulmonary trunk

left pulmonary veins

left ventricle

superior vena cava

right pulmonary veins

left atrium

right atrium

inferior vena cava

right ventricle

Fig. 3.28. Posterior view of the heart.

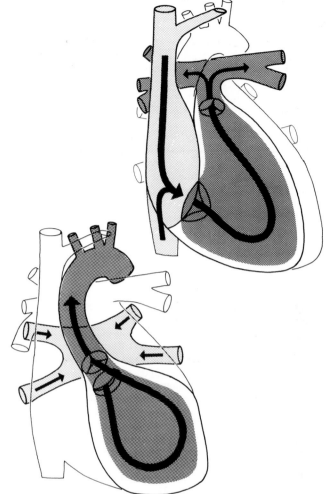

Fig. 3.29. Blood flow through the heart; pulmonary circulation, above; systemic circulation, below.

tricular orifices and the outflow tracts from the ventricles are arranged so that the flow of blood can take place in the desired direction only.

The three surfaces and three borders of the heart usually recognized are the **sternocostal surface** (formed by right atrium plus right ventricle plus apex of left ventricle), **diaphragmatic surface** (right and left ventricles plus the part of the right atrium admitting the inferior vena cava), **posterior surface** or **base** (mainly left atrium, plus a little right atrium), **right border** (entirely right atrium), **left border** (entirely left ventricle), and **inferior border** (right atrium, right ventricle plus apex of left ventricle). The four chambers are separated by grooves on the external surface of the heart, named from their position as atrioventricular or interventricular.

Chambers of the heart

The walls of the four chambers of the heart are lined by an endothelial layer, the **endocardium,** but consist mainly of cardiac muscle, called collectively the **myocardium.** The myocardium of the two atria is continuous as is that of the two ventricles but there is no muscular continuity across the atrioventricular junction, except for the atrioventricular bundle (see below). The junction is occupied by a sheet of fibrous tissue pierced by the right and left atrioventricular orifices. Fibrous tissue also surrounds the pulmonary and aortic orifices and extends into the upper part of the ventricular septum. These fibrous tissues, the **skeleton of the heart,** support the valves and give origin to the cardiac muscle fibres. The principal features of interest in the interior of the chambers of the heart can be summarized as follows.

Right atrium (Fig. 3.30)

Inlets: Superiorly the **superior vena cava,** which has no valve; inferiorly the **inferior vena cava,** which has a rudimentary valve; medially the opening of the **coronary sinus** (draining venous blood from much of the heart wall), which also has a rudimentary valve.

Outlet: the **right atrioventricular orifice** guarded by the valve of the same name.

Morphology: the chamber is divided vertically by a ridge, the **crista terminalis,** on its lateral wall which produces a marking, the **sulcus terminalis,** on the corresponding exterior wall of the atrium. A shallow depression, the **fossa ovalis** (= foramen ovale in developing heart, see page 37) is seen in the septal wall. The prominent upper margin of this is sometimes named as the **annulus ovalis.** The atrial wall receiving the venae cavae, coronary sinus and surrounding the fossa ovalis, i.e. posterior to the crista terminalis, is smooth, the remainder ridged by **musculi pectinati,** muscle bundles running from the crista upwards towards the **right auricle,** a forward projection of the atrium around the base of the aorta. The musculi are particularly well-developed in the auricle.

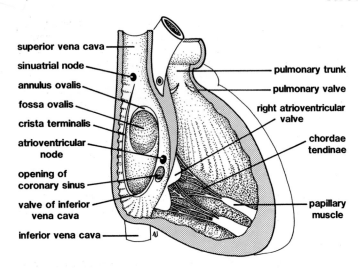

Fig. 3.30. The interior of the right atrium and ventricle from in front.

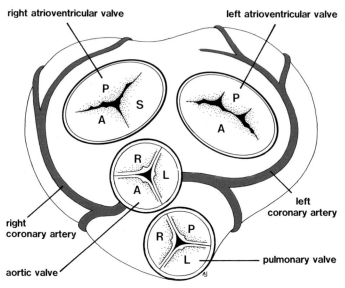

Fig. 3.31. Superior view of the cusps of the heart valves after removal of the atria. A = anterior, L = left, P = posterior, R = right and S = septal.

Right ventricle

Inlet: the **right atrioventricular orifice,** guarded by the correspondingly named valve.

Outlet: the **pulmonary trunk** guarded by the **pulmonary valve.**

Morphology: the **right atrioventricular (tricuspid) valve** is attached to the fibrous atrioventricular ring and has anterior, posterior, and septal cusps (Fig. 3.31). Each cusp is flap-like, consisting of a double layer of endocardium with a fibrous core. The atrial sides of each cusp (in contact with flowing blood) are smooth, the ventricular sides roughened by the insertion of a number of **chordae tendinae** which link the cusps to **papillary muscles** in the ventricular wall (Fig. 3.30). These prevent the valve turning inside out when ventricular pressure exceeds that in the atrium. The pulmonary valve consists of three semilunar cusps, left, right, and posterior attached at their bases to the atrial wall. Each cusp is shaped like a pocket with the concave side facing into the pulmonary trunk. When the ventricle contracts the cusps are pressed against the wall of the artery and offer little resistance to the flow of blood. When the pressure in the ventricle falls below that in the pulmonary artery, the cusps are distended and thus close the valve. Because of their shape the semilunar cusps have great intrinsic strength and require no external bracing. The walls of the ventricle are thicker than those of the atrium with numerous muscle bundles, the **trabeculae carneae,** forming irregular elevations on their internal surfaces. A muscular bundle, the moderator band, crossing the ventricle from septal to anterior wall, carries the right branch of the **atrioventricular bundle** while other bundles project as the papillary muscles. The ventricular walls are smoother towards the pulmonary outlet, a region distinguished as the **infundibulum.**

Left atrium

Inlets: the four pulmonary veins, without valves.

Outlet: the **left atrioventricular orifice,** guarded by its valve.

Morphology: most of the atrial wall is smooth but the walls of the finger-like **auricle** are roughened by muscular ridges.

Left ventricle

Inlet: the **left atrioventricular orifice** guarded by its valve.

Outlet: the **aortic orifice** guarded by the **aortic valve.**

Morphology: the **left atrioventricular (mitral) valve** is similar to the right except in having only two cusps, anterior and posterior (Fig. 3.31), of which the anterior is the larger. Both cusps are flap-like and are supported by chordae tendinae and papillary muscles. The aortic valve has three semilunar cusps similar in structure to those of the pulmonary valve. Above each cusp the aortic wall bulges into an **aortic sinus.** From here originate the **left** (above left cusp) and **right** (above anterior cusp) coronary arteries. The left ventricle is circular in cross-section and in the healthy heart has walls three times the thickness of those of the right ventricle. The bulge of the septal wall of the left ventricle makes the chamber of the right ventricle into a crescent. The ventricular septum is composed principally of muscle apart from a small area in front of the atrioventricular junction where it is fibrous. Trabeculae carneae and papillary muscles are well developed. A moderately smooth area below the aortic opening is named the **aortic vestibule.**

Blood supply to the heart wall (Fig. 3.32)

Arterial supply

The right and left coronary arteries arise from the aorta immediately above the aortic valve where they are assured of a copious supply of well-oxygenated blood, most of the filling taking place during diastole. The **right coronary artery** runs forwards between the right auricle and the pulmonary trunk, descends in the right atrioventricular groove supplying the right atrium and ventricle and continues along the groove to anastomose with the left coronary artery on the posterior side of the heart. One major branch, the **marginal branch,** runs along the inferior border of the heart towards the apex. Another, the **posterior (inferior) interventricular artery,** runs in the posterior (inferior) interventricular groove.

The **left coronary artery,** larger than the right, passes behind and to the left of the pulmonary trunk, enters the left atrioventricular

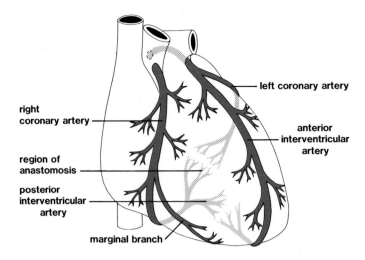

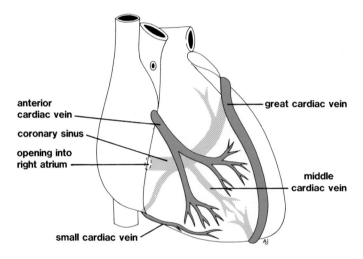

Fig. 3.32. The blood supply of the heart wall. Arteries above, veins below.

groove and follows it until it anastomoses with the right coronary artery on the posterior surface of the heart. An important branch, the **anterior interventricular artery,** runs in the **anterior interventricular groove** to the apex and then ascends in the posterior interventricular groove to anastomose with the right coronary artery. This branch supplies blood to both ventricles.

Potential anastomoses exist between the various branches of the coronary arteries. These are inadequate to bypass a sudden blockage of a large artery.

Venous drainage

About two-thirds of the venous blood from the heart wall drains into the right atrium by veins accompanying the coronary arteries. The remainder drains by small **venae cordis minimae** directly into the heart chambers. The **coronary sinus** in the posterior atrioventricular groove opens into the right atrium near the mouth of the inferior vena cava. It receives: (i) the **great cardiac vein** which begins at the apex of the heart and then accompanies the anterior interventricular

artery in the anterior groove; (ii) the **middle cardiac vein** which runs in the posterior interventricular groove in company with the corresponding artery; and (iii) the **small cardiac vein** which begins at the inferior margin of the heart and then runs in the posterior atrioventricular groove.

The **anterior cardiac vein** often multiple, drains much of the anterior surface of the heart. It traverses the right atrioventricular groove, to open independently into the right atrium.

Nerves of the heart

The heart receives its sympathetic supply through the cardiac branches of the cervical and upper thoracic ganglia of the sympathetic trunk and its parasympathetic supply from cardiac branches of the vagus. These branches join together to form the cardiac plexuses on the base of the heart from which the intrinsic conducting system of the heart is supplied.

Intrinsic conducting system

The conducting system of the heart is made up of specialized impulse-conducting cardiac muscle fibres **(Purkinje fibres).** It functions to control the heart rate and to keep the contraction of atria and ventricles in step. If the conducting system between atria and ventricles is interrupted (complete heart block), the ventricles remain active but beat more slowly than the atria, dropping to around 30 contractions a minute, usually just enough to maintain adequate circulation. The conducting system comprises the following components (Fig. 3.33).

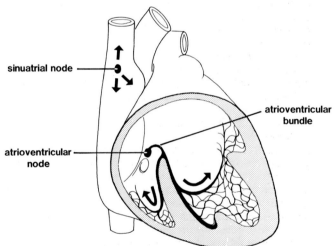

Fig. 3.33. The conducting system of the heart.

1. The **sinuatrial node,** or **pacemaker,** is situated at the upper end of the sulcus terminalis within the wall of the right atrium, just to the right of the point of entry of the superior vena cava (Fig. 3.30). It often occupies the whole thickness of the atrial wall and is well supplied with sympathetic and parasympathetic nerve fibres which form small ganglia adjacent to the node.

2. The **atrioventricular node,** somewhat smaller than the sinuatrial node, is located in the wall of the right atrium immediately above the opening of the coronary sinus.

3. The **atrioventricular bundle** leaves the atrioventricular node and crosses the atrioventricular junction (being the only muscle to do so) behind the septal cusp of the right atrioventricular valve to the ventricular septum. Here it divides into two branches, one for each ventricle. The right branch passes down the right side of the septum to the moderator band, by means of which it crosses to the anterior wall of the right ventricle. Here it splits to form a Purkinje plexus. The left branch pierces the septum and runs down beneath its left surface, often branching into three parts, which again terminate as plexuses of Purkinje fibres among the papillary muscles of the left ventricle.

Action of the conducting system

The following hierachy of control must be appreciated.

1. Cardiac muscle fibres contract rhythmically and synchronously without external stimulation. This occurs in the embryo before developing nerve fibres reach the heart. The first muscles to develop, in the atria, beat faster than those which develop later in the ventricles.

2. The intrinsic muscular contractions are regulated by pacemakers. The normal pacemaker of the heart is the sinuatrial node. From here the impulse passes to the atrioventricular node via the atrial muscle fibres. Some of these run directly from node to node, and may be functionally specialized, although not showing the typical microscopic appearance of Purkinje fibres. The atrioventricular bundle conducts the impulse to the ventricles via its two limbs and Purkinje plexuses.

3. The rate of the pacemaker is regulated by sympathetic and parasympathetic inputs.

Function of the heart

The heart is a muscular pump, filling and emptying during the cardiac cycle. A normal heart beats at about 70 per minute in a resting adult, up to 130 in a newborn child and even faster in a fetus where contractions start as early as the third week of development.

Blood returns continuously to both sides of the heart from the circulatory system. During ventricular contraction (or **systole**) the atrioventricular valves are closed and blood accumulates in the atria and large veins. When the ventricles relax (**diastole**) the atrioventricular valves open and blood flows passively into the ventricles. When the ventricles are nearly full the next cycle of cardiac contraction begins. This is initiated by the sinuatrial node. The impulse spreads rapidly through the myocardium of the atria which contracts from the roots of the great veins towards the atrioventricular orifices, forcing blood into the ventricles and avoiding reflux from the atria into the large veins. When the cardiac impulse reaches the atrioventricular node it is transmitted via the atrioventricular bundle to the muscles of the ventricular walls. The ventricles contract in a wave which passes upwards from the apex towards the aortic and pulmonary orifices. The resultant increase in pressure closes the atrioventricular valves. The papillary muscles are also contracting at this time, taking up slack in the chordae tendinae and preventing the flap-like cusps from turning inside out. Once the intraventricular pressure exceeds that in the large arteries (aorta and pulmonary trunk) the semilunar valves are forced open and blood is ejected from the heart. As soon as the contraction ceases, the intraventricular pressure drops below that of the great vessels and the semilunar valves close. Further relaxation lowers ventricular pressure to below that of the atria, now refilled from the general and pulmonary circulation and the atrioventricular valves open as the cycle begins again.

Auscultation of the heart

There is little point in the dental student memorizing the detailed relationships of the heart to the chest wall, apart from the position of the apex beat (described on page 78). Of more value is a knowledge of how to listen to the heart with a stethoscope. The sounds produced first by closure of the atrioventricular and then of the outflow valves (characterized as 'lub-dub') can be heard over most of the chest wall in the normal subject. There is usually no difficulty in determining which is the first and which is the second heart sound but if in doubt time the heart at the apex beat.

The sounds produced at each of the four valves tend to be heard best at separate specific locations (termed the **sites of maximum propogation**) (Fig. 3.3). These are situated: for the right atrioventricular valve lateral to the left sternal margin in the fifth space, for the pulmonary valve over the second *left* intercostal space (remember the relationship of the origin of the pulmonary trunk to that of the aorta) just lateral to the sternal border, for the left atrioventricular valve at the apex beat and for the aortic valve over the second *right* intercostal space lateral to the sternal border. It must be emphasized that these are not the surface markings of the valves but the sites at which clinical experience has shown their sounds are heard best.

Clinical aspects

Many clinical conditions of the heart are congenital (i.e. defects in development present at birth) and are dealt with in Chapter 2.2 where the development of the heart is considered.

Inadequate supply of blood to the cardiac muscle (myocardial ischaemia) produces severe pain (angina pectoris) over the middle of the sternum, often spreading to one or both arms, the neck, and even the jaw. The pain, believed to be caused by accumulations of metabolites, is transmitted from sensory nerve endings in the myocardium via cardiac branches of the sympathetic trunk and thence to the spinal cord through the dorsal roots of the upper thoracic spinal nerves. It is therefore referred predominantly to the areas of skin supplied by these nerves.

Although coronary arteries anastomose with each other, they are functional end arteries and a sudden blockage of a large branch will lead to necrosis of cardiac muscle (myocardial infarction) supplied by the artery. This is referred to, in lay terms, as a 'heart attack' or 'coronary' and may be immediately fatal or may lead to death after a few days if the necrosed wall ruptures. As the conducting system of the heart receives its blood supply via the coronary arteries, a blockage may interfere with conduction producing arrhythmia or heart block. The usual cause of blockage of the coronary arteries is a degenerative disease of the vessel wall called atherosclerosis.

Damage to the heart valves may lead to stenosis when scarring of the cusps impedes the flow of blood or to incompetence when a valve no longer closes properly. Often the two conditions co-exist. The valvular deformities may be congenital or may be caused by disease, especially rheumatic fever (a disease predominantly of childhood in which antibodies raised by the victim to the invading micro-organisms may attack the tissues of the heart valves especially the atrioventricular). Deformed valves reduce the efficiency of the heart as a pump and may also form a site at which micro-organisms in the blood can be deposited and proliferate (bacterial endocarditis).

The presence of valvular disease can be detected by listening to the heart with a stethoscope since both stenosis and incompetence produce an irregular blood flow with an accompanying murmur. The valves affected and the nature of the deformity can be determined from the site of maximum propogation of the murmur and its timing. For example, incompetence of the left atrioventricular valve will produce a murmur best heard at the apex beat (this being the site of maximum propogation of sounds produced at this valve) and occurring during systole (because the irregular blood flow takes place during contraction of the left ventricle). Stenosis of the left atrioventricular valve will result in a murmur also best heard at the apex beat but occurring during diastole. The sites of maximum propogation and timing of incompetence and stenosis of the other valves should be worked out.

Thrombi (blood clots) may develop within the chambers of the heart. One of the more common sites for this to occur is in the rough-walled auricle of the left atrium, especially when the flow of blood through this chamber is slowed (as happens, for example, in arrythmias). If pieces of clot break loose, they will travel round in the circulation (where they are known as emboli) until they become impacted in a small blood vessel. The effects of emboli depend upon whether or not adequate anastomoses exist in the affected organ to allow the blockage to be bypassed.

OTHER MEDIASTINAL STRUCTURES

Thymus

The thymus gland is a mass of lymphoid tissue which reaches its greatest extent in childhood. It is a flattened bilobed structure with a pink lobulated appearance which lies immediately behind the manubrium sterni. In newborn infants it may extend through the thoracic inlet into the root of the neck. During late childhood the thymus involutes (decreases in size) and by adulthood is scarcely recognizable, present only as a few thymic nodules embedded in fat. Its blood supply is from the inferior thyroid and internal thoracic arteries, its venous drainage into the left brachiocephalic, internal thoracic, and inferior thyroid veins. Lymphatic drainage is to the tracheobronchial, brachiocephalic, and parasternal lymph nodes.

The thymus is necessary in the newborn for the development of peripheral lymphoid tissue; if removed at this stage consequences include wasting and death from infection. In the adult the involuted thymus supplies immunologically uncommitted lymphocytes; its removal, therefore, leads only to a diminished response to new antigens.

Clinical aspects

Because of common embryological origin (see p. 47) a parathyroid gland may accompany the thymus into the superior mediastinum. More often a fibrous band unites thymus with thyroid or parathyroid glands. Tumours of the thymus are rare, but may press on the trachea or superior vena cava.

Oesophagus

The oesophagus (Fig. 3.19) runs from the level of the lower border of the **cricoid cartilage** to the **cardiac orifice** of the stomach, a distance of approximately 25 cm. Its upper end lies in the midline of the neck; it then passes through the mediastinum of the thorax to reach the oesophageal opening of the diaphragm (T10). It has a muscular wall (striated in its upper two-thirds and smooth in its lower

one-third) and is lined by non-keratinized stratified squamous epithelium.

The oesophagus has the following principal relations in the thorax. Anteriorly it is related successively to the trachea, the left main bronchus, the pericardium, and the diaphragm. Posteriorly lie the thoracic vertebrae, the thoracic duct, and, near the diaphragm, the descending aorta. On the left lie the aortic arch and descending aorta, the left recurrent laryngeal nerve, left subclavian artery and thoracic duct. On the right is the azygos vein.

The oesophagus is supplied with blood via the inferior thyroid artery, branches of the descending aorta and ascending branches of the left gastric artery. Venous drainage is into the inferior thyroid veins, the azygos, and left gastric vein. Lymphatic drainage is from the perioesophageal plexus around the oesophagus to deep cervical and posterior mediastinal nodes above and nodes around the left gastric vessels below.

The oesophagus receives a parasympathetic innervation from the vagi and a sympathetic supply from the cervical and thoracic sympathetic ganglia. The parasympathetic innervation of the cervical part of the oesophagus is from the recurrent laryngeal branches of the vagi.

Clinical aspects

The oesophagus is normally indented where it is crossed by the arch of the aorta and the left main bronchus, and at the diaphragmatic hiatus in the thorax. As these are the narrowest points of its lumen, they represent the likely resting places of foreign bodies or sites of damage by swallowed corrosive fluids. The veins draining the upper oesophagus empty into the systemic system which passes directly to the heart, while the left gastric vein, whose tributaries drain the lower part, forms part of the hepatic portal system through which blood from most of the alimentary tract passes to the capillary network in the liver before reaching the heart. Since these two systems anastomose, damage to the capillary bed in the liver (as occurs, for example, in cirrhosis) can lead to diversion of large amounts of blood through the oesophageal vessels. These may respond by forming varicosities (dilation of the veins) which may interfere with the passage of food or rupture causing severe bleeding into the oesophagus.

Rarely the oesophagus may rupture during violent vomiting. The escape of oesophageal contents into the mediastinum may produce a fatal mediastinitis.

Thoracic duct (Fig. 3.34)

This is an important, large lymphatic vessel draining all the lymph from the body except that from the right arm and the right halves of thorax, neck, and head. It is responsible for transporting fatty digestive products (chyle) from the small intestine into the bloodstream. It commences inferiorly at the **cisterna chyli** below the diaphragm, passes through the aortic opening (T12) behind the aorta and ascends behind the oesophagus as far as T5 where it deviates a little to the left and runs up the side of the oesophagus to the neck. In the neck it passes behind the carotid sheath, descends over the left subclavian artery and drains into the commencement of the left brachiocephalic vein. The left jugular, subclavian, and mediastinal lymph trunks usually empty into the thoracic duct, but may drain independently into the great veins.

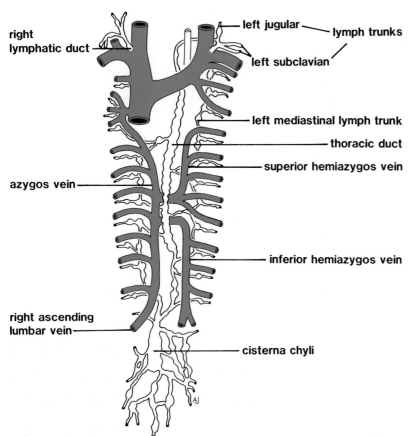

right
lymphatic duct

left jugular ── lymph trunks

left subclavian

left mediastinal lymph trunk

thoracic duct

superior hemiazygos vein

azygos vein

inferior hemiazygos vein

right ascending
lumbar vein

cisterna chyli

Fig. 3.34. The azygos venous system and the thoracic duct.

Lymph from the right arm and right side of the thorax and of the head and neck drains through the smaller **right lymphatic duct** into the right brachiocephalic vein.

Clinical aspects

The thoracic duct may be damaged during major surgery of the neck. If the damage is not made good, lymph may find its way to the surface to produce a chylous fistula in the neck. The thoracic duct may also be damaged as a complication of fractures of the thoracic vertebrae. This may lead to a chylothorax.

Azygos and hemiazygos veins (Fig. 3.34)

The **azygos vein** (an unpaired vessel) is a continuation of the right ascending lumbar vein. It enters the thorax, usually via the aortic opening, but occasionally through the right crus of the diaphragm. It ascends, lying against the right side of the vertebral bodies, to the level of T4 where it arches over the root of the lung to enter the superior vena cava. The azygos vein drains all the right intercostal spaces except the first which drains into the right brachiocephalic vein.

The **hemiazygos veins** are usually two in number. The **inferior hemiazygos vein** is a continuation of the left ascending lumbar vein. It enters the thorax through the left crus of the diaphragm and ascends on the left side of the vertebral bodies. It drains the left lower

three intercostal spaces. The **superior** (or accessory) **hemiazygos vein** descends on the left side of the vertebral column and drains the fourth to eighth left intercostal spaces (the upper three spaces drain into the left brachiocephalic vein). The superior and inferior hemiazygos veins cross in front of the vertebral column to drain into the azygos vein. The azygos system is subject to much variation. Superior and inferior veins may communicate, but still drain individually into the azygos vein, or they may unite and drain via a single cross-connection. The levels of this connection or these connections may also vary. Finally, the superior hemiazygos vein may connect with the vessels draining the upper left intercostal spaces.

Nerves of the thorax

The nerves of the intercostal spaces have already been described. Several other nervous structures are seen in the thorax. We shall describe here only their anatomical appearance and general function; a discussion of the neuronal pathways involved will be found in Section 5.

Sympathetic trunks (Figs. 3.35 and 3.36)

These are found in the posterior mediastinum, one each side of the vertebral column, crossing the neck of the first rib, the heads of ribs 2–10, and the bodies of the 11th and 12th vertebrae. They then pass behind the medial lumbosacral arches of the diaphragm to the abdo-

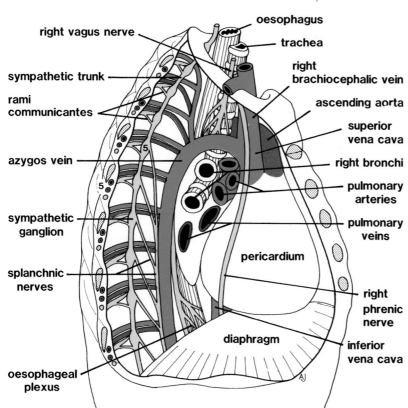

right vagus nerve
oesophagus
trachea
sympathetic trunk
right brachiocephalic vein
rami communicantes
ascending aorta
superior vena cava
azygos vein
right bronchi
pulmonary arteries
pulmonary veins
sympathetic ganglion
pericardium
splanchnic nerves
right phrenic nerve
diaphragm
inferior vena cava
oesophageal plexus

Fig. 3.35 Right side of the mediastinum. In the interests of clarity the posterior intercostal arteries to the upper two intercostal spaces (branches of the superior intercostal artery, itself a branch of the costocervical trunk) and the posterior intercostal vein to the first space (often a tributary of the brachiocephalic vein) are not shown. The first intercostal nerve, which is very small, is also not shown.

men. The thoracic trunk is beaded by 12 **ganglia,** one for each spinal nerve. Often the ganglion of the first nerve is incorporated with the inferior cervical ganglion to form the **stellate ganglion. White** and **grey rami communicantes** run posteriorly from each ganglion to join the corresponding spinal nerve. The first five thoracic ganglia send branches to the heart and great vessels, lungs, and oesophagus. The lower seven send branches which are grouped into three nerve trunks, the greater (T5–9), lesser (T10–11), and least (T12) splanchnic nerves, to the abdominal viscera. These lie medial to the trunks on the borders of the thoracic vertebrae as they pass towards the abdomen through the crura of the diaphragm.

Vagus nerves

The right and left nerves are best considered individually as they are somewhat asymmetrical. The right vagus (Fig. 3.35) crosses in front of the subclavian artery, gives off its recurrent laryngeal branch, and enters the thorax behind the brachiocephalic vein, then descends in contact with the trachea and passes behind the root of the lung where it sends branches to the pulmonary plexus. It then passes on to the posterior surface of the oesophagus and joins the oesophageal plexus.

The **left vagus** (Fig. 3.36) enters the thorax between left subclavian and common carotid arteries, crosses the left side of the aortic arch (where it is itself crossed by the phrenic nerve), runs behind the root of the left lung, where it contributes to the pulmonary plexus, and then joins the oesophageal plexus on the anterior surface of the oesophagus. As the nerve crosses the aortic arch it gives off the left recurrent laryngeal nerve which passes below the arch, behind the

ligamentum arteriosum, and then ascends on the side of the trachea.

Through the pulmonary and oesophageal plexuses the two vagi supply the lungs and oesophagus. The right vagus also gives off cardiac branches in the thorax (both vagi give cardiac branches in the cervical part of their course). From the oesophageal plexus posterior and anterior vagal trunks are formed, each containing fibres from both vagi. These trunks enter the abdomen through the oesophageal opening, with the relationship to the oesophagus indicated by their names, and supply the abdominal viscera.

Phrenic nerves

The phrenic nerves are derived from the ventral rami of C3–5 and supply the diaphragm, which originates embryologically in the neck region (see p. 43). The nerve on each side passes downwards on the anterior scalene muscle to the thoracic inlet which it enters between the subclavian artery and vein. From then on the relationships are asymmetrical on the two sides. The **right phrenic nerve** (Fig. 3.35) descends successively on the right side of the brachiocephalic vein, superior vena cava, and pericardium to reach the diaphragm which it traverses through the caval opening to supply the diaphragm on its lower surface. The left phrenic (Fig. 3.36) descends on the left side of the left subclavian artery, aortic arch (and left vagus nerve), and pericardium. It pierces the muscular part of the diaphragm in front of the central tendon. As well as supplying the muscle of the diaphragm, the phrenic nerves are sensory to the mediastinal and diaphragmatic pleura, to the fibrous and parietal layer of the serous pericardium and to the peritoneum on the inferior surfaces of the diaphragm.

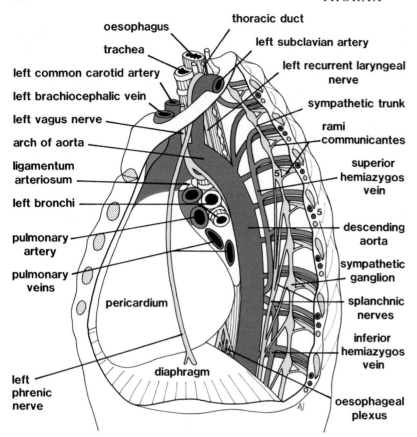

Fig. 3.36 Left side of the mediastinum. In the interests of clarity the posterior intercostal arteries to the upper two intercostal spaces (branches of the superior intercostal artery, itself a branch of the costocervical trunk) and the posterior intercostal vein to the first space (often a tributary of the brachiocephalic vein) are not shown. The first intercostal nerve, which is very small, is also not shown.

Great vessels

Large veins of the thorax (Fig. 3.37)

1. **Brachiocephalic veins** and **superior vena cava**. The right brachiocephalic vein is formed at the root of the neck by the union of the **right subclavian** and **right internal jugular veins** just above the first rib. The left brachiocephalic is formed similarly. The veins pass down behind the manubrium sterni and in front of the large branches of the aorta to unite as the superior vena cava, a little above the level of the sternal angle. The left brachiocephalic vein is longer and runs in a more horizontal direction than the right vein. The superior vena cava passes downwards to the right atrium, being joined posteriorly by the **azygos vein**.

2. **Inferior vena cava**. The inferior vena cava pierces the diaphragm at the level of T8 and almost immediately empties into the right atrium.

3. **Pulmonary veins**. These leave each lung and drain oxygenated blood into the left atrium.

Large arteries of the thorax (Fig. 3.37)

1. **Aorta.** The **thoracic aorta** is conveniently divided into ascending and descending parts, united by the arch of the aorta. The **ascending aorta** leaves the left ventricle and runs upwards and forwards to the level of the sternal angle. Its only branches are the left and right coronary arteries. The **arch of the aorta** lies behind the manubrium

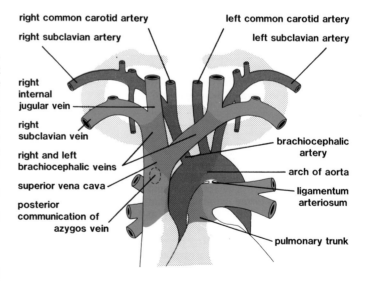

Fig. 3.37. Great vessels of the thorax.

sterni and runs upwards, backwards, and to the left in front of the trachea, then turns downwards and to the left behind the left main bronchus. The **brachiocephalic artery** leaves the ascending part of the aortic arch and runs upwards to the right of the trachea where it divides, behind the right sternoclavicular joint, into **right subclavian** and **right common carotid** arteries. On the left side the **common carotid** and **subclavian** arteries arise separately from the upper surface of the arch and run along the left side of the trachea to the neck, with the subclavian artery behind the common carotid. Each subclavian artery gives off vertebral, internal thoracic, thyrocervical, and costo-cervical branches.

The **descending aorta** runs downwards from the aortic arch to leave the thorax through the aortic opening behind the diaphragm. In the thorax, the descending aorta has many branches, grouped as follows:

Nine pairs of **posterior intercostal arteries** (to the lower nine spaces).

One pair of **subcostal arteries** which run below the twelfth ribs.

Paired **pericardial, oesophageal,** and **bronchial** arteries.

2. **Pulmonary trunk**. The pulmonary trunk leaves the right ventricle and runs upwards, backwards, and to the left. Close to the concavity of the arch of the aorta it divides into left and right pulmonary arteries. The right pulmonary artery runs behind the ascending aorta and superior vena cava to the root of the right lung. The left pulmonary artery runs in front of the descending aorta to the root of the left lung.

The bifurcation of the pulmonary trunk and concave side of the aortic arch are united by the fibrous **ligamentum arteriosum**. The left recurrent laryngeal nerve loops around the lower border of the arch of the aorta behind the ligamentum.

Clinical aspects

Portions of the walls of the great vessels may be weakened by a variety of causes, so that they partially give way under the pressure of the enclosed blood and balloon outwards as aneurisms. Aneurism of the arch of the aorta may compress the trachea, oesophagus, recurrent laryngeal nerve, or sympathetic chain. An aorta damaged by atheroma may develop a dissecting aneurism with blood coursing between the layers of the aortic wall, often blocking off branches as it does so. Aneurisms, being due to weakness of the vessel walls, tend to rupture, fatally.

5

Chest radiographs

X-rays have useful abilities (a) to pass through the tissues of the body to a variable extent and (b) to blacken photographic film. If a body, or part of a body, is placed between a source of X-rays and a flat photographic film in a light-tight box (**cassette**), the film (when suitably developed) will be dark where the X-rays have reached it and less dark where some part of the body has interrupted their progress. Thus dense structures (bone, heart, fluid) appear white and less dense structures (air in lungs) will appear black. Remember in viewing radiographs that they give a two-dimensional impression of three-dimensional structures.

The most useful views of the thorax are:

1. posterior/anterior (the source of X-rays is posterior, the cassette anterior);
2. lateral (left or right);
3. oblique.

The posterior/anterior (P/A) radiograph (Plate 1, Fig. 3.38)

The first check in viewing any P/A chest radiograph should be that the patient was correctly orientated. If the chest was properly positioned relative to the X-ray source and cassette, the sternal ends of the clavicles should be equidistant from the vertebral spines and the thoracic cage should appear symmetrical. Remember, of course, that the patient may have a deformed chest.

Superficial soft tissues

The nipples of both sexes may be superimposed on the lung fields, and the outline of the breasts may be seen in females.

Bony thorax

The thoracic vertebrae can be seen only imperfectly, as they are masked by the shadows of heart and diaphragm. The costotransverse joints should be examined as far down as possible and compared with their fellows on the opposite side. Ribs should always be counted to avoid missing a cervical or lumbar rib. Costal cartilages are usually not seen, but may be variably ossified (and thus visible) especially in older patients. The clavicles are clearly visible, as are the medial borders of the scapulae (the patient will have been asked to bring the shoulders as far forward as possible, thus moving

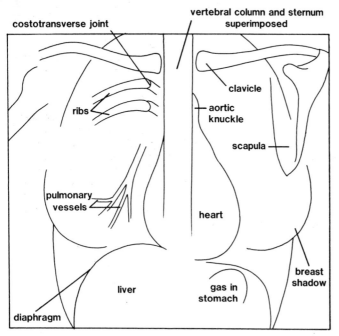

Fig. 3.38. Key to Plate 1.

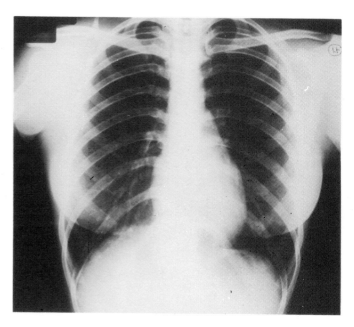

Plate 1. Posterior/anterior radiograph of thorax.

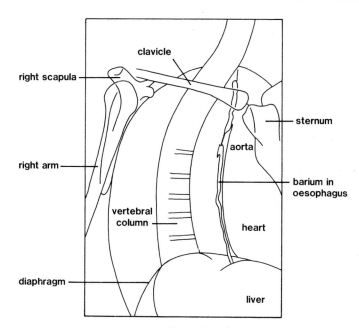

Fig. 3.39. Key to Plate 2.

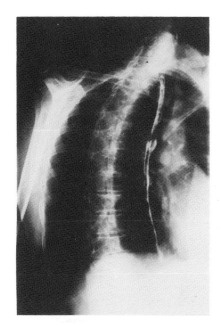

Plate 2. Lateral oblique radiograph of thorax. Oesophagus outlined by barium.

the scapulae as far laterally as possible to avoid obstructing the centre of the field).

Diaphragm

The domes of the diaphragm can be seen on each side. Under the right dome is the solid mass of the liver, under the left any gas bubbles present in the stomach may be seen. The plain P/A film may be taken on inspiration or expiration: the position of the diaphragm (and associated structures) will, of course, be different in each case.

Trachea

The air-filled trachea is seen in the midline as a dark area superimposed on the lower cervical and upper thoracic vertebrae.

Lungs

The roots of the lungs are clearly visible due to the presence of pulmonary vessels, lymphatics and lymph nodes, and the main bronchi. Smaller pulmonary blood vessels can be seen radiating from the dense lung root into the much darker lung fields. Seen end on, these vessels (and the smaller bronchi) form small white rings. Small bronchioles are not seen. A **bronchogram** can be produced by injecting a radio-opaque dye into the main bronchus.

Mediastinum

Note the shape of the outline of the heart and great vessels; a normal heart rarely occupies more than half the width of the thoracic cage. The width/length ratio of the heart will decrease on deep inspiration and in infants the heart is altogether more globular. Remember that some conditions may cause a shift of the mediastinum to right or left. The right border of the outline of the heart is formed by the right atrium and the left border by the left ventricle (Fig. 3.27). At the upper end of the left border is a bulge produced by the left pulmonary artery and left atrium. Above this, the mediastinal outline projects as the aortic knuckle produced by the arch of the aorta.

Oblique and lateral radiographs (Plate 2, Fig. 3.39)

These give a much clearer view of some structures, notably the heart, because the image of the spine is no longer superimposed. Lateral views are useful in visualizing the upper digestive tract, especially after a barium swallow. In this technique the patient is given a suitably flavoured paste of barium sulphate (the only insoluble, and hence non-poisonous, salt of barium) to swallow. Serial X-rays will reveal the course of barium to the stomach, the outline of the oesophagus and those structures (such as the posterior border of the left atrium) to which it is related.

Section 4

Head and neck

1

Skull

The skull encloses and protects the brain, forms the skeleton of the upper parts of the alimentary and respiratory systems, and provides protective capsules for the organs of sight, hearing, and smell. It is so intimately related to the teeth and soft tissues of the oral region that a detailed knowledge of its anatomical structure and of its growth and development is essential for the dental student. The following account is intended to be read in conjunction with personal examination of a dried skull.

The skull minus the lower jaw is called the **cranium** (strictly speaking the terms 'skull' and 'cranium' are not, therefore, synonymous but in practice they are frequently used as though they are). The cranium can be subdivided into the **braincase**, enclosing the brain, and the **upper facial skeleton**, forming the **orbits, nasal cavity,** and **upper jaw**. The upper facial skeleton and lower jaw together make up the **facial skeleton.**

The plate of bone forming the floor of the braincase is termed the **cranial base**. The under surface of its anterior part gives attachment to the upper facial skeleton. The roof and side walls of the braincase are called the **cranial vault**. A strong bar of bone, the **zygomatic arch**, runs on each side from the lower part of the lateral surface of the cranial vault to the side of the upper facial skeleton.

After the first year of postnatal life the lower jaw consists of a single bone, the **mandible**. The mandible articulates with the under surface of the middle part of the cranial base by the right and left **temporomandibular joints.**

The joints between the bones of the upper facial skeleton and of the vault of the braincase are fibrous in nature and are termed **sutures**. The joints in the central regions of the cranial base consist of hyaline cartilage and are termed **synchondroses**. After birth neither the sutures nor the synchondroses allow movement but both are important growth sites. At the time of birth the sutures of the vault are sufficiently flexible to allow some overriding of adjacent bones (called moulding) which allows the head, usually the first part to be born, to pass more readily through the birth passage. In many cases the sutures and synchondroses are named from the participating bones (e.g. the zygomaticomaxillary suture and sphenoccipital synchondrosis) but in some instances are named from their shape (e.g. lambdoid suture) or position (e.g. coronal suture).

For the practice of dentistry an understanding of the cranium as a whole, rather than of the individual bones, is required and this aspect is emphasized in the following account. The maxilla, however, is of such great practical importance that it is described in the disarticulated state. There are three other bones which you may find helpful to study in the disarticulated state because they occupy key positions in the cranium. These are the sphenoid, ethmoid, and temporal bones and they are described individually in the final section of this chapter. The mandible, being attached to the cranium at only the temporomandibular joints, is necessarily treated as a separate bone.

BRAINCASE

The division of the braincase into vault and cranial base has a developmental and evolutionary as well as a structural basis. As described in the embryology section, the vault is a derivative of the dermal shield of the primitive vertebrate skull. The cranial base, on the other hand, represents the ventral part of the braincase of the primitive skull in which the bones are preceded by a cartilaginous stage. As would be expected from this evolutionary history, the bones of the vault ossify in membrane, and the joints between them are fibrous, whereas the bones of the cranial base ossify in cartilage and are united by cartilaginous joints.

Vault

Bones and sutures

The vault of the braincase is made up of the **frontal**, paired **parietals**, the **squamous** part of the **occipital**, the **greater wings** of the **sphenoid**, and the **squamous** parts of the paired **temporal bones**. When sectioned these bones can be seen to have an inner and an outer lamina (**table**) of compact bone separated from each other by an internal layer of cancellous bone (the **diploë**). Within the spaces of this cancellous bone is red marrow which retains its blood-forming function until old age.

The forehead region is formed by the frontal bone which curves upwards and backwards from the **supraorbital margins** to meet the parietal bones at the **coronal suture**. On the external ectocranial surface of the frontal bone immediately above the medial part of each supraorbital margin is a smooth elevation called the **superciliary arch**. It forms the eyebrow ridge in the living subject. At the junction of the lateral two-thirds and medial one-third of the supraorbital margin is the supraorbital notch (sometimes a foramen).

In immature skulls a suture, termed **frontal** or **metopic**, is present in the median plane of the frontal bone dividing it into right and left halves and indicating its development from two ossification centres. In the majority of individuals the frontal suture fuses during early childhood but in a few it persists, in whole or in part, into adult life.

The supraorbital part of the frontal bone contains the two **frontal paranasal air sinuses**. These are described on page 120. Projecting posteriorly from the main part of the frontal bone are the horizontal **orbital parts** of the bone. They form the roofs of the orbits and are described on pages 111 and 115.

The right and left parietal bones make up the greater part of the vault. They articulate with each other in the median plane at the **sagittal suture**. Anteriorly they articulate with the frontal bone at the coronal suture and posteriorly with the squamous part of the occipital bone at the **lambdoid suture**. Laterally each parietal bone extends downwards to form part of the lateral wall of the vault. Inferior to the

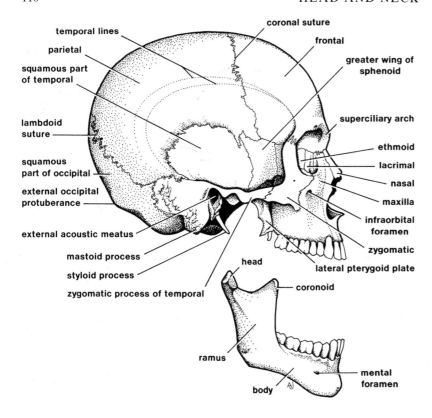

temporal lines

parietal

squamous part
of temporal

lambdoid
suture

squamous
part of occipital

external occipital
protuberance

external acoustic meatus

mastoid process

styloid process

zygomatic process of temporal

coronal suture

frontal

greater wing of
sphenoid

superciliary arch

ethmoid

lacrimal

nasal

maxilla

infraorbital
foramen

zygomatic

lateral pterygoid plate

head

coronoid

ramus

body

mental
foramen

Fig. 4.1. Lateral view of the skull.

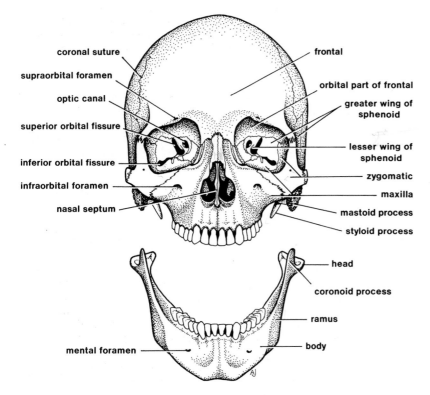

coronal suture

supraorbital foramen

optic canal

superior orbital fissure

inferior orbital fissure

infraorbital foramen

nasal septum

frontal

orbital part of frontal

greater wing of
sphenoid

lesser wing of
sphenoid

zygomatic

maxilla

mastoid process

styloid process

head

coronoid process

ramus

body

mental foramen

Fig. 4.2. Frontal view of the skull.

parietal bone the lateral wall of the vault is completed by the greater wing of the sphenoid and the squamous part of the temporal bone. The greater wing, squamous temporal, frontal and parietal bones meet in the temple region at the **pterion,** an irregular H-shaped arrangement of sutures (see Fig. 4.1). The pterion is crossed on its internal surface by the anterior branches of the middle meningeal artery and vein. The lateral wall of the vault ends inferiorly at a pronounced ridge, the **infratemporal crest,** on the greater wing of the sphenoid and squamous part of the temporal. From this ridge the bones turn medially to form the roof of the **infratemporal fossa** (p. 114).

Foramina

The bones of the vault are pierced by a number of small foramina which transmit emissary veins, connecting the intracranial dural venous sinuses with extracranial veins, and also, in some cases, small arterial branches to the meninges. The most constant are the **parietal foramen** (situated close to the sagittal suture on the posterior part of the parietal) and the **mastoid foramen** (located on the mastoid part of the temporal bone above the mastoid process).

Muscle markings

On the lateral aspect of the external surface of the vault are the **superior** and **inferior temporal lines.** These begin anteriorly as a single line which is continuous with the prominent ridge on the part of the frontal that articulates with the zygomatic bone. The two lines diverge as they pass posteriorly and then arch together, about 1 cm apart, across the frontal and parietal bones. Posteriorly the superior temporal line fades away but the inferior line becomes more prominent and curves downwards and forwards across the squamous part of the temporal to become continuous with the posterior root of the zygomatic arch. The area on the lateral wall of the vault bounded by the superior temporal line is called the **temporal fossa.** The roof of the fossa is formed by the temporal fascia which is attached superiorly to the superior temporal line and inferiorly to the upper border of the zygomatic arch. The temporal muscle takes

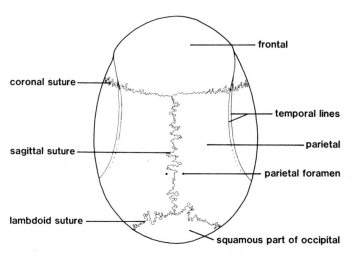

Fig. 4.3. Superior view of the skull.

coronal suture

sagittal suture

lambdoid suture

frontal

temporal lines

parietal

parietal foramen

squamous part of occipital

origin from the inferior temporal line and the area of bone which it encloses on the lateral wall of the cranial vault.

The occipital region of the vault has a number of ridges marking the attachment of the extensor (nuchal) musculature of the neck. In the midline is the **external occipital crest** which begins at the posterior margin of the foramen magnum and ascends on the squamous part of the occipital bone to end at a prominence termed the **external occipital protuberance.** On each side the **nuchal lines** curve laterally from the external occipital protuberance towards the mastoid process of the temporal bone. The **inferior nuchal line** runs laterally from the external occipital crest some distance below the superior line.

Internal features

In addition to the inner aspects of the bones, sutures, and foramina already described, the principal features to be seen on the internal, or endocranial, surface of the cranial vault are the markings produced by vascular structures.

Running in the median plane is the **sagittal sulcus,** a groove produced by the superior sagittal sinus (one of the dural venous sinuses draining blood from the brain and cerebrospinal fluid from the subarachnoid space). It begins on the inner surface of the frontal bone and runs posteriorly, widening progressively as it does so, to end close to the **internal occipital protuberance,** a prominence on the internal aspect of the occipital bone located opposite the external occipital protuberance. On each side of the sagittal sulcus are several irregular depressions. These mark the position of the arachnoid granulations through which cerebrospinal fluid drains into the venous blood in the superior sagittal sinus and associated venous lakes.

The inner surface of each parietal bone, lateral to the sagittal sulcus, is marked by a system of irregular but quite deeply cut grooves produced by the branches of the middle meningeal blood vessels. These are described further on page 113.

Cranial base

With the cranial vault removed it is possible to see the whole of the superior or endocranial surface of the cranial base. It is subdivided into three regions – the **anterior, middle,** and **posterior cranial fossae.** When the cranium is viewed from below the inferior surface of the anterior region is hidden by the attached upper facial skeleton.

Anterior cranial fossa

The anterior fossa forms the anterior third of the cranial base as seen in superior view. It houses the frontal lobes of the cerebral hemispheres.

The lateral regions of the floor of the fossa are made up of the **orbital parts of the frontal bone** and the **lesser wings of the sphenoid,** the under surfaces of which roof the orbital cavities. The posterior borders of the lesser wings provide the posterior boundary of the lateral parts of the fossa. Medially each lesser wing bears a prominent projection termed the **anterior clinoid process.**

The orbital parts of the frontal bone are separated from each other by a narrow gap occupied by the **cribriform plate of the ethmoid.** Behind the cribriform plate the central part of the fossa is completed by the part of the **body of the sphenoid** located between the lesser wings. Between the cribriform plate and the body of the sphenoid is the **sphenoethmoidal joint** which is initially cartilaginous but becomes

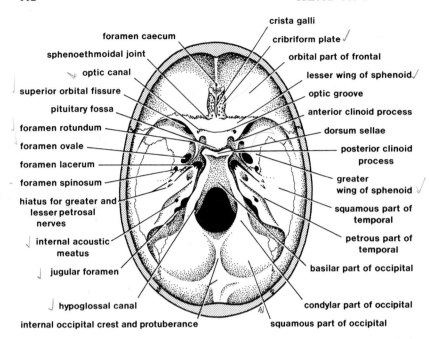

Fig. 4.4. Superior view of the cranial base.

fibrous soon after birth. The posterior boundary of the fossa in this region is provided by the anterior border of the **optic groove**.

The inferior surfaces of the cribriform plate and of the front part of the body of the sphenoid together form the roof of the nasal cavity. The cribriform plate is pierced by numerous fine foramina for the transmission of the olfactory nerves. Projecting upwards from its midline is the **crista galli**, a prominent crest of bone which gives attachment to the anterior edge of a fold of dura mater called the falx cerebri. Just in front of the crista galli is the **foramen caecum**, usually a blind-ended canal but occasionally transmitting an emissary vessel connecting the veins of the nose with the superior sagittal sinus. On each side of the crista galli is the narrow **nasal slit**.

Opening on the line of the suture between the cribriform plate and the orbital part of the frontal are the **anterior** and **posterior ethmoidal canals**. The former transmits the anterior ethmoidal nerve and vessels from the orbit to the anterior cranial fossa; the latter transmits the posterior ethmoidal vessels only. The anterior ethmoidal nerve and vessels pass from the anterior cranial fossa into the nasal cavity through the nasal slit.

Middle cranial fossa

The middle fossa is bounded in front by the posterior borders of the lesser wings of the sphenoid and the anterior margin of the optic groove and behind by the superior borders of the **petrous parts of the temporal bones** and, between these latter elements, by the **dorsum sellae**, a prominent projection on the endocranial surface of the body of the sphenoid. The central region of the fossa is short anteroposteriorly and is formed by the **body of the sphenoid**. The lateral regions are much more extensive and each is formed by the corresponding **greater wing of the sphenoid**, the anterior surface of the petrous temporal and the inferior part of the squamous temporal

bone. The fossa lodges the temporal lobes of the cerebral hemispheres and the pituitary gland.

The endocranial surface of the body of the sphenoid bears a deep depression, the **pituitary** (or **hypophysial) fossa**, which houses the pituitary gland (or hypophysis cerebri). In front of the pituitary fossa is the optic groove. Followed laterally this groove leads, on each side, to the **optic canal** situated between the roots of the lesser wing and transmitting the optic nerve and ophthalmic artery to the orbit. In the cranial cavity the fibres of the optic nerve undergo a partial decussation (crossing over) to form the optic chiasma. This lies just above the optic groove. Between the pituitary fossa and the optic groove is a rounded swelling, the **tuberculum sellae**. Posterior to the fossa is the dorsum sellae, the superolateral angles of which are produced to form the **posterior clinoid processes**. From its fancied resemblance to a Turkish saddle, this area of the sphenoid is termed the **sella turcica**.

The greater wings project laterally and superiorly from each side of the body of the sphenoid. As well as providing part of the floor of the middle cranial fossa they also form a small part of the lateral walls of the cranial vault. Between the greater and lesser wings is the **superior orbital fissure** through which the middle cranial fossa communicates with the orbit. It transmits the oculomotor, trochlear, and abducent nerves, the ophthalmic division of the trigeminal nerve and the superior and inferior ophthalmic veins.

The medial part of each greater wing is pierced by three foramina. The most anterior is the **foramen rotundum**. This runs directly forwards into the pterygopalatine fossa and transmits the maxillary division of the trigeminal nerve, the nerve supply to the upper jaw and teeth. Some distance posterior to foramen rotundum is the **foramen ovale** which opens downwards into the infratemporal fossa. Through it passes the mandibular division of the trigeminal nerve, supplying the lower jaw and teeth, as well as the lesser petrosal

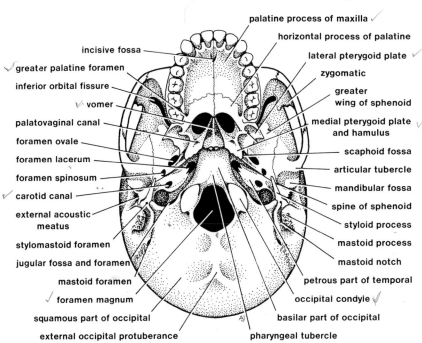

palatine process of maxilla
horizontal process of palatine
incisive fossa
lateral pterygoid plate
greater palatine foramen
zygomatic
inferior orbital fissure
greater wing of sphenoid
vomer
palatovaginal canal
medial pterygoid plate and hamulus
foramen ovale
scaphoid fossa
foramen lacerum
articular tubercle
foramen spinosum
mandibular fossa
carotid canal
spine of sphenoid
external acoustic meatus
styloid process
stylomastoid foramen
mastoid process
jugular fossa and foramen
mastoid notch
mastoid foramen
petrous part of temporal
foramen magnum
occipital condyle
squamous part of occipital
basilar part of occipital
external occipital protuberance
pharyngeal tubercle

Fig. 4.5. Inferior view of the cranial base.

nerve (which may have its own, separate foramen) and accessory meningeal artery. Immediately postero-lateral to foramen ovale is the **foramen spinosum** which transmits the middle meningeal vessels, the main arterial and venous channels to the meninges, and the nervus spinosus, a meningeal branch of the mandibular division of the trigeminal nerve. Occasionally other foramina may be present for small emissary veins.

The middle meningeal vessels, after entering the cranial cavity through the foramen spinosum, run laterally for a short distance and then divide into anterior and posterior branches. The anterior branch runs upwards across the cerebral surface of the pterion. The posterior branch runs upwards and backwards onto the posterior part of the parietal bone. The course of these vessels is marked by grooves on the bones.

Medial to the foramen ovale is a large opening with jagged edges. This is the **foramen lacerum.** It is bounded by the apex of the petrous part of the temporal bone and the body and greater wing of the sphenoid. Opening into its posterior wall is the **carotid canal,** a large sinuous channel traversing the petrous bone and transmitting the internal carotid artery. From its anterior wall the **pterygoid canal** runs forwards to open into the pterygopalatine fossa. It transmits the nerve of the pterygoid canal. At a level below these two openings the foramen lacerum is closed by a plug of cartilage pierced by only one or two small emissary veins.

Immediately behind the foramen lacerum the anterior surface of the petrous bone is marked by a shallow concavity, the **trigeminal impression,** which lodges the trigeminal ganglion contained within a recess of the dura mater called the trigeminal cave.

Lateral to the trigeminal impression the anterior surface of petrous bone bears a narrow groove which runs from a small hiatus in the bone forwards and medially towards the foramen lacerum. The **hiatus and groove** transmit the **greater petrosal nerve,** a branch of the facial nerve given off within the petrous bone. This nerve crosses the foramen lacerum, where it is joined by the deep petrosal nerve containing sympathetic fibres from the nerve plexus on the internal carotid artery, and then passes through the pterygoid canal (where it is called the nerve of the pterygoid canal) to reach the pterygopalatine fossa. A second **hiatus** and **groove** for the **lesser petrosal nerve,** can usually be identified anterolateral to those for the greater petrosal nerve. The lesser petrosal, a branch of the tympanic plexus which is located on the wall of the middle-ear cavity within the petrous bone, runs towards the foramen ovale through which, in most cases, it passes to the exterior of the skull.

The inferior surface of the cranial base in the region of the middle cranial fossa is very irregular. Projecting downwards on either side, from the junction of the body and greater wing of the sphenoid, are the **pterygoid processes.** Each consists of a large **lateral** and a smaller **medial pterygoid plate** which diverge posteriorly to enclose the **pterygoid fossa.** The inferior one-third of the anterior border of the pterygoid process articulates with the posterior border of the perpendicular plate of the palatine bone. The upper two-thirds of the anterior border are free and here a narrow gap, the **pterygomaxillary fissure,** leads medially into the pterygopalatine fossa (Fig. 4.13).

The lateral surface of the lateral pterygoid plate provides the origin for the lower head of the lateral pterygoid muscle and its medial surface the origin for the main part of the medial pterygoid muscle.

The posterior border of the medial pterygoid plate is related above to the auditory tube while below it gives attachment to the superior constrictor muscle (part of the wall of the pharynx). At its upper extremity the posterior border divides to enclose the shallow

scaphoid fossa which gives origin to the anterior fibres of the tensor veli palatini muscle, the tensor of the soft palate. The lower end of the posterior border projects as the hook-like **hamulus**. This process gives attachment to the pterygomandibular raphe and to fibres of the superior constrictor muscle. The tendon of the tensor veli palatini muscle curves around its lower surface. Projecting medially from the upper part of the medial pterygoid plate is the **vaginal process**, a thin lamina of bone which covers the lateral part of the inferior surface of the body of the sphenoid.

Between the medial pterygoid plates of the right and left sides is the posterior nasal aperture divided into two by the median **vomer** bone. The nasopharynx is located immediately behind the posterior nasal aperture. The body of the sphenoid bone, which occupies the central region of this part of the cranial base, forms the roof of the nasopharynx and of the posterior part of the nasal cavity. Its inferior surface is largely obscured in inferior view by the **alae of the vomer** and the vaginal processes of the medial pterygoid plates.

The inferior surface of the vaginal process is traversed by a shallow anteroposterior groove which is converted anteriorly into the **palato-vaginal canal**. The canal opens into the pterygopalatine fossa and transmits the pharyngeal branch of the pterygopalatine ganglion.

The **infratemporal fossa** lies lateral to the pterygoid process. It contains many soft structures of interest to the dental student including the pterygoid musculature, the mandibular division of the trigeminal nerve, the maxillary artery and the pterygoid plexus of veins. It is bounded in front by the posterior surface of the maxilla, above by the inferior surface of the greater wing of sphenoid, medially by the lateral pterygoid plate and laterally by the ramus of the mandible. The fossa has no bony floor or posterior wall although, with the soft parts present, its posterior boundary is usually taken to be the styloid apparatus and carotid sheath. It communicates with the temporal fossa through the gap between the zygomatic arch and the side wall of the braincase.

Opening into the infratemporal fossa are the foramen ovale, foramen spinosum, pterygomaxillary fissure, and inferior orbital fissure (note that the foramen rotundum cannot be seen in the roof of the infratemporal fossa – it runs forwards to open into the ptery-gopalatine fossa). The first three of these openings have already been described. The **inferior orbital fissure** is located between the upper margin of the posterior wall of the maxilla and the greater wing of the sphenoid. It connects the orbit with the infratemporal fossa laterally and with the pterygopalatine fossa medially. It transmits the maxillary nerve (which becomes the infraorbital nerve once it has entered the orbit), zygomatic nerve, infraorbital vessels, and frequently connecting channels between the inferior ophthalmic vein and the pterygoid plexus of veins.

Just posterior to foramen spinosum the inferior surface of the greater wing of the sphenoid bears an irregular downward projection, the **spine of the sphenoid**. This gives attachment to the spheno-mandibular ligament.

The posterior border of the greater wing of the sphenoid articulates with the anterior surface of the petrous part of the temporal bone. The articulation runs medially, with a slight anterior inclination, from the spine of the sphenoid to the foramen lacerum. Following the course of the articulation on the inferior surface of the cranial base is a groove which begins laterally at an opening in the petrous bone (this opening can be found between the foramen spinosum and the inferior opening of the carotid canal, in the angle between the petrous and squamous parts of the temporal bone – see the description of the disarticulated temporal bone, pages 127–9). The cartilaginous part of the **auditory tube** occupies this groove. It is continuous laterally with the bony part of the tube, which is located within the petrous bone and communicates with the tympanic cavity. The function of the auditory tube is to equalize air pressure between the tympanic cavity and the exterior (i.e. on both sides of the eardrum). The auditory tube is also known as the Eustachian or pharyngotympanic tube.

The inferior surface of the petrous bone is very irregular. Its apex is separated from the body of the sphenoid by the foramen lacerum. Some distance posterolateral to this foramen is the circular lower opening of the carotid canal. Behind this opening is a deep depression termed the **jugular fossa**. On the ridge separating the carotid canal from the jugular fossa is the small opening of the **canaliculus for the tympanic nerve** (Fig. 4.23).

The inferior surface of the cranial base in this region is completed laterally by the squamous and tympanic parts of the temporal bone. As already described, the major part of the squamous bone is situated in the lateral wall of the cranial vault. Inferiorly, however, the squamous turns medially to contribute to the cranial base posterior to the lateral part of the greater wing of the sphenoid. Here its inferior surface bears the superior articular facet of the temporo-mandibular joint (Fig. 4.23). The anterior part of this articular surface is provided by the **articular tubercle**, a transverse eminence which is also known as the anterior root of the zygomatic process of the squamous bone. The anterior limit of the articular surface is marked on the dried skull by a faint curved line running transversely across the anterior part of the articular tubercle. Behind the tubercle is a concavity, the **mandibular fossa**. The anterior part of this fossa forms the remainder of the articular surface. The posterior wall of the fossa is provided by the tympanic part of the temporal bone and is non-articular. The posterior boundary of the articular surface is formed by the **squamotympanic fissure** which lies in the depth of the mandibular fossa separating the squamous and tympanic parts of the temporal bone. The lateral part of the posterior edge of the articular surface projects downwards to form the **postglenoid tubercle**.

The **tympanic part of the temporal bone** is a curved plate of bone which as well as providing the posterior wall of the mandibular fossa forms the anterior and inferior boundaries of the **external acoustic meatus**. It partly ensheaths the **styloid process**, a downwardly projecting bony process which is usually broken or missing altogether in the dried skull. The styloid process gives attachment to the stylohyoid and stylomandibular ligaments and the styloid musculature.

A small lip of bone can usually be seen projecting downwards through the medial part of the squamotympanic fissure (Fig. 4.23). This is the anterior edge of the **tegmen tympani**, part of the petrous bone. Between this lip of bone and the tympanic plate is the opening of the **canaliculus for the chorda tympani**, the latter an important branch of the facial nerve.

Posterior cranial fossa

This is the largest and deepest of the three cranial fossae. It houses the cerebellum and brainstem. Its central zone, the **clivus**, is formed by the **body of the sphenoid**, posterior to the dorsum sellae, and the **basilar part of the occipital bone**. In the immature skull these elements are separated by the **sphenoccipital synchondrosis**. This cartilaginous joint begins to fuse in the early teens and has completely disappeared in the adult skull. The lateral parts of the fossa are formed by the posterior surfaces of the petrous bones and the **condylar** and **squamous parts of the occipital bone.** The floor of the fossa is pierced in the midline by the **foramen magnum.** This is traversed by the medulla oblongata (plus meninges), spinal roots of the accessory nerves, vertebral arteries, and a number of other structures (see Chapter 4.2).

Between the petrous temporal bone and the basilar and condylar parts of the occipital bone is the **petro-occipital fissure.** The anteromedial part of the fissure is closed in life by cartilage. The posterolateral end of the fissure is widened to form the **jugular foramen** which transmits the glossopharyngeal, vagus, and accessory nerves and the sigmoid and inferior petrosal venous sinuses. The surface of the petrous temporal bone forming the anterolateral wall of the foramen is hollowed out into a deep depression, the **jugular fossa.** Lateral to the jugular foramen the petrous and the condylar part of occipital meet at a fibrous joint, the **petro-occipital suture.**

Opening on to the posterior surface of the petrous bone, some distance above the jugular foramen, is the **internal acoustic meatus.** It transmits the vestibulocochlear nerve and the motor and sensory roots of the facial nerve.

Just posterior to the junction of its basilar and condylar parts (i.e. some distance medial to the jugular foramen), the occipital bone is pierced by the **hypoglossal canal.** The internal opening of this canal is situated in the anterolateral wall of the foramen magnum. The canal opens on the inferior surface of the skull lateral to the occipital condyle and transmits the hypoglossal nerve and a meningeal branch of the ascending pharyngeal artery.

Behind the foramen magnum the squamous part of the occipital bears a median ridge, the **internal occipital crest,** which gives attachment to a fold of dura mater called the falx cerebelli. It ends above at the **internal occipital protuberance.** A shallow groove, marking the course of the transverse venous sinus, curves away from the protuberance on each side. Laterally the groove turns to run first downwards and medially and then turns forwards to reach the jugular foramen. This part of the groove is occupied by the sigmoid sinus, a continuation of the transverse sinus.

The most obvious feature on the inferior surface of the posterior part of the cranial base is the **foramen magnum.** On either side of the foramen are the downwardly projecting **occipital condyles.** These provide the surfaces by which the skull articulates with the first cervical vertebra (the **atlas**) at the synovial **atlanto-occipital joints.** As already noted the hypoglossal canal opens lateral to the condyle. Further laterally still are the inferior opening of the jugular foramen and the jugular fossa. Posterolateral to the jugular foramen is the prominent **mastoid process of the temporal bone** which gives insertion to the sternocleidomastoid muscle. Immediately medial to the mastoid process is a deep cleft, the **mastoid notch,** from which the posterior belly of the digastric muscle takes origin. Between the mastoid and styloid process is the **stylomastoid foramen** through which the facial nerve leaves the skull. A short distance anterior to the foramen magnum is a small median elevation, the **pharyngeal tubercle.** It gives attachment to the uppermost fibres of the superior constrictor muscle.

FACIAL SKELETON

Upper facial skeleton

The upper facial skeleton comprises the upper jaw and the bony framework around the nasal and orbital cavities. Apart from the ethmoid bone and inferior conchae, which ossify in the cartilage of the nasal capsule, the facial bones are derivatives of the dermal shield and palate of primitive vertebrates and ossify, as would be expected, in membrane. The joints between the dermal bones are fibrous.

Orbit

The orbital cavities are pyramidal recesses containing the eyeballs, together with their associated muscles, vessels, and nerves, the lacrimal apparatus and nerves and vessels passing through to reach the face. Each has a base (the orbital opening), an apex, a roof and floor, and medial and lateral walls. The long axis of the orbit is directed forwards and laterally.

The greater part of the roof of the orbit is formed by the inferior surface of the **orbital part of the frontal bone.** Posteriorly, close to the apex, a small part of the roof is provided by the inferior surface of the **lesser wing of the sphenoid.** The lateral wall is formed by the **orbital surfaces of the zygomatic bone and greater wing of the**

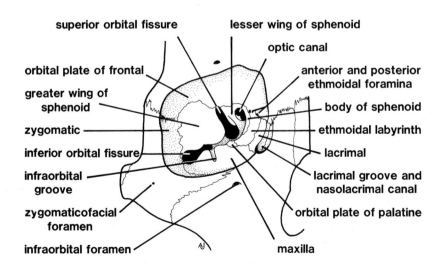

superior orbital fissure

lesser wing of sphenoid

optic canal

orbital plate of frontal

anterior and posterior ethmoidal foramina

greater wing of sphenoid

body of sphenoid

zygomatic

ethmoidal labyrinth

inferior orbital fissure

lacrimal

infraorbital groove

lacrimal groove and nasolacrimal canal

zygomaticofacial foramen

orbital plate of palatine

infraorbital foramen

maxilla

Fig. 4.6. Frontal view of the orbit.

sphenoid. The lateral wall separates the orbital cavity from the temporal fossa anteriorly and from the middle cranial fossa posteriorly. The floor of the orbit is occupied by the thin plate of bone forming the upper surface of the **body of the maxilla.** Over most of its extent this plate of bone also provides the roof of the maxillary paranasal air sinus, which occupies the maxillary body. At the posteromedial corner of the orbital floor is a small triangular area formed by the **orbital plate of the palatine bone.** The medial orbital wall is very thin and is frequently damaged in the dried skull. The bones forming the medial wall are, from before backwards, the **frontal process of the maxilla, the lacrimal, the orbital plate of the ethmoidal labyrinth,** and the **body of the sphenoid.**

The lateral wall and roof are separated posteriorly by the **superior orbital fissure,** lying between the greater and lesser wings of the sphenoid. It transmits the nerves to the muscles moving the eyeballs, the ophthalmic division of the trigeminal nerve and ophthalmic veins. The lateral wall and floor are similarly separated by the **inferior orbital fissure,** in this case bordered by the maxilla and greater wing of sphenoid. In its posteromedial part the inferior fissure communicates with the pterygopalatine fossa while its anterolateral part communicates with the infratemporal fossa. Leading forwards across the floor of the orbit from the medial part of the inferior orbital fissure is the **infraorbital groove.** This traverses the orbital floor and becomes roofed over anteriorly to form a canal which opens on the front of the maxilla at the **infraorbital foramen.** Groove, canal, and foramen transmit the infraorbital nerve, the continuation of the maxillary nerve, which enters the orbit through the inferior orbital fissure. Immediately above the medial end of the superior orbital fissure is the **optic canal** lying between the roots of the lesser wing of the sphenoid. The optic nerve and ophthalmic artery pass into the orbit from the cranial cavity through this canal.

Anteriorly the medial orbital wall bears the **lacrimal groove** which houses the lacrimal sac. The groove is bounded in front by the anterior lacrimal crest on the frontal process of the maxilla and behind by the posterior lacrimal crest on the lacrimal bone. The suture between the maxilla and the lacrimal can be seen in the floor of the groove. Leading downwards from the groove is the **nasolacrimal canal** which traverses the maxilla to open into the inferior meatus of the nasal cavity. The canal transmits the nasolacrimal duct through which tears are drained from the lacrimal sac to the nose. The suture between the upper border of the orbital plate of the ethmoid and the orbital part of the frontal is interrupted by the **anterior** and **posterior ethmoidal foramina.**

The orbital surface of the zygomatic bone, in the lateral wall of the orbit, is pierced by two foramina. These lead into canals which open at the **zygomaticofacial foramen** on the lateral surface of the bone and the **zygomaticotemporal foramen** on the surface of the bone facing into the temporal fossa.

Nasal cavity

This is an irregularly shaped cavity lying between the bony palate below and the floor of the anterior cranial fossa above. Superiorly it is situated between the orbits; inferiorly its lateral boundaries are formed principally by the maxillae. The cavity is high and deep but compressed from side to side. It is divided into right and left halves by the **nasal septum.** The bony part of the septum does not reach as far as the **anterior nasal aperture** which is therefore undivided in the dried skull. In life the septum is completed anteriorly by cartilage.

The **posterior nasal aperture** on the other hand is divided into two by the back edge of the bony septum. In order to see the internal structure of the nasal cavity you will need to examine a skull sectioned in the median plane.

The roof of the nasal cavity is formed by the **nasal bones** anteriorly, by the **cribriform plate of the ethmoid** in its intermediate part and by the **body of the sphenoid** posteriorly. Its floor is provided by the **bony palate** (made up of the **palatine processes of the maxillae** in front and **horizontal plates of the palatine bones** behind) which separates the nasal and oral cavities. Each maxillary palatine process is pierced anteriorly, close to the septum, by an **incisive canal** which transmits the nasopalatine nerve and the terminal branch of the greater palatine artery. The canals of the two sides open inferiorly into the **incisive fossa,** a funnel-shaped depression on the oral surface of the palate.

The lateral wall is very irregular. Its main structural elements are the **maxilla** and the **labyrinth of the ethmoid** (a knowledge of the disarticulated maxilla and ethmoid is helpful in understanding the details of the lateral nasal wall: see pages 117–18 and 126–7) but the **nasal, lacrimal,** and **palatine bones** and the **inferior nasal concha** also contribute to its formation (see Figs 4.7 and 4.8). In general terms the maxilla forms the anterior and inferior parts, the palatine the posterior part and the ethmoidal labyrinth the superior part of the lateral wall. The nasal and lacrimal bones provide small contributions to the anterosuperior part of the lateral wall. The inferior concha projects into the nasal cavity, from its articulation with the maxilla and palatine, as a scroll-like plate of bone.

The nasal surface of the maxilla, in the disarticulated state (Fig. 4.10), can be seen to comprise a smoothly curved area anteroinferiorly, the prominent **frontal process** anterosuperiorly and a roughed area pierced by a large opening, the **maxillary hiatus,** into the maxillary sinus posteriorly. Immediately behind the frontal process is the deep **nasolacrimal groove.** In the articulated skull much of the posterior and superior parts of the nasal surface of the maxilla are involved in articulations with the perpendicular plate of the palatine, ethmoidal labyrinth, inferior concha, and lacrimal which reduce the maxillary hiatus to a number (sometimes only one) of small openings located on the lateral wall of the nasal cavity above the inferior concha.

The lacrimal bone is small and quadrilateral. Its orbital surface, as already described, forms a small part of the medial wall of the orbit in the region of the lacrimal groove while its nasal surface forms the lateral wall of the nasal cavity between the frontal process of the maxilla and the ethmoidal labyrinth. An inferior prolongation descends medial to the nasolacrimal groove, articulating with the edges of the groove to convert it into the nasolacrimal canal. Below the lacrimal bone the inferior concha articulates with the edges of the groove to complete the canal. It will be apparent from the arrangement of these articulations that the nasolacrimal canal begins at the lacrimal groove in the medial wall of the orbit and opens into the lateral wall of the nose below the inferior concha.

Posterior to the lacrimal bone the superior part of the lateral nasal wall is provided by the **medial plate of the ethmoidal labyrinth.** Projecting into the nasal cavity from the medial plate are two curved laminae, the **superior** and **middle nasal conchae.** Below the middle concha the labyrinth bears a rounded swelling termed the **ethmoidal bulla.** Contained within the labyrinth, between its medial and orbital plates, are the **ethmoidal air cells** which open into the nasal cavity above and below the middle concha. As already noted the orbital plate of the labyrinth forms an extensive area of the medial orbital

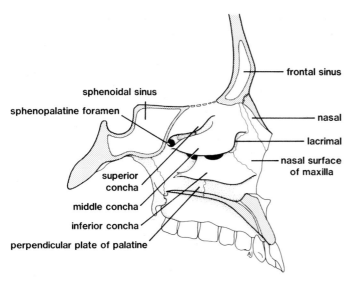

Fig. 4.7. The lateral wall of the nasal cavity.

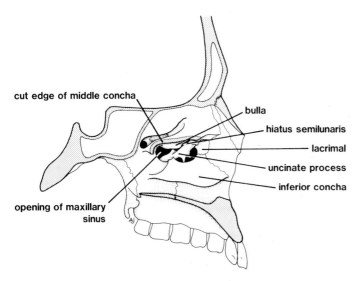

Fig. 4.8. As in Fig. 4.7 except that the middle concha has been resected to show the structures of the middle meatus.

(representing the reduced maxillary hiatus) is situated in the posterior part of the hiatus semilunaris. Frequently additional openings can be seen in the dried skull both above and below the uncinate process though these may be closed by mucous membrane in the living subject. The **frontal sinus** opens through the **frontonasal canal** into the anterior part of the hiatus semilunaris usually via the **ethmoidal infundibulum**, although in some skulls the canal opens directly into the anterosuperior part of the middle meatus (see p. 127).

The palatine bone consists of **horizontal** and **perpendicular plates** (or processes) arranged, as seen in frontal view, at right angles to each other in the manner of the letter L. The horizontal plate projects medially to contribute to the posterior part of the palate. The perpendicular plate articulates with the roughened posterior area of the medial surface of the maxilla to form the posterior third or so of the lateral nasal wall and, in so doing, covers over the posterior part of the maxillary hiatus. The superior part of the perpendicular plate projects above the maxilla to articulate with the body of the sphenoid which forms the roof of the nasal cavity in this region. Here the perpendicular plate intervenes between the nasal cavity and the pterygopalatine fossa and is pierced by the **sphenopalatine foramen**, through which nasal branches of the pterygopalatine ganglion and maxillary artery pass from the pterygopalatine fossa into the nose.

The inferior nasal concha, a separate bone, is a curved plate which projects into the nasal cavity below the middle concha. Its superior border articulates along a curved line with the bones forming the lateral nasal wall. It provides the medial wall of the lower part of the nasolacrimal canal and covers over the inferior part of the maxillary hiatus.

The conchae incompletely divide the nasal cavity into three passages, or **meatus** – the **superior meatus** between the superior and middle conchae, the **middle meatus** between the middle and inferior conchae, and the **inferior meatus** between the inferior concha and the palate. Each meatus is in open communication anteriorly, posteriorly, and medially with the remainder of the nasal cavity. The area of the lateral wall above the superior concha is termed the **sphenoethmoidal recess**.

The structures opening into the lateral wall of the nose are: (i) the **sphenoidal air sinus** into the sphenoethmoidal recess; (ii) the **posterior ethmoidal air cells** into the superior meatus; (iii) the **frontal** and **maxillary sinuses**, and the **anterior** and **middle ethmoidal air cells** into the middle meatus; and (iv) the **nasolacrimal canal** into the inferior meatus. Immediately posterior to the superior meatus is the sphenopalatine foramen, bounded by the perpendicular plate of the palatine bone and the body of the sphenoid. In life it is closed by mucous membrane.

The bony nasal septum extends from the roof of the nasal cavity to its floor. It is a thin sheet of bone formed by the **vomer** and the **perpendicular plate of the ethmoid**. It frequently deviates considerably from the median plane.

The upper jaw and bony palate

The upper jaw is made up of the two maxillae. Each consists of a **body** and four **processes.** The body is large and roughly pyramidal in shape. Its interior is hollowed out by the **maxillary paranasal air sinus** (detailed on page 120). The upper (orbital) surface of the body occupies the floor of the orbit, the anterior surface forms the curved external surface of the upper jaw, the posterior (infratemporal) surface provides the anterior wall of the infratemporal fossa and the

wall. Inferiorly it articulates with the superior part of the nasal surface of the maxilla. From the anterior part of its inferior border a long and irregularly shaped bar of bone, the **uncinate process,** curves downwards and backwards across the anterior part of the maxillary hiatus to articulate with the inferior concha (Fig. 4.8).

Between the uncinate process and the ethmoidal bulla is a curved gap, the **hiatus semilunaris.** The opening of the maxillary sinus

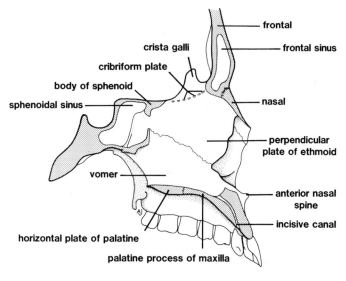

Fig. 4.9. The nasal septum.

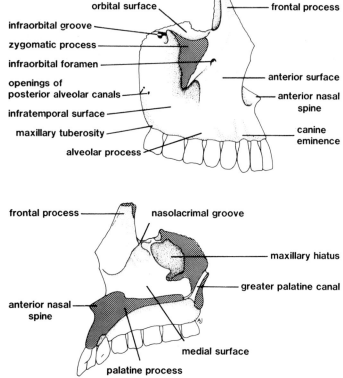

Fig. 4.10. The right maxilla in lateral (above) and medial (below) view.

medial (nasal) surface, as already described, is a major structural component in the wall of the nasal cavity.

Above the incisor teeth the anterior surface has a shallow depression termed the **incisive fossa** (not to be confused with the incisive fossa seen on the oral surface of the bony palate; see below). Further laterally is the deeper **canine fossa** which is separated from the incisive fossa by the **canine eminence** produced by the root of the canine tooth. Above the canine fossa is the **infraorbital foramen.** The anterior surface ends medially at the anterior nasal aperture. At the inferior margin of this aperture the maxillae of the two sides form a median projection, the **anterior nasal spine.**

Above the molar teeth the anterior surface is continuous with the boldly convex infratemporal surface which faces posterolaterally. The lateral part of the infratemporal surface provides the anterior wall of the infratemporal fossa. The surface ends below at a prominent rounded eminence, the **maxillary tuberosity,** located behind the last molar tooth. More medially the lower part of the infratemporal surface articulates with the pyramidal process of the palatine bone (the pyramidal process projects posterolaterally from the junction of the perpendicular and horizontal plates of the palatine to intervene between the maxilla and pterygoid process) while the upper part forms the anterior wall of the pterygopalatine fossa. Some distance above the tuberosity on the posterior maxillary surface can be seen the openings of a number of **posterior alveolar canals,** through which the posterior alveolar neurovascular bundles reach the upper molar teeth and associated structures. Running across the orbital surface of the maxilla is the infraorbital groove and canal. Opening from the canal is the **sinuous canal** which, though small, is important because it transmits the branch of the infraorbital nerve to the anterior teeth. It leaves the lateral side of the infraorbital canal, runs downwards and forwards for a short distance and then curves medially close to the anterior wall of the maxillary sinus to reach the margin of the anterior nasal aperture. It then continues downwards, following the lower margin of the aperture, to reach the incisor and canine teeth.

The nasal surface of the maxilla has been described in the section on the lateral wall of the nose.

The four maxillary processes are: (i) the **zygomatic process** which projects laterally from the body, at the junction of its anterior and infratemporal surfaces, to form the anterior part of the zygomatic arch; (ii) the **frontal process** which projects upwards to articulate with the frontal bone and enters into the medial wall of the orbit and lateral wall of the nose as well as forming the bridge of the nose behind the nasal bone; (iii) the **palatine process** which projects medially to articulate with its fellow of the opposite side – the two processes together forming the anterior three-quarters of the bony palate; (iv) the **alveolar process** which projects downwards and contains the sockets (alveoli) for the roots of the upper teeth. The alveolar process ends posteriorly at the tuberosity.

The **bony palate** (the term **hard palate** is used to describe the bony palate plus its covering of mucous membrane; the bony palate thus forms the skeleton of the hard palate) provides the floor of the nasal cavity and the roof of the mouth. Its anterior three-quarters are formed by the **palatine processes of the maxillae** and its posterior one-quarter by the **horizontal plates of the palatine bones.** Two sutures cross the palate – the **median suture** between the elements of the right and left sides and the **transverse suture** between the palatine processes of the maxillae and the horizontal plates of the palatines. On the oral surface, the **incisive fossa** can be seen in the midline, a short distance behind the central incisors. It receives the lower

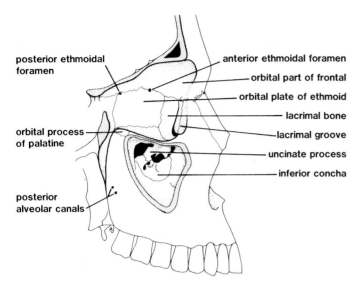

Fig. 4.11. The upper jaw and orbit in lateral view. The lateral wall of the orbit and part of the maxilla have been removed.

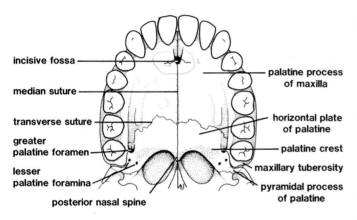

Fig. 4.12. Inferior view of the bony palate.

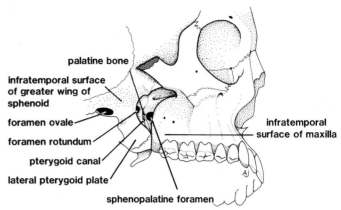

Fig. 4.13. The right pterygopalatine fossa seen through the pterygomaxillary fissure. The skull is tilted so that the fossa is viewed somewhat from below. The width of the pterygomaxillary fissure is exaggerated so that the openings of the pterygoid canal and foramen rotundum can be seen. The opening of the palatovaginal canal is hidden from view but lies just medial to that of the pterygoid canal.

The zygomatic arch

The arch is formed by the **zygomatic process of the maxilla, the zygomatic bone,** and the **zygomatic process of the squamous part of the temporal,** in that order from anterior to posterior. The temporal fascia is attached to its sharp upper border. The masseter muscle arises from its inferior border and medial surface.

The pterygopalatine fossa

Between the upper parts of the infratemporal surface of the maxilla and the anterior border of the pterygoid process is a narrow triangular gap, the **pterygomaxillary fissure.** This leads medially from the infratemporal fossa into the **pterygopalatine fossa,** a small pyramidal space located just below the apex of the orbit. It is bounded in front by the infratemporal surface of the maxilla, behind by the root of the **pterygoid process** and adjacent part of the **greater wing of the sphenoid,** and medially by the upper part of the perpendicular plate of the palatine. Below the fossa is closed by the articulation of the pterygoid process with the perpendicular plate of the palatine bone. Laterally is the pterygomaxillary fissure. The fossa opens above through the posteromedial end of the inferior orbital fissure into the orbit.

Three canals open on the posterior wall of the fossa – the **foramen rotundum, pterygoid canal,** and **palatovaginal canal** (Fig. 4.13). The foramen rotundum runs forwards from the middle cranial fossa, the pterygoid canal leads from the anterior border of the foramen lacerum and the palatovaginal canal traverses the undersurface of the vaginal process of the medial pterygoid plate, between it and the palatine bone. The medial wall of the fossa is pierced by the **sphenopalatine foramen,** located between the body of the sphenoid and the perpendicular plate of the palatine. It provides a communication between the pterygopalatine fossa and the nasal cavity. Inferiorly, at the junction of the anterior and posterior walls of the pterygopalatine fossa is the opening of the **greater palatine canal.** This runs downwards, in the articulation between the nasal surface of the maxilla and the lateral surface of the perpendicular plate of the palatine, to

openings of the two incisive canals which communicate above with the corresponding halves of the nasal cavity. Medial to the last molar tooth on each side are the **greater** and **lesser palatine foramina.** These are the inferior openings of the greater palatine canal which runs down from the pterygopalatine fossa. They transmit nerves and vessels of the same name. Leading forwards from the greater palatine foramen is a groove of variable distinctness which lodges the greater palatine neurovascular bundle in its course in the palate. The posterior border of the palate has a median projection, termed the **posterior nasal spine.** A short distance anterior to the posterior border is the transverse **palatine crest.** In many skulls the bone either side of the median suture is heaped up to form a ridge. When pronounced this ridge is called the **palatine torus.**

open on the palate at the greater and lesser palatine foramina.

The principal contents of the pterygopalatine fossa are the maxillary nerve, pterygopalatine ganglion, and terminal portion (third part) of the maxillary artery. The maxillary nerve enters the fossa through the foramen rotundum and then passes forwards and laterally across the upper part of the fossa and through the inferior orbital fissure to enter the orbit, where it is known as the infraorbital nerve. Attached to the maxillary nerve by two ganglionic branches is the pterygopalatine ganglion. This is an important parasympathetic relay station. Preganglionic neurons enter the ganglion through the nerve of the pterygoid canal. The postganglionic neurons, together with sensory neurons derived from the maxillary nerve, are distributed in the branches of the ganglion. The latter are described on page 180, all that need be noted here are the greater and lesser palatine nerves which descend through the greater palatine canal to the palate, the nasal branches which enter the nasal cavity through the sphenopalatine foramen and the pharyngeal branch which leaves the fossa through the palatovaginal canal and passes backwards to the nasopharynx. The branches of the pterygopalatine ganglion are accompanied by similarly named branches of the third part of the maxillary artery.

The paranasal air sinuses

Several of the cranial bones are hollowed out by air-containing spaces which communicate with the nasal cavity. In life these cavities are lined by respiratory mucous membrane which is often involved in upper respiratory tract infections – sinusitis following a 'head cold' is a common experience. The sinus located within the maxilla may also be involved in dental infections and in dental surgical procedures.

The paranasal air sinuses are characteristic features of the skull of placental mammals. Probably the first to evolve was the maxillary sinus since this is the only one found in primitive placental mammals such as insectivores and bats. Most other modern mammals have additional sinuses. In some species, especially the large herbivores, these are so extensive that practically every cranial bone is pneumatized. In man sinuses are found in the frontal and sphenoid bones and in the ethmoidal labyrinth, as well as in the maxilla. They are irregularly shaped cavities and vary greatly in size and shape from one individual to another and between sides in the same individual. They enlarge considerably during adolescence and continue to grow, although more slowly, throughout adult life.

The function of the paranasal sinuses is uncertain. One view is that they serve to reduce the weight of the head. In fact the saving, so far as man is concerned, is small although in species where pneumatization is extensive it may be sufficiently great to be of functional significance. Another possibility is that they serve as resonators modifying the voice and certainly in man blockage of the sinuses by secretions can greatly modify its character. Yet a further possibility is that the sinuses have an insulating effect, preventing heat loss from the nasal cavity. None of these suggestions is totally convincing, at least so far as man is concerned, and it may well be that the sinuses are really functionless being, as it were, just spaces left between the mechanically important parts of the skull.

Maxillary sinus

The body of the adult maxilla is occupied by a large sinus. It is roughly pyramidal in shape with its base adjacent to the lateral wall of the nose and its apex extending laterally into the zygomatic process. In the disarticulated bone, the base is deficient over the area of the **maxillary hiatus** but in the complete skull this deficiency is

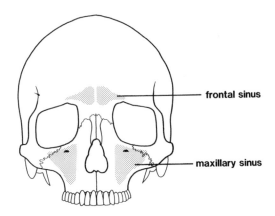

Fig. 4.14. Outlines of the maxillary and frontal sinuses. Note that the maxillary sinus does *not* extend into the zygomatic bone – this is an optical illusion resulting from the fact that the suture between the maxilla and the zygomatic bone runs posterolaterally from its position on the anterior surface of the facial skeleton; the posterior part of the maxillary body extends lateral therefore to the line of the suture.

narrowed down by the articulation of the neighbouring bones. As a result the sinus opens into the posterior part of the hiatus semilunaris of the middle meatus of the nose by one or more small apertures of which all but one are usually closed by mucous membrane in life. The communication between the sinus and nasal cavity is quite high on the medial wall of the sinus so that drainage cannot be achieved by gravity but is dependent upon the action of the cilia of the lining epithelium.

The walls of the sinus are very thin, especially those corresponding to the nasal, orbital, anterior, and infratemporal surfaces of the maxilla. In consequence a tumour of the epithelium lining the sinus may push its way into the nose, orbit, cheek or infratemporal fossa.

The inferior wall of the sinus, which is underlain by the alveolar process, appears to be more rugged but even here the bone intervening between the cavity and the roots of the upper molar teeth may be very thin or even absent (when only mucous membrane covers the roots). Dental infection may thus spread into the sinus and extraction of upper molar teeth may result in a communication, called an oroantral fistula, being established between the mouth and the sinus.

The infraorbital nerve, as it traverses the orbital plate of the maxilla, frequently produces a ridge which bulges into the cavity of the sinus. The posterior wall of the sinus is pierced by the alveolar canals which transmit the posterior superior alveolar nerves and blood vessels. These pass down to the molar teeth beneath the mucous membrane lining the sinus. In some cases the neurovascular bundles are contained within canals in the bony wall of the sinus. The sinuous canal, transmitting the anterior superior alveolar nerve, passes close to the anterior wall of the sinus.

The maxillary sinus used to be called the maxillary antrum. You will still meet this name in the clinical context.

Frontal sinus

The frontal bone above the orbits is hollowed out by two frontal sinuses. These are irregularly shaped cavities which extend, to a variable extent, backwards into the roof of the orbit and upwards into the frontal region. They are separated from each other by a septum which often deviates considerably from the median plane. As a result the two sinuses are frequently of unequal size.

In the majority of skulls the frontal sinus opens through the frontonasal canal into the anterior part of the hiatus semilunaris of the middle meatus of the corresponding side via the infundibulum in the ethmoidal labyrinth (p. 127). In the remainder the canal opens directly into the anterosuperior part of the middle meatus.

Sphenoidal sinus

The body of the sphenoid bone contains the right and left sphenoidal sinuses. These are large irregular cavities separated from each other by a septum which is usually deflected to one side or other of the median plane. They open into the sphenoethmoidal recess of the same side.

Ethmoidal air cells

Each ethmoidal labyrinth is hollowed out by a variable number of thin-walled air cells. They are divided into three groups on the basis of their openings into the nasal cavity: (i) the posterior group which opens into the superior meatus, usually by a single orifice; (ii) the middle group, which occupies the bulla and opens by one or more orifices above this elevation; (iii) the anterior group which opens by one or more orifices into the frontonasal canal and ethmoidal infundibulum.

Mandible

The mandible consists of a curved **body,** which is horseshoe-shaped when viewed from above, and two vertical **rami** which project upwards one from each posterior end of the body.

At birth the right and left halves of the mandible are united in the midline of the chin region by a fibrocartilaginous joint, the **symphysis menti.** During the first year of postnatal life this joint is obliterated by fusion of the two halves of the mandible.

The mandible ossifies predominantly in membrane although parts of the ramus ossify in secondary cartilage. It develops in the mesoderm of the mandibular arch lateral to Meckel's cartilage, the primary cartilage of this arch. It represents one of the dermal bones (the dentary) of the primitive vertebrate lower jaw.

Body

The body has **external (buccal or labial)** and **internal (lingual) surfaces.** The external surface is marked by a vertical ridge in the median plane below the interproximal space between the central incisor teeth. This indicates the line of fusion of the symphysis menti. Inferiorly this ridge runs into a raised area termed the **mental protuberance,** the presence of which gives the human chin its characteristic shape. Laterally the protuberance may present a somewhat more prominent area on each side. This is the **mental tubercle.** Running backwards and upwards from the mental tubercle is a faint ridge, the **oblique line.** Below the last molar tooth the ridge becomes more prominent before becoming continuous with the anterior border of the ramus. Immediately above the oblique line, in the region of the premolar teeth, is the **mental foramen.** This transmits the mental branches of the inferior alveolar nerve and blood vessels which themselves run in the **mandibular canal** within the body of the mandible. Note that the canal leading inwards from the foramen runs forwards and downwards and that the foramen itself has sharp anterior and inferior

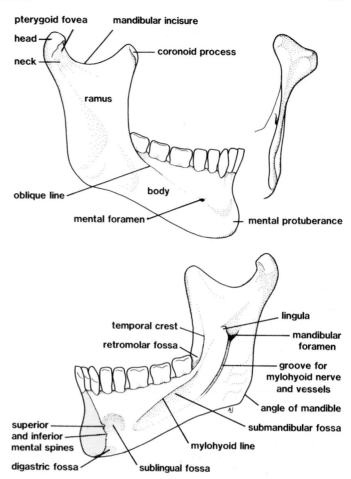

Fig. 4.15. Lateral (above) and medial (below) views of the mandible. Also shown (to the right above) is the posterior border of ramus, neck, and head of the mandible.

borders but smooth posterior and superior borders, indicating that the mental branches run backwards and somewhat upwards.

The internal surface of the body bears an oblique ridge, the **mylohyoid line,** which begins a short distance below the last molar tooth as a prominent crest and runs forwards and downwards to end by becoming indistinct in the region below the canine and incisor teeth. Below the mylohyoid line is a concave area, termed the **submandibular fossa,** which lodges the submandibular salivary gland. Running forwards from the ramus into the submandibular fossa is the shallow **mylohyoid groove** which fades out anteriorly. This marks the course of the mylohyoid branches of the inferior alveolar nerve and vessels. The area above the mylohyoid line has a smooth somewhat convex form and in life is covered over most of its extent by the fused mucous membrane and periosteum (mucoperiosteum) of the lower gum. Immediately above the line, in the region below the premolar teeth, is the shallow **sublingual fossa** for the salivary gland of the same name. The inferior part of the internal surface below the incisor teeth bears two small elevations, the **superior** and **inferior mental spines** for attachment of the genial muscles.

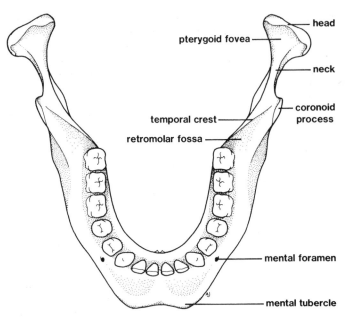

Fig. 4.16. Superior view of the mandible.

The upper part of the body of the mandible is formed by the **alveolar process.** This contains the sockets for the roots of the lower teeth and in life is covered, on both buccal and lingual surfaces, by the mucoperiosteum of the lower gum.

The inferior border of the body is marked, a little to each side of the midline, by the small, roughened **digastric fossa** for attachment of the anterior belly of the digastric muscle.

Ramus

The ramus is a quadrilateral plate of bone. Its lateral surface is flat with a roughened area in its posteroinferior part marking the insertion of the masseter muscle. The medial surface has a less regular appearance. Approximately at its centre is the **mandibular foramen** which transmits the inferior alveolar nerve and blood vessels. This opening leads into the mandibular canal which runs downwards and forwards into the body of the mandible and then continues directly forwards just below the roots of the teeth (see pages 190–1 for variations in its arrangement). Projecting over the foramen from its anterior border is a thin plate of bone, termed the **lingula.** The **mylohyoid groove** begins at the lower border of the mandibular foramen, just behind the lingula, whence it runs downwards and forwards onto the body of the mandible. The area posteroinferior to the mylohyoid groove is roughened for insertion of the medial pterygoid muscle. The region where the inferior and posterior borders of the ramus meet is termed the **angle of the mandible.**

Surmounting the superior border of the ramus are the **coronoid** and **condylar processes,** separated from each other by the wide **mandibular incisure.** The coronoid process is a triangular plate of bone which projects upwards and forwards in front of the mandibular incisure. On the medial aspect of the coronoid process is a faint ridge, the **temporal crest,** which becomes more prominent as it is traced downwards towards the margin of the alveolar bone medial to the last molar tooth. Between the temporal crest and the anterior

border of the ramus is the **retromolar fossa.** The superior and anterior margins of the coronoid process and the retromolar fossa provide the area of insertion of the temporalis muscle.

The condylar process is expanded to form the **head of the mandible.** In life the superior and posterior surfaces of the head are covered with fibrocartilage and articulate with the **articular surface of the squamous part of the temporal** at the synovial **temporomandibular joint.** The head is cylindrical in shape being expanded from side to side but narrow from front to back. Its long axis is not quite in the transverse plane but is directed somewhat posteriorly and superiorly as well as medially. The constricted part of the condylar process below the head is termed the **neck of the mandible.** Its anterior aspect has a shallow depression, the **pterygoid fovea,** into which part of the lateral pterygoid muscle is inserted.

HYOID BONE

Although the hyoid bone is not strictly speaking part of the skull it is convenient to describe it with this part of the skeleton because many of its muscular and ligamentous connections are with the cranial base and mandible with which it forms a functional unit.

The hyoid is a U-shaped bone located in the anterior part of the upper neck, a short distance below the inferior border of the mandible and above the larynx. It has no direct articulations with other skeletal elements being held in position by its numerous muscular and ligamentous connections. It consists of a **body** and two **greater cornua** (or **horns**) and two **lesser cornua.**

The hyoid bone ossifies in the ventral parts of the cartilages of the second and third pharyngeal arches. The cartilage of the second arch is represented in the adult by the lesser cornu and upper part of the body (the dorsal part of the cartilage forms the stapes, styloid process, and stylohyoid ligament) while the third arch cartilage is represented by the greater cornu and lower part of the body.

The body constitutes the anterior part of the hyoid bone. Its anterior surface is slightly roughened for attachment of suprahyoid (geniohyoid, mylohyoid, and anterior part of hyoglossus) and

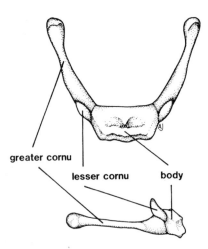

Fig. 4.17. Superior (above) and lateral (below) views of the hyoid bone.

infrahyoid (sternohyoid and omohyoid) muscles. The posterior surface is smooth being in contact with a bursa which separates it from the thyrohyoid membrane (a fibrous sheet which descends from the upper margin of the posterior surface of the body and the medial margins of the greater cornua to the upper borders of the thyroid cartilage).

A greater cornu projects backwards from each lateral extremity of the body. Near the junction are the attachments of the stylohyoid muscle and the fibrous sling for the digastric muscle. The middle constrictor and the posterior part of the hyoglossus muscle are attached to the upper border, the thyrohyoid muscle to the lateral border and the thyrohyoid membrane to the medial border of the greater cornu. Posteriorly the greater cornu ends in a tubercle.

Each lesser cornu is a small, upward projecting process attached to the junction of the body and greater cornu by fibrous tissue. The stylohyoid ligament descends from the tip of the styloid process to the apex of the lesser cornu.

CLINICAL ASPECTS

The skull may be involved in any of the generalized diseases of the skeletal system, including the osteodystrophies and the effects of nutritional deficiencies and endocrine disorders. It may in addition be involved in congenital deformations of the head and be the site of either primary or secondary tumours and of localized infections. It is also frequently fractured in severe traumatic injuries to the head. Apart from congenital abnormalities and fractures, most of these conditions are of pathological rather than anatomical interest and are not considered further in the present text. The commoner congenital abnormalities of the head are described in Chapter 2.3, leaving just the anatomical aspects of skull fractures to be discussed here.

Head injuries are a relatively common feature of modern life. The majority is associated with such violent incidents as road and sporting accidents and criminal assaults. In all such cases the possibility that the skull has been fractured must be borne in mind. Skull fractures are also a common type of war injury.

The injury may involve the cranial vault, cranial base, upper facial skeleton, or mandible and may be single or multiple. Fractures of the cranial vault occur most frequently in regions, such as the pterion, where the bone is thin. The break may be either in the form of a split starting at the site of the trauma and travelling along the line of least resistance, or a depressed fracture in which an area of bone is displaced inwards. A serious complication of fractures of the vault is intracranial bleeding resulting from tearing of the blood vessels. The vessels involved may be the dural venous sinuses and their tributaries or, if the injury is in the region of the pterion, the middle meningeal artery or vein. The resulting haemorrhage is into the extradural or subdural spaces (see p. 139).

The bone of the cranial base, except for the petrous part of the temporal bone, is relatively thin and is frequently involved in split fractures spreading from the cranial vault. The proximity of important structures results in numerous clinical manifestations which vary according to the precise site of the fracture. Fractures of the anterior cranial fossa may involve the roof of the orbit, the roof of the nose, and the frontal, sphenoidal, and ethmoidal sinuses. Bleeding into the orbit may produce a black eye and the subconjunctival haemorrhage. Fractures involving the nasal cavity and paranasal air sinuses may be accompanied by bleeding into the nose or mouth. If the meninges have been torn, cerebrospinal fluid may leak into the nose or air into the cranial cavity. Possible long-term effects of fractures of the anterior cranial fossa include anosmia, caused by damage of the olfactory nerves at the cribriform plate, or blindness produced by damage to the optic nerve in the optic canal. Fractures of the middle cranial fossa may be accompanied by bleeding or the leakage of cerebrospinal fluid into the mouth or into the middle ear and external acoustic meatus and may be followed by facial paralysis and deafness due to damage to the facial and vestibulocochlear nerves. Fractures of the posterior fossa may similarly be accompanied by clinical manifestations resulting from involvement of the glossopharyngeal, vagus, accessory, or hypoglossal nerves.

Fractures of the upper facial skeleton are of a wide variety of types. They may be relatively simple involving a single bone, or may be extensive and result in massive dislocation of the facial skeleton. Amongst the simpler injuries are fractures of the nasal bones and nasal septum and of the alveolar process of the maxilla. These are usually produced by blows to the front of the face. Occasionally during extraction of an upper second or third molar the alveolar process and tuberosity may break, sometimes with exposure of the maxillary sinus. Blows to the side of the face may result in a fracture of the zygomatic arch, with or without displacement. A potentially more serious injury is when the lateral orbital wall is involved since this can cause damage to the extraocular muscles and to the suspension of the eyeball. The consequent impaired movement and displacement of the eyeball results in double vision (diplopia).

More complex injuries of the facial skeleton include subzygomatic fractures (Le Fort type I), pyramidal fractures (Le Fort type II) and suprazygomatic fractures (Le Fort type III). The positions of the fracture lines in these injuries are shown in Fig. 4.18. In the type I injury the fracture line passes through both maxillae, at a level above the apices of the teeth and the hard palate, and into the lower part of the lateral wall of the nose. The fracture passes through the perpendicular plates of the palatines and usually involves as well the bony elements of the nasal septum. As a result the whole lower portion of the upper jaw, including the tooth-bearing parts and the hard palate, is detached from the rest of the facial skeleton.

The type II injury results in the detachment of a pyramidal-shaped segment of the facial skeleton, the fracture line passing above the apices of the roots of the posterior upper teeth and upwards through the lateral parts of the bodies of the maxillae, through the lacrimals (or ethmoidal labyrinths) and then across the frontal processes of the maxillae and the nasal bones. Again the lateral walls and septum of the nose are involved but at a higher level than in the type I fracture.

The type III fracture crosses the nasal bones, close to the frontonasal suture, the frontal processes of the maxillae and then runs posteriorly on each side along the medial wall of the orbit through the lacrimal bone and the orbital plate of the labyrinth. The fracture line usually passes below the optic canal to the posteromedial end of the inferior orbital fissure. It continues from the anterolateral end of the fissure across the lateral wall of the orbit through the orbital part of the zygomatic bone. A further fracture line passes vertically from the inferior orbital fissure across the pterygopalatine fossa and through the pterygoid process of the sphenoid. The zygomatic arches are also fractured. Hence virtually the whole of the upper facial skeleton is detached from the remainder of the cranium.

Obviously injuries of sufficient magnitude to produce the Le Fort type fractures will be associated with considerable damage to neighbouring soft tissues with much haemorrhage, oedema, and pain. In the type II and III fractures the involvement of the ethmoid region

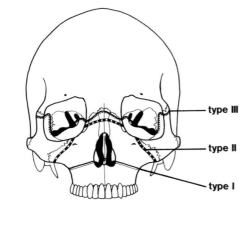

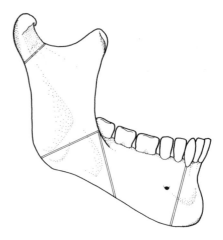

Fig. 4.19. Commoner sites for fractures of the mandible.

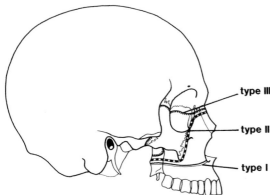

Fig. 4.18. Le Fort type I, II, and III fractures.

may result in tearing of the meninges and consequent leakage of cerebrospinal fluid.

Fractures of the mandible occur more frequently than do those of the upper facial skeleton. The common sites are indicated in Fig. 4.19. In many cases the injury is bilateral. Fractures of the condylar process are usually the result of a blow to the chin. They may be within or outside the capsule of the temporomandibular joint. The degree of displacement depends upon whether or not the periosteum and the capsule and ligaments of the joint are torn.

Fractures of the angle of the mandible may run downwards and backwards or downwards and forwards (see Fig. 4.19). In the former case the pull of the masseter, temporalis, and medial pterygoid muscles (all attached to the ramus) will pull the upper fragment in a superior and medial direction, causing considerable dislocation. In the latter case the impaction of the bone ends prevents such dislocation taking place.

Fractures of the body of the mandible are frequently located in the canine region, partly because the length of the root of the canine tooth weakens the bone in this position and partly because lateral compression, due to a blow on the side of the jaw, will cause it to break at the site of maximum convexity which is located in the neighbourhood of this tooth. A not uncommon occurrence is for the breakage to involve the body of the mandible on the side of the blow and the condylar process on the opposite side.

SPHENOID, ETHMOID, AND TEMPORAL BONES

Although the emphasis should be on understanding the skull as a whole, some knowledge of the structure of the disarticulated sphenoid, ethmoid and temporal bones is helpful because these three bones occupy key positions in important regions of the cranium.

Sphenoid

This is the key bone of the middle cranial fossa and also enters into the walls of the orbit, nasal cavity and infratemporal fossa. It consists of (i) a **central body,** (ii) two **greater wings,** (iii) two **lesser wings,** and (iv) two **pterygoid processes.**

The sphenoid ossifies from numerous centres, mostly within the cartilage of the cranial base. The principal exceptions are the lateral parts of the greater wings and the pterygoid processes which ossify intramembranously.

Body

The body is cuboidal in shape and is hollowed out by the two **sphenoidal air sinuses.** It articulates in front with the cribriform plate of the ethmoid and behind with the basilar part of the occipital. The superior surface of the body is marked by several important features. In anteroposterior sequence these are the **optic groove,** the **pituitary fossa,** and the **dorsum sellae.** The superior angles of the dorsum sellae project to a variable degree as the **posterior clinoid processes.** The anterior border of the pituitary fossa frequently bears two small lateral tubercles, the **middle clinoid processes.**

The anterior surface of the body, below the articulation with the cribriform plate, bears a median ridge, the **sphenoidal crest.** In the complete skull this articulates with the posterior edge of the perpendicular plate of the ethmoid. Either side of the sphenoidal crest are the openings of the sphenoidal sinuses. The area lateral to each opening articulates with the ethmoidal labyrinth. The sinus thus opens into the sphenoethmoidal recess. The smooth area of the anterior surface, between the opening of the sinus and the sphenoidal crest, provides the posterior part of the roof of the nasal cavity.

The inferior surface of the body projects in the median plane to form the **rostrum.** This articulates with the groove in the upper

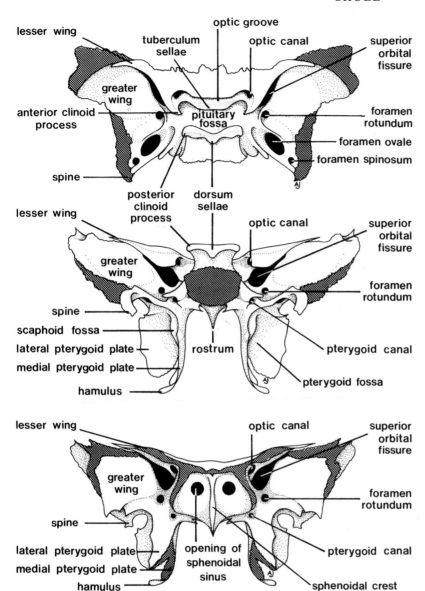

Fig. 4.20. Superior (above), posterior (middle), and anterior (below) views of the sphenoid bone. Areas of articulation shown in cross-hatching.

border of the vomer, between its two alae. Posteriorly the lateral part of the inferior surface is covered by the vaginal process of the medial pterygoid plate.

Greater wings

The greater wings project laterally and upwards from the sides of the body. Each has a superior (cerebral), lateral, and orbital surface.

The superior surface forms the floor of the lateral part of the middle cranial fossa and is pierced by foramina rotundum, ovale, and spinosum and occasional additional foramina.

The lateral surface is convex and is divided into upper (temporal) and lower (infratemporal) parts by the **infratemporal crest.** The infratemporal surface is pierced by the **foramina ovale** and **spinosum** and bears the **spine of the sphenoid.**

The orbital surface faces forwards and somewhat medially. A horizontal ridge divides the surface into a large upper area, forming the posterior part of the lateral orbital wall, and a small lower area which provides the upper part of the posterior boundary of the pterygopalatine fossa. The latter area is pierced medially by the anterior opening of the **foramen rotundum.**

The greater wing has several margins. With the help of a dried skull, trace them out as follows. The common border of the superior and lateral surfaces makes sutural connections at its tip (i.e. in the region of the pterion) with the frontal and parietal bones and further posteriorly with the squamous part of the temporal bone. This border ends posteriorly at the spine of the sphenoid. From here the posterior border, also common to the superior and lateral surfaces, runs medially to the body of the sphenoid. In its lateral part the posterior margin enters into a cartilaginous joint with the petrous part of the temporal bone while medially it forms the anterior boundary of the **foramen lacerum.** Below the pterion a common border is shared between the orbital and lateral surfaces. In its upper part this articulates with the zygomatic bone. In its lower part the border turns medially to form the lower margin of the orbital surface and the upper boundary of the inferior orbital fissure. Medial to the pterion the common border is between the orbital and superior surfaces. Laterally this border articulates with the orbital plate of the frontal while medially it provides the inferior border of the superior orbital fissure.

Lesser wings

The lesser wings project from the upper part of the body anterior to the attachments of the greater wings. They are triangular in shape with anterior and posterior margins and a lateral tip. The superior surface forms a small, posterior part of the anterior cranial fossa. The inferior surface provides the superior boundary of the superior orbital fissure and a small area of the posterior part of the orbital roof. The anterior margin articulates with the orbital plate of the frontal. The posterior margin is smooth and rounded forming the posterior boundary of the anterior cranial fossa. It ends medially at a projection, the **anterior clinoid process.**

The lesser wing is attached to the body of the sphenoid by two **roots** between which lies the **optic canal.**

Pterygoid processes

The pterygoid process of each side is attached to the inferior surface of the sphenoid bone in the region where the greater wing fuses with the body. It descends perpendicularly and consists of **medial** and **lateral pterygoid plates** which are fused anteriorly. The two plates diverge posteriorly to enclose the **pterygoid fossa.** Just below the body of the sphenoid the pterygoid process is pierced by the **pterygoid canal.**

The anterior border of the pterygoid process, formed by the fused medial and lateral plates, is smooth in its upper part where it provides the posterior boundaries of the pterygopalatine fossa and pterygo-maxillary fissure. Inferiorly the two plates diverge leaving a fissure into which fits the pyramidal process of the palatine bone. Adjacent to this fissure the anterior border is roughened for articulation with the perpendicular plate of the palatine bone.

The lateral pterygoid plate is an extensive but thin lamina. Its lateral surface forms the medial wall of the infratemporal fossa and provides the area of origin for the inferior head of the lateral pterygoid muscle. The medial surface forms the lateral boundary of the ptery-goid fossa and gives attachment to the main part of the medial pterygoid muscle.

The medial pterygoid plate is narrower but more robust than the lateral plate. Its medial surface forms the lateral boundary of the nasal aperture and its lateral surface the medial wall of the pterygoid fossa. Superiorly the medial plate extends medially across the inferior surface of the body of the sphenoid as the **vaginal process.** On the inferior surface of this process is a groove which becomes converted to the **palatovaginal canal** by the articulation with the palatine bone. The posterior border of the medial pterygoid plate is sharp over its lower two-thirds, where it gives origin to the superior constrictor muscle, but rather blunter over its upper one-third, where it gives attachment to the pharyngobasilar fascia (a component of the wall of the nasopharynx) which is pierced by the auditory tube

which thus lies against the blunter part of the posterior border of the plate. At its upper end the posterior border splits to enclose the small **scaphoid fossa,** the area of origin of part of the tensor veli palatini muscle. Immediately above and medial to the scaphoid fossa is the posterior opening of the pterygoid canal. The lower end of the posterior border forms a laterally curving process, the **pterygoid hamulus.** This gives attachment to the pterygomandibular raphe. The tendon of tensor veli palatini curves around the hamulus in a groove on its anterior (inferior) border.

Ethmoid

Although a relatively small bone, the ethmoid contributes to the anterior cranial fossa, the roof and lateral walls of the nasal cavity, the nasal septum, and the medial walls of the orbits. A knowledge of its structure helps understanding of these important regions.

The ethmoid consists of the **perpendicular plate,** the **cribriform plate,** and the two **labyrinths.** It ossifies in the cartilage of the nasal capsule.

Perpendicular plate

The perpendicular plate is a thin lamina of bone which occupies the upper part of the bony nasal septum. It possesses four margins (Fig. 4.9). The superior margin is attached to the inferior surface of the cribriform plate in the midline. The anterosuperior margin articulates with the frontal and nasal bones. The posterior margin articulates in its upper part with the crest of the sphenoid and in its lowest part with the superior border of the vomer. The anteroinferior surface is free in the dried skull but in life provides the attachment for the cartilage forming the anterior part of the nasal septum.

Cribriform plate

The cribriform plate lies horizontally, occupying the notch between the orbital parts of the frontal. It thus provides both the floor of the central part of the anterior cranial fossa and the roof of the middle part of the nasal cavity. The perpendicular plate descends from its lower surface. A stout triangular plate, the **crista galli,** projects upwards from the midline of the cribriform plate to give attachment to the falx cerebri. The cribriform plate is pierced on either side of the crista galli by numerous foramina for the olfactory nerves. A narrow gap in the cribriform plate, termed the **nasal slit,** lies immediately adjacent to the crista galli on each side.

Labyrinths

Each labyrinth consists in essence of two vertical laminae, the **medial** and **orbital (lateral) plates,** separated from each other by a number of thin-walled **ethmoidal air cells.** Although each labyrinth is, therefore, quite wide in its tranverse dimension, it is relatively fragile. The orbital plate forms part of the medial wall of the orbit, articulating above with the orbital part of the frontal, below with the orbital surface of the maxilla and orbital plate of the palatine, in front with the lacrimal and behind with the sphenoid. Projecting downwards and backwards from the anterior part of the orbital plate is the thin curved **uncinate process,** which helps form the lateral· wall of the middle meatus.

The medial plate forms the upper part of the lateral wall of the nasal cavity. It is attached above to the lateral border of the inferior surface of the cribriform plate. The lower edge of the plate projects into the nasal cavity medial to the lower part of the lateral nasal wall

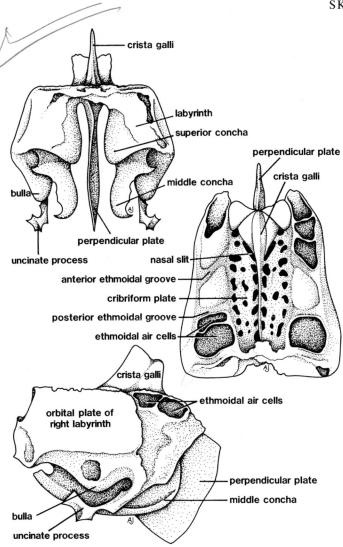

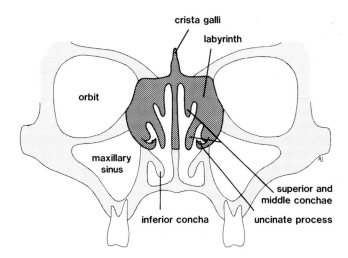

Fig. 4.21. Posterior (above), superior (middle), and lateral (below) views of the ethmoid bone.

Fig. 4.22. Diagrammatic representation of the relationships of the ethmoid bone in coronal section.

as a horizontal, rolled ridge, the **middle nasal concha.** Approximately halfway between its upper and lower borders the medial plate bears a prominent horizontal ridge which projects into the nasal cavity as the **superior nasal concha.** Above the superior concha is the spheno-ethmoidal recess while between the superior and middle conchae is the superior meatus. The middle concha forms the roof of the middle meatus, the lateral wall of which is completed by the uncinate process and the nasal surface of the maxilla.

The superior surface of the labyrinth articulates with the corresponding edge of the ethmoidal notch of the orbital part of the frontal bone. A number of air cells which open onto this surface are thus completed and two grooves which run transversely across the superior surface are converted into the **anterior** and **posterior ethmoidal canals.** The posterior surface articulates with the anterior surface of the body of the sphenoid and the orbital plate of the palatine,

again completing the air cells which open on that surface. The anterior surface articulates with the lacrimal and frontal bones and the frontal process of the maxilla. As already described the inferior margin of the medial plate projects, as the middle concha, into the nasal cavity. Lateral to the middle concha, between the medial and orbital plates, the inferior surface of the labyrinth is deeply concave. It forms the roof and upper lateral wall of the middle meatus and bears a rounded swelling, the **ethmoidal bulla.** At the lateral edge of this concave under surface (i.e. at the inferior margin of the orbital plate) the labyrinth articulates with the maxilla. The uncinate process projects from the orbital plate, curving downwards and backwards across the nasal surface of the maxilla, and helps close the maxillary hiatus. The curved gap between the bulla and the uncinate process is called the **hiatus semilunaris.**

The interior of the labyrinth is occupied by a series of air cells, of variable size and number. These are divided into three groups on the basis of their openings into the nasal cavity. The **anterior group** (up to about ten in number) opens into the ethmoidal infundibulum; the **middle group** (usually three in number) occupies the ethmoidal bulla and opens into the middle meatus above the bulla; the **posterior group** (up to seven in number) opens into the superior meatus. In the disarticulated ethmoid some of the air cells have incomplete walls, opening onto the superior and posterior surfaces of the labyrinth. In the intact skull these are completed by articulating bones. Traversing the anterior part of the labyrinth is the **ethmoidal infundibulum,** a short curved canal which begins below at the anterior end of the hiatus semilunaris of the middle meatus and in most cases opens above on the superior surface of the labyrinth. This upper opening of the infundibulum communicates with the frontal sinus which thus drains into the middle meatus. In the remaining cases the infundibulum ends blindly above and the frontal sinus opens directly into the middle meatus.

Temporal

This is a composite bone consisting of four fused elements – the **periotic, squamous, tympanic,** and **styloid** – which remain separate or only partly fused in many mammals. Each has a separate evolutionary and developmental history. The periotic ossifies in the cartilage of the auditory capsule. The squamous is an intramembranously ossifying element which was originally part of the dermal armour shield. The tympanic is also a dermal bone and is represented in non-mammals by the angular, one of the numerous bones of the lower jaw. The styloid ossifies in the dorsal part of the cartilage of the hyoid arch. Contained within the periotic are the **middle ear** (or **tympanic) cavity** and the **cavity for the internal ear**. Traversing the middle-ear cavity are the three ossicles, **malleus, incus,** and **stapes,** which convey vibrations from the ear drum to the internal ear. All three ossicles are cartilage-replacing bones, the malleus and incus ossifying in the cartilages of the mandibular arch and representing the articular and quadrate (lower and upper jaw elements respectively) of non-mammals while the stapes ossifies in the cartilage of the hyoid arch, dorsal to the styloid ossification, and is equivalent to the single ear ossicle of reptiles and amphibia and the jaw support of fishes.

In the human temporal bone the periotic is usually described as two separate components, the **petrous** and **mastoid** parts.

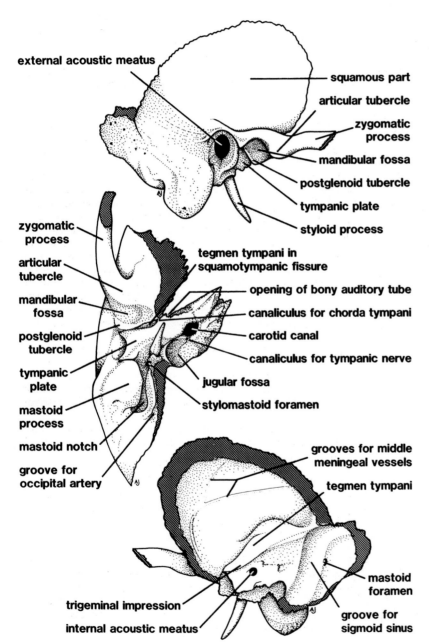

external acoustic meatus

squamous part

articular tubercle

zygomatic process

mandibular fossa

postglenoid tubercle

tympanic plate

styloid process

zygomatic process

articular tubercle

mandibular fossa

postglenoid tubercle

tympanic plate

mastoid process

mastoid notch

groove for occipital artery

tegmen tympani in squamotympanic fissure

opening of bony auditory tube

canaliculus for chorda tympani

carotid canal

canaliculus for tympanic nerve

jugular fossa

stylomastoid foramen

grooves for middle meningeal vessels

tegmen tympani

mastoid foramen

trigeminal impression

internal acoustic meatus

groove for sigmoid sinus

Fig. 4.23. Lateral (above), inferior (middle), and medial (lower) views of the right temporal bone. Areas of articulation are in cross-hatching.

Petrous part

This part of the temporal bone houses the tympanic and internal ear cavities. As its name suggests it is composed of very hard bone. It lies entirely within the cranial base, wedged between the sphenoid and occipital bones with its apex directed anteromedially. It has anterior, posterior, and inferior surfaces.

The anterior surface forms part of the middle cranial fossa (Fig. 4.4). Just posterolateral to the apex (and to foramen lacerum in the articulated skull) it is marked by the **trigeminal impression** which lodges the trigeminal ganglion housed within the trigeminal cave. Posterolateral to the trigeminal impression much of the anterior surface is formed by a plate of bone called the **tegmen tympani**. This is a new addition to the mammalian skull which developed as an outgrowth from the periotic (which originally enclosed just the internal ear) to help surround and protect the tympanic cavity. The tegmen tympani has two small openings from which grooves may be traced leading forwards and medially. The more posteromedial of the openings is the **hiatus for the greater petrosal nerve** and the more anterolateral the **hiatus for the lesser petrosal nerve**. The anterior edge of the tegmen tympani projects downwards between the squamous and tympanic parts of the temporal. On the under surface of the cranial base this downturned edge can be seen as a lip of bone in the medial part of the squamotympanic fissure, dividing it into a posterior petrotympanic and an anterior petrosquamous part. The petrotympanic fissure leads into the tympanic cavity. Its medial end is widened to form the **canaliculus for the chorda tympani** through which that branch of the facial nerve escapes from the tympanic cavity to the exterior of the skull.

The posterior surface of the petrous bone forms part of the posterior cranial fossa, the superior border of the bone providing the boundary between middle and posterior fossae. Approximately in the centre of the posterior surface is the opening of the **internal acoustic meatus**.

The inferior surface makes up part of the under surface of the cranial base. It is very irregular and has a large, circular opening which leads into the **carotid canal** and behind this the deep **jugular fossa** which houses the superior bulb of the internal jugular vein. The ridge separating the carotid opening from the jugular fossa is pierced by the **canaliculus for the tympanic branch of the glossopharyngeal nerve**. Just in front of the opening of the carotid canal, in the angle between the petrous and squamous parts, is the opening of the bony part of the **auditory tube**. This leads into the anterior part of the tympanic cavity. With the soft tissues in place the tube is continued medially in cartilage to open into the nasopharynx.

The anterior border articulates laterally with the squamous part of the temporal bone at the petrosquamosal suture and medially with the greater wing of the sphenoid at a cartilaginous joint. The posterior border articulates by a cartilaginous joint with the occipital bone. Immediately adjacent to the jugular fossa the petrous and occipital bones are separated by a wide gap, the **jugular foramen**. The apex of the petrous bone forms the posterolateral boundary of the **foramen lacerum** and is here pierced by the inner opening of the carotid canal.

Mastoid part

This is the most posterior part of the temporal bone and bears on its external aspect a conical projection, the **mastoid process** to which is attached the sternocleidomastoid muscle. Medial to the process is a deep groove, the **mastoid notch**, for the attachment of the posterior belly of the digastric muscle. Further medially still is a shallow groove in which runs the occipital artery. The endocranial surface is marked by a deep, curved groove for the sigmoid sinus.

The mastoid part articulates by its superior border with the parietal bone and by its posterior border with the occipital bone. Anteriorly it is fused with the squamous and petrous parts.

Squamous part

The squamous part of the temporal bone is a large plate of bone which forms the lower part of the side wall of the cranial vault and a small area of the lateral part of the cranial base.

The temporal surface is smooth and forms much of the temporal fossa from which the temporalis muscle takes origin. Projecting forwards from the temporal surface is the **zygomatic process** which articulates anteriorly with the zygomatic bone to form the zygomatic arch.

The cerebral surface is marked by a number of depressions, corresponding to the convolutions of the temporal lobes of the cerebral hemispheres, and by grooves for the posterior branches of the middle meningeal vessels.

The inferior aspect of the squamous part bears the superior articular surface of the temporomandibular joint formed by the **articular tubercle** and the anterior part of the **mandibular fossa**. The fossa is transversely widened and is bounded in front by the articular tubercle and completed behind by the tympanic part of the temporal bone. Located in the depth of the fossa, between the squamous and tympanic, is the squamotympanic fissure. Only the squamous (i.e. anterior) part of the fossa is articular, the tympanic plate being excluded from the temporomandibular joint by the attachment of the capsule to the anterior lip of the squamotympanic fissure. Laterally the posterior edge of the articular surface is downturned to form a lip of bone called the **postglenoid tubercle**. Medially the squamotympanic fissure is divided, as already described, into petrotympanic and petrosquamous portions by the lip of the tegmen tympani.

The articular tubercle is sometimes described as the anterior root of the zygomatic process (the posterior root being the ridge of bone which continues from the zygomatic process above the external acoustic meatus).

The posterosuperior border of the squamous part articulates with the parietal bone and the anteroinferior border with the greater wing of the sphenoid bone.

Tympanic plate

This is a curved plate of bone which is fused with the petrous, mastoid, and squamous parts to complete the external acoustic meatus. It partly ensheaths the base of the styloid process.

Styloid process

The styloid process is a slender, curved bony projection of variable length. It is usually broken in the dried skull. Its upper part is ensheathed by and fused with the tympanic plate. The process gives attachment to the styloid muscles and the stylohyoid and stylomandibular ligaments. Between the styloid and mastoid processes is the stylomastoid foramen through which the facial nerve leaves the skull.

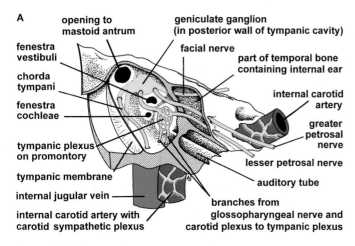

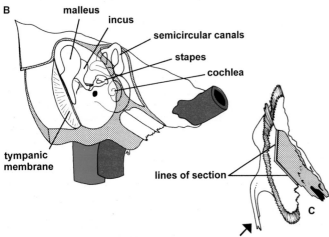

Fig. 4.24. A is a view of the right tympanic cavity obtained by sectioning the temporal bone along the lines shown in C (which is a superior view of the right temporal bone) and looking at the detached (i.e. hatched) portion from in front and from the lateral side—the arrow in C shows the direction of viewing. In A the three ossicles have been removed but would stretch across the tympanic cavity from the tympanic membrane to the fenestra vestibuli as shown in B.

Tympanic cavity

Although the organs of hearing are not involved, at least intentionally, in the practice of dentistry, a general idea of the structure of the tympanic cavity is necessary to understand the course of the facial nerve and its branches, all structures of considerable vocational importance.

The tympanic cavity is a mediolaterally compressed space within the petrous bone. In its lateral wall is the ear drum or tympanic membrane which separates the cavity from the external acoustic meatus. The medial wall is formed by the bony partition separating the tympanic cavity from the internal ear. This wall has two openings, the **fenestra vestibuli** and **fenestra cochleae**. Vibrations are transmitted from the ear drum to the internal ear by the three ossicles. The malleus is attached to the drum by its **manubrium** (handle) and articulates with the **head of the incus**. The incus articulates with the **head of the stapes** and the **footplate of the stapes** occupies the fenestra vestibuli. The fenestra cochleae is not closed by bone and provides a release mechanism for the pressure changes in the fluids of the internal ear produced by the vibrations of the footplate at the fenestra vestibuli. Pressure within the middle-ear cavity is maintained at atmospheric level by means of the auditory tube which connects the anterior part of the cavity with the nasopharynx. The vibrations of the ossicles are damped by two small muscles, the tensor tympani (attached to the manubrium of the malleus) and the stapedius (attached to the stapes).

Running in the medial wall, first posteriorly above fenestra vestibuli and then inferiorly to end at the **stylomastoid foramen,** is the bony **canal for the facial nerve**. The facial nerve enters this canal from the internal acoustic meatus, making an abrupt posterior turn (the **genu**) in so doing. Close to this point the facial nerve is swollen to form the geniculate ganglion. The greater petrosal nerve branches off the facial nerve here and leaves the petrous bone through the hiatus of the same name to enter the middle cranial fossa. Just before the facial nerve leaves the facial canal through its lower opening, the stylomastoid foramen, it gives off the chorda tympani nerve. This runs in a bony canal across the narrow posterior wall of the tympanic cavity to reach the lateral wall. Here the chorda tympani leaves the bony canal to run forwards across the ear drum between its fibrous and mucous layers, close to the manubrium of the malleus. It then enters the canaliculus for the chorda tympani which passes downwards and forwards to open at the medial end of the petrotympanic fissure.

Just in front of the fenestra cochleae, on the medial wall of the tympanic cavity, is a bulge, termed the **promontory,** which overlies the basal turn of the cochlea (part of the internal ear). The mucous membrane over the promontory contains a plexus of fine nerve fibres called the **tympanic plexus**. It is formed from the tympanic branch of the glossopharyngeal nerve, branches from the geniculate ganglion of the facial nerve and sympathetic branches from the carotid plexus. It supplies the mucous membrane lining the tympanic cavity and also gives rise to the lesser petrosal nerve which leaves the petrous bone through a hiatus located anterolateral to that for the greater petrosal nerve.

The tympanic cavity is lined with mucous membrane, bearing a ciliated columnar epithelium.

2

Interior of cranial cavity

MENINGES

The cerebral meninges are three layers of membrane that lie between the bone of the braincase and the external surface of the brain. They are continuous at the foramen magnum with similar layers of membrane surrounding the spinal cord. The outermost layer, the **dura mater**, lies immediately adjacent to the braincase. The innermost layer, the **pia mater**, is intimately applied to the surface of the brain. Between these two is the intermediate layer or **arachnoid mater**. The pia and arachnoid mater are referred to together as the **leptomeninges**.

Layers

Dura mater

Conventionally, the dura mater is described as consisting of an outer, or **endosteal**, and an inner, or **meningeal**, layer. Except where they separate to enclose the venous sinuses and meningeal blood vessels these two layers are, in fact, united. The endosteal layer provides the periosteum of the internal surface of the braincase to which it is tightly adherent. At the margins of the foramina leading out of the cranial cavity it is continuous with the periosteum on the external surface of the braincase.

The meningeal layer is of a tough, fibrous nature. It provides tubular sheaths for the cranial nerves as they leave the cranial cavity through the foramina in the cranial base. Outside the skull these sheaths fuse with the epineurium of the nerves except in the case of the optic nerve where the sheath passes along its whole length to fuse with the sclera of the eyeball. At certain places the meningeal layer is expanded to form double-layered folds which project into the cranial cavity. These folds are four in number and are termed the **falx cerebri**, **tentorium cerebelli**, **falx cerebelli**, and **diaphragma sellae**.

Pia mater

The pia consists of a delicate layer of richly vascular connective tissue. It closely invests the surface of the brain at all points, even in the deepest fissures and invaginates the walls of the ventricles of the brain to form the **choroid plexuses**, structures concerned with the production of cerebrospinal fluid. The pia gives a covering to each of the cranial nerves which blends with the epineurium.

Arachnoid mater

The arachnoid is a delicate membrane lying against the internal surface of the meningeal layer of the dura mater. The two are separated by a narrow gap, the **subdural space**, containing a thin film of tissue fluid. Between the arachnoid and the pia is a rather wider gap, the **subarachnoid space**. Fine strands of arachnoid tissue extend across the subarachnoid space which is filled with cerebrospinal fluid. The size of the space varies, being much narrower over convexities of the brain than it is over fissures and other depressions. On the under surface of the brain are several large expansions of the subarachnoid space termed the **basal cisterns** (Fig. 4.26). These include the **cerebellomedullary cistern** (or **cisterna magna**) occupying the angle between the cerebellum and the posterior surface of the medulla, the **pontine cistern** between the front of the pons and the cranial base, the **interpeduncular cistern** between the dorsum sellae and the cerebral peduncles, and a number of smaller cisterns.

The arteries and veins of the brain travel in the extracerebral part of their course within the subarachnoid space. The cranial nerves cross the subarachnoid space and pick up sheaths of arachnoid tissue as they pierce the arachnoid membrane. These sheaths extend as far as the exit of the nerves from the skull where they fuse with the epineurum, apart from the optic nerve where the arachnoid sheath, located within the dural sheath, extends to the back of the eyeball.

In certain areas the arachnoid herniates through the meningeal layer of the dura mater to protrude into the venous sinuses and associated venous lakes. Some of these herniations are very small and are called **arachnoid villi**. Others are considerably larger and are termed **arachnoid granulations**. Villi and granulations are especially numerous in the vicinity of the superior sagittal sinus. They are concerned with the absorption of the cerebrospinal fluid into the bloodstream.

Dural processes

Falx cerebri

This is a double-layered fold of the dura mater located in the median plane in the longitudinal fissure between the two cerebral hemispheres. Anteriorly it is attached to the crista galli while posteriorly it is continuous with the superior surface of the tentorium cerebelli. Between these limits its convex upper border is attached to the endocranial surface of the cranial vault where it is continuous with the meningeal layer of the dura. At this attachment the two leaves of the falx are separated by the **superior sagittal venous sinus**. The concave lower border of the falx is free and contains the **inferior sagittal venous sinus**. Between the superior and inferior sagittal sinuses the two leaves of the falx are firmly united to form a strong, inelastic membrane. At its posterior line of attachment the leaves of the falx are continuous, on each side, with the upper leaf of the tentorium cerebelli and are here separated by the **straight sinus**.

Tentorium cerebelli

The tentorium projects into the cranial cavity between the cerebellum and occipital lobes of the cerebral hemispheres, lying in the

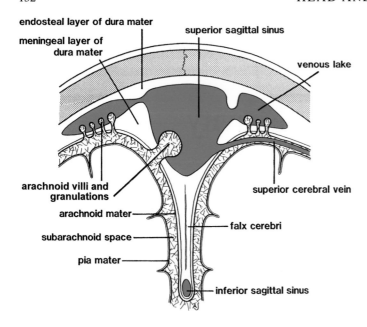

Fig. 4.25. Coronal section to show the arrangement of the meninges. The section is through the region adjacent to the sagittal suture of the cranial vault and includes the falx cerebri, a fold of the meningeal layer of the dura which extends into the fissure between the two cerebral hemispheres.

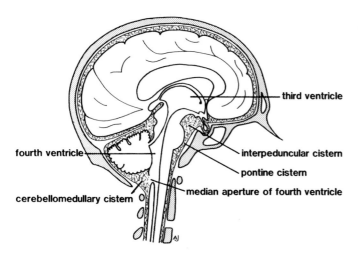

Fig. 4.26. Median section through the cranial cavity to show the basal cisterns.

horizontal plane at right angles to the falx cerebri. Its two leaves are continuous, on each side, with the meningeal dura along the upper and lower lips of the groove for the **transverse venous sinus**, the superior border of the petrous part of the temporal bone (where they are separated by the **superior petrosal sinus**) and the lateral edge of the dorsum sellae as far as the posterior clinoid process. The attached, outer margin is therefore long and convex. The free inner

margin is concave and much shorter. Between the free margin and the dorsum sellae is an opening, the **tentorial incisure**, occupied by the midbrain.

At the apex of the petrous part of the temporal bone the free and attached borders of the tentorium cross each other, the attached border ending at the posterior clinoid process but the free border continuing forwards to the anterior clinoid process (see Fig. 4.28). Anterior to the point where it crosses the attached border, the free border lies in the roof of the cavernous sinus.

Near the apex of the petrous bone the lower layer of the tentorium is evaginated forwards across the superior border of the petrous bone to form a small outpouching, the **trigeminal (Meckel's) cave**, between the endosteal and meningeal layers of the dura of the middle cranial fossa in the region of the trigeminal impression, (see Fig. 4.29). It contains the roots and posterior part of the ganglion of the trigeminal nerve.

Falx cerebelli

This is a small curved fold of dura mater which projects into the cranial cavity below the tentorium. It lies in the median plane, occupying the posterior notch on the cerebellum. It is continuous with the inferior layer of the tentorium and with the meningeal layer of the dura on the occipital bone.

Diaphragma sellae

The diaphragma sellae is a circular fold of dura which forms the roof of the sella turcica, completely covering the pituitary gland apart from a small central opening for the pituitary stalk.

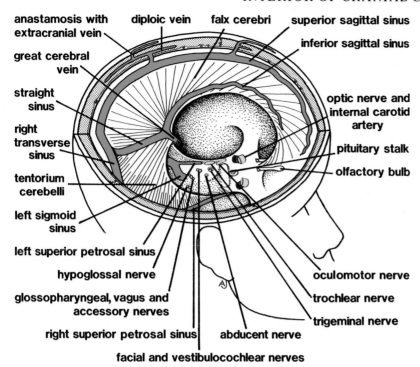

anastamosis with extracranial vein

diploic vein

falx cerebri

superior sagittal sinus

inferior sagittal sinus

great cerebral vein

straight sinus

right transverse sinus

tentorium cerebelli

left sigmoid sinus

left superior petrosal sinus

hypoglossal nerve

glossopharyngeal, vagus and accessory nerves

right superior petrosal sinus

facial and vestibulocochlear nerves

optic nerve and internal carotid artery

pituitary stalk

olfactory bulb

oculomotor nerve

trochlear nerve

trigeminal nerve

abducent nerve

Fig. 4.27. Superolateral view of the interior of the cranial cavity with the brain removed but the dural processes intact.

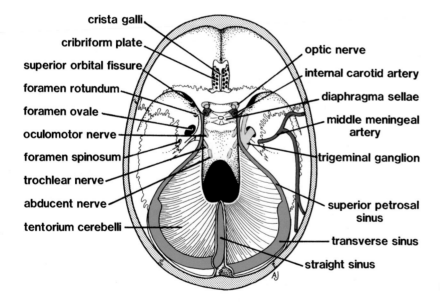

crista galli

cribriform plate

superior orbital fissure

foramen rotundum

foramen ovale

oculomotor nerve

foramen spinosum

trochlear nerve

abducent nerve

tentorium cerebelli

optic nerve

internal carotid artery

diaphragma sellae

middle meningeal artery

trigeminal ganglion

superior petrosal sinus

transverse sinus

straight sinus

Fig. 4.28. Superior view of the tentorium cerebelli.

Nerve and blood supply of dura mater

Nerve supply

The meningeal nerves of the anterior cranial fossa are branches of the **ethmoidal nerves.** The dura of the middle cranial fossa is innervated by **meningeal branches of the maxillary and mandibular nerves.** The meningeal branch of the maxillary nerve is given off within the cranial cavity just before the main trunk of the nerve enters the foramen rotundum. The meningeal branch (nervus spinosus) of the mandibular nerve arises immediately below the foramen ovale and enters the cranial cavity through the foramen spinosum. The dura of the posterior cranial fossa is innervated by ascending branches from **the upper cervical spinal nerves.** These enter the cranial cavity through the foramen magnum, jugular foramen and hypoglossal

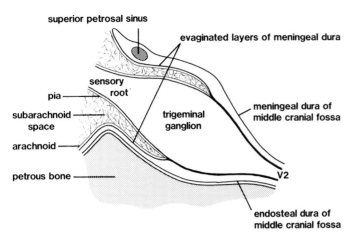

Fig. 4.29. Anteroposterior section through the trigeminal cave. The meningeal layer of the dura mater is evaginated forwards across the superior border of the petrous bone to form a pocket, the trigeminal cave, between the endosteal and meningeal layers of the dura mater of the middle cranial fossa. The cave is occupied by the posterior part of the trigeminal ganglion; the roots of the nerve enter through the mouth of the cave. The cave is lined by arachnoid and pia mater.

canal, some of the filaments running within the sheaths of the vagus and hypoglossal nerves.

The meningeal nerves contain sensory and postganglionic sympathetic fibres. The latter may have a vasomotor function.

Blood supply

The arteries to the dura mater are numerous, most of the blood going to the endosteal layer. The principal supply to the supratentorial part is through the **middle meningeal artery**, a branch of the maxillary artery, which enters the cranial cavity through the foramen spinosum. It then runs laterally across the floor of the middle cranial fossa, between the endosteal and meningeal layers of the dura, and divides into anterior and posterior branches. The anterior branch ascends across the pterion towards the vertex of the cranial vault. The posterior branch runs backwards towards the posterior part of the cranial cavity. These arteries are accompanied throughout their course by **meningeal veins** which tend to lie between the artery and the bone of the cranium and are responsible for the grooves in the latter. The middle meningeal veins drain into the sphenoparietal sinus and also through the foramen spinosum and foramen ovale into the pterygoid plexus of veins located in the infratemporal fossa.

Other arteries supplying the supratentorial dura mater include the **accessory meningeal artery** (a branch of the maxillary artery entering the cranial cavity through the foramen ovale) and meningeal branches of the ophthalmic, ethmoidal, and internal carotid arteries.

The subtentorial dura mater is supplied by meningeal branches of the vertebral arteries.

Venous sinuses of dura mater

Apart from the inferior sagittal and straight sinuses, these venous channels lie between the endosteal and meningeal layers of the dura mater. Like other veins they are lined by endothelium but contain no valves and have walls devoid of muscular tissue. They receive blood from the brain (through the cerebral veins), from the bones of the braincase (via the diploic veins) and from the meninges.

Superior sagittal sinus

The superior sagittal sinus lies between the two leaves of the falx cerebri at their attachment to the cranial vault (Figs 4.25 and 4.27). It begins in the anterior part of the falx and passes posteriorly growing progressively larger as it does so. In the posterior part of its course it grooves the endocranial surface of the cranial vault. Extending laterally from the sinus are a variable number of **venous lakes**. These lie alongside the sinus between the two layers of the dura. Projecting into them are numerous arachnoid granulations. Opening into the superior sagittal sinus are the superior cerebral veins draining blood from the superior, lateral and medial surfaces of the cerebral hemispheres.

At the internal occipital protuberance the superior sagittal sinus turns, usually to the right but occasionally to the left, to become the transverse sinus of that side.

Inferior sagittal sinus

This is situated between the two leaves of the falx cerebri at its inferior, free margin (Fig. 4.27). It begins just above the crista galli, enlarges as it runs posteriorly and ends at the attachment of the falx to the tentorium cerebelli by opening into the straight sinus. It receives blood from the falx.

Straight sinus

The straight sinus runs posteriorly in the junction of the falx cerebri and the tentorium cerebelli (Fig. 4.27). As well as draining the inferior sagittal sinus it receives the great cerebral vein (containing blood from the deep parts of the cerebral hemispheres). The sinus ends at the internal occipital protuberance by turning to become, in most cases, the left transverse sinus. In those instances where the superior sagittal sinus opens into the left transverse sinus, the straight sinus is continuous with the transverse sinus of the right side.

Transverse sinus

The transverse sinus draining the superior sagittal sinus is usually the larger. From its commencement at the internal occipital protuberance the transverse sinus of each side passes laterally between the two leaves of the tentorium cerebelli in its attached margin, grooving the endocranial surface of the occipital bone (Fig. 4.28). At the junction of petrous and mastoid parts of the temporal bone the transverse sinus curves downwards to become the sigmoid sinus. It receives inferior cerebral, cerebellar, and diploic veins and, near its continuation with the sigmoid sinus, the superior petrosal sinus.

Sigmoid sinus

The sigmoid sinus curves downwards and forwards from its continuation with the transverse sinus to the jugular foramen, producing a deep groove on the endocranial surface of the mastoid part of the temporal bone (Fig. 4.30). In the posterior part of the jugular foramen it expands to form the jugular bulb which is continuous below with the internal jugular vein.

Cavernous sinus

The right and left cavernous sinuses lie each side of the body of the sphenoid (Figs 4.30 and 4.31). In cross-section they have a spongy

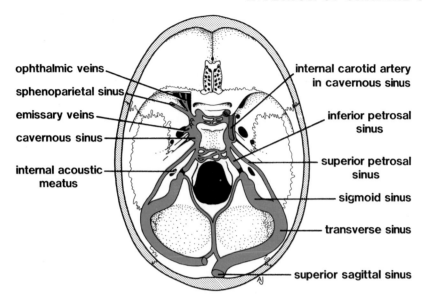

ophthalmic veins

sphenoparietal sinus

emissary veins

cavernous sinus

internal acoustic
meatus

internal carotid artery
in cavernous sinus

inferior petrosal
sinus

superior petrosal
sinus

sigmoid sinus

transverse sinus

superior sagittal sinus

Fig. 4.30. Superior view of the venous sinuses of the cranial base with the tentorium cerebelli removed.

appearance resulting from the presence of numerous fibrous trabeculae crossing their cavities. Each sinus is located between the endosteal layer of the dura mater covering the lateral aspect of the body of the sphenoid and a layer of meningeal dura which extends laterally from the side wall of the pituitary fossa and dorsum sellae, to form the roof of the sinus between the anterior and posterior clinoid processes, and then descends to the floor of the middle cranial fossa, so forming the lateral wall of the sinus. The walls of the sinus are traversed by the internal carotid artery, the nerves to the extraocular muscles and the first two divisions of the trigeminal nerve.

The cavernous sinus receives blood from the middle cerebral vein (draining the lateral surface of the hemisphere), the sphenoparietal sinus (from the dura mater over the temporal region), and the superior and inferior ophthalmic veins (from the orbit). Before entering the sinus, the inferior ophthalmic vein communicates with the pterygoid plexus of veins through the inferior orbital fissure. The cavernous sinus also communicates directly with the pterygoid plexus by emissary veins transmitted through the foramen ovale (or the emissary sphenoidal foramen if present). The sinus drains into the superior and inferior petrosal sinuses.

Several important structures are related to the cavernous sinus. (i) The **internal carotid artery** curves upwards from the opening of the carotid canal to enter the posterior part of the sinus. It runs forwards on the side of the body of the sphenoid between the endosteal layer of the dura and the endothelial lining of the sinus, then curves upwards to pierce the roof of the sinus just medial to the anterior clinoid process. (ii) The **abducent nerve** pierces the meningeal layer of the dura lateral to the dorsum sellae. It then runs upwards between the two layers of the dura and turns forwards across the superior border of the petrous part of the temporal bone to pass in the medial wall of the cavernous sinus between the internal carotid artery and the endothelium lining the cavernous sinus. Anteriorly it leaves the wall of the sinus to enter the orbit through the superior orbital fissure. (iii) The **ophthalmic** and **maxillary divisions of the trigeminal nerve** leave the trigeminal ganglion and run forwards between the reflected

meningeal layer of the dura forming the lateral wall of the cavernous sinus and the lining endothelium. The ophthalmic nerve is the more superior of the two and divides into its three branches (lacrimal, frontal, and nasociliary) while still in the wall of the sinus. These enter the orbit through the superior orbital fissure. The maxillary nerve leaves the cranial cavity through the foramen rotundum. (iv) The **trochlear nerve** enters the roof of the cavernous sinus and then runs forwards in its lateral wall, above the ophthalmic nerve, to pass into the orbit through the superior orbital fissure. (v) The **oculomotor nerve** enters the roof of the sinus in front of the trochlear nerve. It also runs forwards in the lateral wall of the sinus but inclines somewhat downwards crossing medial to the trochlear nerve and the branches of the ophthalmic nerve. While still within the wall of the sinus the oculomotor nerve divides into superior and inferior rami which enter the orbit through the superior orbital fissure.

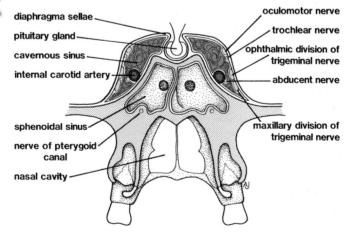

diaphragma sellae

pituitary gland

cavernous sinus

internal carotid artery

sphenoidal sinus

nerve of pterygoid
canal

nasal cavity

oculomotor nerve

trochlear nerve

ophthalmic division of
trigeminal nerve

abducent nerve

maxillary division of
trigeminal nerve

Fig. 4.31. Coronal section through the cavernous sinuses.

Superior petrosal sinus

The superior petrosal sinus drains out of the posterior part of the cavernous sinus (Fig. 4.30). It runs across the roots of the trigeminal nerve to reach the superior border of the petrous bone along which it then runs between the two layers of the attached margin of the tentorium cerebelli. It ends by entering the junction of the transverse and sigmoid sinuses.

Inferior petrosal sinus

The inferior petrosal sinus also leaves the posterior part of the cavernous sinus (Fig. 4.30). It passes downwards, between the two layers of the dura, along the petro-occipital fissure to enter the anterior part of the jugular foramen. Having traversed the foramen it joins the internal jugular vein a short distance below the cranial base.

Clinical aspects

Infections of the meninges

Inflammation of the pia and arachnoid mater is called meningitis. It is most frequently caused by infection with micro-organisms. The infection may spread from a nearby focus (such as a brain abscess) or a penetrating wound or it may be blood-borne. It usually involves the spinal as well as the cerebral part of the leptomeninges.

The outstanding features of meningitis are headache, fever, and the signs of spinal meningeal irritation (neck rigidity and resistance to knee extension with the hip flexed).

Infections of the venous sinuses

Several of the venous sinuses have anastomotic channels connecting them with extracranial veins. These are particularly numerous in the case of the cavernous sinus which communicates with the veins of the face through the superior ophthalmic vein and with the pterygoid plexus through emissary vessels and through the connections of the inferior ophthalmic vein. Infection may thus spread from the face or from the area drained by the pterygoid plexus (which includes most of the dental structures) into the cavernous sinus where it may result in an infected thrombosis. This may produce, in turn, a retrograde thrombosis of the middle cerebral vein which is usually fatal. It will also affect the cranial nerves passing through the walls of the cavernous sinus. The abducent nerve is the most frequently involved resulting in paralysis of the lateral rectus muscle.

INTRACRANIAL COURSE OF CRANIAL NERVES

There are twelve bilaterally paired cranial nerves. As they leave the brain they acquire a sheath of pia mater then travel in the subarachnoid space to their exits from the skull. Each nerve receives a further sheath as it passes through the arachnoid layer. The pia and arachnoid sheaths blend with the epineurium of the nerves close to their exits from the skull. As they emerge through the foramina in the base of the skull the nerves receive a final coat from the meningeal layer of the dura. This fuses with the epineurium a short distance outside the skull. The only major departure from this arrangement is found in the case of the optic nerve where, as might be expected for what is really an extended tract of the brain, the sheaths surround the nerve throughout its extracranial course.

Anterior cranial fossa (cranial nerve I)

Lying immediately above the cribriform plate are the right and left **olfactory bulbs** (Fig. 4.27). Olfactory sensory fibres pass as numerous fine filaments, constituting the **olfactory nerve** (cranial nerve I), from the mucous membrane lining the nose, through the foramina of the cribriform plate, to end in the bulb of the corresponding side. Between the meningeal and endosteal layers of the dura in the region of the cribriform plate is a small gap termed the supracribrous recess. The olfactory nerves cross this space in minute evaginations of the meningeal layer of the dura and of the leptomeninges. Also running within the supracribrous recess are the anterior ethmoidal nerve and vessels. The latter structures pass from the anterior ethmoidal canal across the cribriform plate to enter the nasal cavity through the nasal slit located alongside the crista galli.

Middle cranial fossa (cranial nerves II to V)

The **optic nerve** (II) runs from the **optic chiasma** to the eyeball. The optic chiasma (Figs 4.32 and 5.34, p. 248) connects the optic nerves of the two sides and consists of fibres from the nasal half of each retina crossing to the opposite side. The chiasma lies just above and behind the optic groove in close relationship to the pituitary gland. Each optic nerve runs anterolaterally from the chiasma to enter the orbit through the optic canal. The **optic tracts** continue posteriorly from the chiasma to the lateral geniculate bodies (nuclei within the brain). Each tract contains fibres from the temporal half of the retina of the same side and fibres which have crossed in the chiasma from the nasal half of the retina of the opposite side. The tracts, chiasma, and nerves lie within the subarachnoid space ensheathed within a layer derived from the pia mater. As the nerve passes through the optic canal it receives further coats from the arachnoid mater and the meningeal layer of the dura. These three layers continue forwards around the optic nerve to the posterior wall of the eyeball. The optic nerve is thus surrounded by a cuff consisting of dura, arachnoid, and pia and containing a subarachnoid space filled with cerebrospinal fluid. In raised intracranial pressure the nerve is squeezed producing distension of the optic disc (the area where the optic nerve enters the retina). This condition, called papilloedema, can be seen with the aid of an ophthalmoscope.

The **oculomotor** (III) and **trochlear** (IV) nerves leave the brainstem at the level of the midbrain. The oculomotor nerve emerges from the medial side of the cerebral peduncle (a paired swelling on the ventral aspect of the midbrain) and passes forwards in the subarachnoid space between the posterior cerebral and superior cerebellar arteries (Figs 4.32 and 5.11, p. 230) to enter the roof of the cavernous sinus. The trochlear nerve is unique in that it is the only cranial nerve to emerge from the dorsal surface of the brainstem. It curves forwards around the cerebral peduncle and then runs forwards to enter the roof of the cavernous sinus behind the oculomotor nerve. The oculomotor and trochlear nerves leave the cranial cavity through the superior orbital fissure.

The **trigeminal nerve** (V) is the largest cranial nerve and is of particular importance in the practice of dentistry because it provides the sensory supply to a wide area of the head, including the teeth and their supporting structures, and also innervates muscles involved in jaw movements. It leaves the ventral surface of the pons as a large **sensory** and a small **motor root** (Figs 4.32 and 5.11). The two roots run forwards, with the motor root lying medially, and pass into the middle cranial fossa by crossing the superior border of the petrous part of the temporal bone just lateral to its apex. The superior petrosal sinus passes above the roots at this point. The meningeal layer of dura is invaginated about the two roots to form the trigeminal cave which lies between the meningeal and endosteal layers of the dura on the floor of the middle cranial fossa immediately lateral to the apex of the petrous bone (Fig. 4.29). Within the cave the sensory root is swollen to form the trigeminal ganglion. The invaginated dura fuses with connective tissue covering the ganglion so that only the posterior half of the ganglion lies within the trigeminal cave. The cave is lined by the leptomeninges.

The **ophthalmic** and **maxillary divisions** of the trigeminal nerve leave the upper part of the ganglion and pass forwards into the lateral wall of the cavernous sinus. The branches of the ophthalmic nerve leave the cranial cavity through the superior orbital fissure and the maxillary nerve through the foramen rotundum. The **mandibular division,** the largest of the three, emerges from the lower part of the ganglion and after a very short intracranial course passes through the foramen ovale into the infratemporal fossa. The motor root passes below the ganglion, closely applied to its surface, and fuses with the mandibular division in the foramen. Hence all the motor fibres in the trigeminal nerve enter the mandibular nerve.

Surgical access to the trigeminal ganglion may be required in the treatment of conditions such as trigeminal neuralgia (p. 257). The anterior half of the ganglion and the three emerging divisions of the nerve lie in front of the trigeminal cave and can be approached between the endosteal and meningeal layers of the dura across the floor of the middle cranial fossa.

Posterior cranial fossa (cranial nerves VI to XII)

The **abducent nerve** (VI) leaves the brainstem at the junction of pons and medulla close to the midline (Figs 4.32 and 5.11). It runs upwards through the pontine cistern and pierces the meningeal dura mater lateral to the dorsum sellae. It continues upwards and then turns sharply forwards across the superior border of the petrous bone to enter the medial wall of the cavernous sinus. It leaves the cranial cavity through the superior orbital fissure. The nerve has a long course within the subarachnoid space and may be affected by raised intracranial pressure. The resulting medial squint (produced by paralysis of the lateral rectus muscle) is termed a **false localizing sign** because, although pressure is raised throughout the cranial cavity, the squint gives the impression of a lesion located specifically in the region of the abducent nerve.

The **facial** (VII) and **vestibulocochlear** (VIII) nerves leave the junction of pons and medulla lateral to the origin of the abducent nerve, with the facial nerve lying the more medially of the two (Figs 4.32 and 5.11). The facial nerve consists of a large motor root and a small sensory root, the latter sometimes referred to as **nervus intermedius** since it lies between the motor root and the vestibulocochlear nerve. All these nervous structures pass laterally to enter the internal acoustic meatus where the roots of the facial nerve are situated anterior to the vestibulocochlear nerve. At the lateral termination of the meatus the roots of the facial nerve enter the facial canal in the petrous bone. The vestibulocochlear nerve splits into vestibular and cochlear branches while still within the meatus. These branches pierce the plate of bone closing the lateral end of the meatus to gain access to the internal ear. Within the meatus the meningeal and endosteal layers of the dura are fused and the two nerves are sur-

rounded by the leptom...

The **glossopharyngeal** ... **root of the accessory** (XI) ... the anterolateral surface o... inferior cerebellar peduncle ... the occipital bone to leave th... foramen. The **spinal root of th...** series of rootlets emerging from ... of the cervical spinal cord. It runs u... through the foramen magnum (wh... arachnoid space) and unites with th... ...ar foramen.

The jugular foramen is divided into t... ...ents by two septa formed by the meningeal layer of th... ...ater. The glossopharyngeal nerve and inferior petrosal sin... traverse the anterior compartment, the vagus and accessory nerves pass through the middle compartment, and the posterior compartment is occupied by the sigmoid sinus.

The **hypoglossal nerve** (XII) arises by a series of rootlets from the anterior surface of the medulla between the pyramid and olive (Fig. 5.11). The rootlets are gathered into two bundles which pierce the dura separately opposite the hypoglossal canal and fuse to form a single trunk after their passage through the canal.

BLOOD VESSELS OF BRAIN

The brain is supplied with blood by two **internal carotid arteries** and two **vertebral arteries**. The internal carotid and vertebral systems connect with each other on the under surface of the brain by a circle of anastomotic vessels termed the **circulus arteriosus** (or **circle of Willis**). The venous return from the brain is generally into the nearest venous sinus of the dura mater.

During their intracranial course the arteries and veins of the brain run within the subarachnoid space. The arteries tend to lie deep in the sulci of the cerebral hemispheres while the veins travel more superficially over the gyri.

Arteries

The arteries supplying the brain are thin-walled, the tunica adventitia (the outermost fibrous coat) in particular being poorly developed or absent. Unlike the arteries supplying other organs, the cerebral arteries undergo repeated subdivision before they enter the brain. As a result the surface of the brain is covered by numerous, fine arteries which are readily ruptured.

Internal carotid artery

Having traversed the cavernous sinus, the internal carotid artery emerges through its roof medial to the anterior clinoid process and then turns to run posteriorly below the optic nerve to the anterior perforated substance (an area on the inferior surface of the cerebral hemisphere lateral to the optic chiasma) where it divides into **anterior** and **middle cerebral arteries.** Just above the point where it leaves the cavernous sinus the internal carotid artery gives off the **ophthalmic artery** which runs anterolaterally to enter the orbit through the optic canal. A short distance before its termination the internal carotid gives rise to the **posterior communicating artery.** This runs backwards above the oculomotor nerve to anastomose with the posterior cerebral artery.

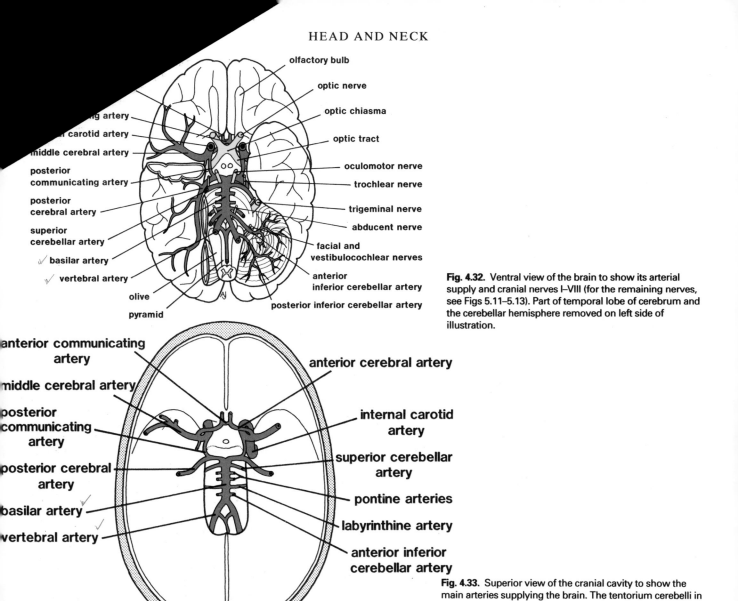

olfactory bulb

optic nerve

optic chiasma

optic tract

oculomotor nerve

trochlear nerve

trigeminal nerve

abducent nerve

facial and
vestibulocochlear nerves

anterior
inferior cerebellar artery

posterior inferior cerebellar artery

...ng artery

...carotid artery

middle cerebral artery

posterior
communicating artery

posterior
cerebral artery

superior
cerebellar artery

basilar artery

vertebral artery

olive

pyramid

Fig. 4.32. Ventral view of the brain to show its arterial supply and cranial nerves I–VIII (for the remaining nerves, see Figs 5.11–5.13). Part of temporal lobe of cerebrum and the cerebellar hemisphere removed on left side of illustration.

anterior communicating
artery

middle cerebral artery

posterior
communicating
artery

posterior cerebral
artery

basilar artery

vertebral artery

anterior cerebral artery

internal carotid
artery

superior cerebellar
artery

pontine arteries

labyrinthine artery

anterior inferior
cerebellar artery

Fig. 4.33. Superior view of the cranial cavity to show the main arteries supplying the brain. The tentorium cerebelli in place. On the right-hand side the roof of the cavernous sinus has been removed.

The anterior cerebral artery passes forwards and medially above the optic nerve to the longitudinal fissure separating the two cerebral hemispheres. Here it comes into close proximity with its fellow of the opposite side to which it is joined by the short **anterior communicating artery**. The anterior cerebral arteries then turn to run upwards and backwards, above the corpus callosum, across the medial surfaces of the corresponding hemispheres to their posterior extremities.

The middle cerebral artery, larger than the anterior branch, passes along the lateral cerebral sulcus to supply the lateral surface of the cerebral hemisphere.

Vertebral system

The **vertebral artery** is a branch of the subclavian artery. It ascends through the neck, in the foramina in the transverse processes of the upper six cervical vertebrae, winds around the lateral mass of the atlas and enters the cranial cavity through the foramen magnum. Here it pierces the dura and arachnoid mater and runs in the subarachnoid space upwards and medially in front of the rootlets of the hypoglossal nerve to join the artery of the opposite side at the lower border of the pons.

The artery so formed is the **basilar**. It ascends within the pontine cistern to the upper border of the pons where it divides into right and left **posterior cerebral arteries**.

Within the cranial cavity the vertebral artery gives rise to **spinal** branches which pass downwards to the spinal canal, a **posterior inferior cerebellar** branch to the cerebellum and **medullary** branches to the medulla oblongata. Arising from either side of the basilar artery are **pontine** branches, a **labyrinthine** branch to the internal ear, **anterior inferior** and **superior cerebellar** branches and the posterior cerebral artery.

Circulus arteriosus

The circulus is formed by the posterior cerebral arteries, posterior communicating arteries, internal carotid arteries, anterior cerebral arteries, and anterior communicating artery (see Fig. 4.33). It lies within the interpeduncular cistern surrounding the optic chiasma and pituitary stalk. The communicating vessels are small and are usually inadequate to maintain sufficient circulation to the brain if one or other of the internal carotid arteries is suddenly blocked. They are, however, capable of expanding if the blockage occurs more slowly so that an adequate cerebral blood supply may be maintained even if one or more of the feeders into the circulus should become completely occluded.

Veins

The veins returning blood from the brain are extremely thin-walled, possessing no muscular layer, and have no valves. They open into the venous sinuses of the dura mater. The cerebral veins comprise two groups, external and internal, draining respectively the outer and inner parts of the cerebral hemispheres. The **superior external veins** drain the superolateral and medial aspects of the hemispheres and open into the superior sagittal sinus. The **middle external vein** returns blood from the lateral surface of the hemisphere and opens into the cavernous sinus. The **inferior external veins** are small vessels which drain the inferior surface of the hemispheres and join the superior and middle external veins and the **basal vein**. The latter begins at the anterior perforated substance by the union of **anterior cerebral** (draining an area equivalent to that supplied by the artery of the same name), **deep middle cerebral** (draining the insula, see page 239) and **striate veins** (from the interior of the cerebral hemispheres) and opens into the great cerebral vein.

Right and left **internal cerebral veins** drain the choroid plexuses of the third and lateral ventricles. Below the posterior part of the corpus callosum they join together to form the **great cerebral vein**. This latter vessel runs upwards around the posterior edge of the corpus callosum, receives the right and left basal veins, and then joins the straight sinus.

The veins draining the cerebellum and brainstem open into the adjacent venous sinuses.

Clinical aspects – intracranial haemorrhage

Intracranial haemorrhage may occur either within or outside the brain. The former type of haemorrhage is discussed on page 244.

Intracranial haemorrhage occurring outside the brain may be into the extradural, subdural, or subarachnoid space. The extradural space, located between the endosteal and meningeal layers of the dura mater, is absent in many areas because of the fusion of the two dural layers. Haemorrhage into this space (extradural haemorrhage) is relatively uncommon and is usually the result of tearing of meningeal vessels or venous sinuses consequent upon fracture of the braincase. Because of the thinness of the bone and the proximity of the meningeal vessels, blows to the region of the pterion are particularly liable to lead to bleeding into the extradural space.

The subdural space is normally only a potential gap between the meningeal layer of the dura and the arachnoid mater. Bleeding into this space (subdural haemorrhage) is not, however, an uncommon event. It is usually the consequence of tearing of one or more of the superior cerebral veins at the point where they enter the superior sagittal sinus. Although the cerebral veins run for most of their extracerebral course in the subarachnoid space they traverse the arachnoid, subdural space, and meningeal layer of the dura to reach the venous sinus. In blows to the head the brain may be suddenly moved within the cranial cavity through a sufficient distance to tear the cerebral veins close to the point at which they are fixed by their passage through the dura mater. Blood then enters the subdural space.

The principal clinical features of extradural and sudural haemorrhage are the results of compression of the brain caused by the raised intracranial pressure. Their rate of onset is extremely variable.

Most haemorrhages into the subarachnoid space follow rupture of a congenital aneurism of one or other of the arteries comprising the circulus arteriosus. The principal clinical features of subarachnoid haemorrhage are those of meningeal irritation (extravasated blood being a powerful irritant).

CEREBROSPINAL FLUID

Cerebrospinal fluid is secreted into the ventricles of the brain by the choroid plexuses. It leaves the ventricular system by passing through the median and lateral apertures in the roof of the fourth ventricle and so enters the cerebellomedullary cistern. The fluid flows upwards into the subarachnoid space through the tentorial incisure and over the lateral aspects of the cerebral hemispheres. It re-enters the bloodstream through the arachnoid villi and granulations associated with the superior sagittal venous sinus and its venous lakes. There is no active flow of cerebrospinal fluid in the vertebral canal, the constituents in the spinal fluid being maintained at appropriate levels by the process of diffusion. Cerebrospinal fluid is a clear, colourless liquid maintained at a pressure of 50–150 mm of water. It contains inorganic salts similar to those in blood plasma and small amounts of protein and glucose. It also contains a few lymphocytes.

The principal functions of the cerebrospinal fluid are to provide mechanical support and nutrition for the central nervous system. It is also important in defending the central nervous system and meninges against infection.

The character of the fluid may change greatly in diseases of the central nervous system and meninges. The number of white blood cells rises in infections of these structures, the predominant cell type depending on the nature of the infecting organism. Bleeding into the cerebrospinal fluid, as occurs in subarachnoid haemorrhage, results in the presence of red blood cells. A rise in protein content occurs in many conditions including tumours of the brain and spinal cord. The pressure of the cerebrospinal fluid is increased, a condition known as **raised intracranial pressure**, in the presence of space-occupying lesions (such as tumours) within the cranial cavity or vertebral canal.

Alterations in the character of the cerebrospinal fluid are clearly of value in diagnosing neurological disease. A sample of fluid for examination can be obtained by means of a lumbar puncture (p. 224).

3

Superficial structures of head and neck

SURFACE ANATOMY

Facial appearance varies markedly from one individual to another. Part of this variation reflects differences in the contours of the skull but of greater importance are the disposition of the soft tissues, the amount and arrangement of the hair and the play of the muscles of facial expression. These muscles are also responsible for the rapid changes in facial appearance which occur in the individual in response to alterations in mood and emotions and which are of such great importance in the social life of our species.

The appearance of the head also changes greatly with age. Before puberty the braincase completes much more of its growth than does the facial skeleton. In consequence the face remains relatively small and the facial features undeveloped giving the characteristic 'childish' appearance. With the onset of the adolescent growth spurt there is an acceleration of growth in the facial skeleton, unaccompanied by any corresponding acceleration in the braincase, as a result of which the head rapidly attains its adult proportions and the facial features become more strongly emphasized. The sex differences in facial appearance become fully established during adolescence because of the differential effects of the sex hormones in boys and girls on the growth of the facial skeleton and on such features as the development of muscle and fat and the growth of hair.

Facial appearance changes less rapidly in adult life. Up to middle age there is usually some increase in the heaviness of the features resulting from continued small amounts of growth in the facial skeleton and the accumulation of fat. In old age the face tends to develop a shrunken appearance. This results partly from some loss of bone from the facial skeleton but of much greater significance are the wasting of the muscles of the face, the changes in the skin, hair, and connective tissue that accompany advancing age, and, in many individuals, the loss of some or all of the teeth.

Despite all these variations the surface relationships of the major structures of the head and neck change little after infancy. Before describing these it will probably be helpful to give a brief survey of the general arrangement of the structures of the head and neck.

The head comprises the braincase and face. Posteriorly the neck extends up to the floor of the braincase (i.e. to the posterior part of the cranial base and the occipital region of the vault of the skull). Anteriorly the face intervenes and the neck ends at the level of the **mylohyoid muscles** which stretch like a diaphragm from the hyoid bone to the medial surface of the mandibular body and form the mobile lower boundary of the floor of the mouth.

The neck is supported by the cervical part of the vertebral column.

Attached to the back of the column is the large mass of **extensor vertebral muscles**. Attached to the front is the smaller **flexor vertebral musculature** and on each side are the **lateral vertebral muscles** running from the cervical vertebrae to the first and second ribs. In front of the flexor musculature are the viscera of the neck. Most anteriorly in the median plane are the **larynx** and its downward continuation the **trachea**. Between these and the flexor muscles is the **pharynx** leading downwards into the **oesophagus**. Either side of the midline viscera are the **carotid sheaths**, each containing the **carotid artery, internal jugular vein,** and **vagus nerve**. Closely applied to the front and sides of the upper part of the trachea is the **thyroid gland**.

Above the larynx is the **hyoid bone**. This is attached by muscles to the mandible and base of skull above and to the sternum and scapula below.

Running obliquely across each side of the neck from the mastoid process to the sternum and clavicle is the strap-like **sternocleido-mastoid muscle**. Lying superficial to the extensor muscles on the back of the neck is a sheet of muscle formed by the upper parts of the **trapezius muscles** of the two sides.

The **subcutaneous tissue (superficial fascia)** of the head and neck is variable in its degree of development but tends, in general, to be rather thinner and contain less fat than in the trunk. It is particularly dense in the scalp where it consists of a layer of strong connective tissue uniting skin and deep fascia. It is virtually absent from the external ears. In the face, scalp, and anterior part of the neck the subcutaneous layer contains sheets of muscle, the **muscles of facial expression** and related groups, which act to move the skin and which represent part of the skin-twitching musculature found over most of the body in lower mammals.

The **deep fascia** is well developed in the neck where it forms an investing layer, situated immediately beneath the subcutaneous tissue and arranged like a cylinder around the deeper structures, and also provides sheaths for many of the muscles and viscera. The deep fascia is also strongly developed in the scalp where it is called the **epicranial aponeurosis**. Over most of the face the deep fascia is absent.

In studying the surface features of the head and neck it is best to choose a young adult subject without facial hair. Start your examination at the root of the neck where, following the instructions given on pages 77 and 79, you should identify the **clavicles, suprasternal notch** and **acromion** and **spinous processes of the scapulae.** Running obliquely upwards from the junction of the middle and lateral thirds of the clavicle to the **superior nuchal line** on the occipital region of the skull is the lateral margin of the upper part of the **trapezius muscle.** You

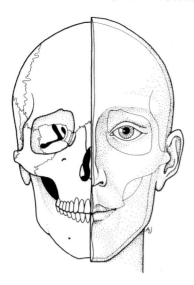

Fig. 4.34. Relationship between the skull and the surface features of the face.

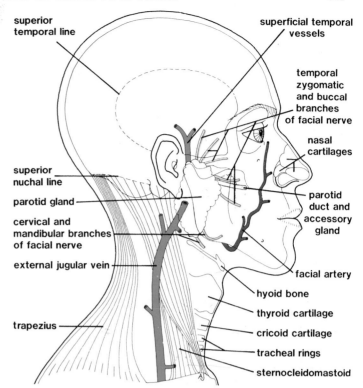

Fig. 4.35. To show the surface markings of some of the structures of the head and neck.

should be able to see or feel the lower part of this margin, especially if the shoulders are raised, but superiorly the muscle thins considerably and its edge may not be identifiable.

Two rounded ridges can be seen passing up the back of the neck either side of the midline. These are produced by the **semispinalis muscles,** part of the extensor group of vertebral muscles. The **sternocleidomastoid muscle** can be made to stand out by turning the head towards the opposite side against resistance. Note its lower attachments to the sternum and medial one-third of the clavicle and its upper attachment to the **mastoid process** which forms a readily visible and palpable bony landmark behind the lobe of the ear. Between the posterior border of the sternocleidomastoid muscle and the lateral edge of trapezius is a triangular area, called the **posterior triangle,** with its base at the middle one-third of the clavicle and its apex just behind the mastoid process.

The **deep cervical lymph nodes** lie alongside the **internal jugular vein** deep to the sternocleidomastoid muscle. A few **superficial cervical nodes** are arranged about the **external jugular vein** which crosses the superficial aspect of the muscle. This vein can usually be seen as a narrow elevation running from the region behind the angle of the mandible to the clavicle lateral to the sternocleidomastoid attachment. The cervical lymph nodes are not normally palpable but may become so in infections in their areas of drainage or if infiltrated by metastases from malignant tumours.

The **platysma** is a broad sheet of muscle which is situated in the subcutaneous tissues over the upper part of the thorax, side of the neck and lower part of the face. It can be demonstrated by forcefully drawing down the lower lip and angle of the mouth when its anterior portion will be seen to wrinkle the skin below the mandible. The muscle is variable in its degree of development and may be absent.

In the lower part of the posterior midline of the neck the **spinous processes** of the **seventh cervical** and **first thoracic vertebrae** are easily recognized. The spinous processes of the remaining cervical vertebrae can be felt by deep pressure in the groove between the semispinalis muscles. At the top of this groove is the easily palpable **external occipital protuberance** of the occipital bone.

The **laryngeal prominence of the thyroid cartilage** lies in the anterior midline of the neck at the level of C5. It is usually much more conspicuous in adult men than in women and children, hence its more familiar name of 'Adam's apple'. If you run your finger down the anterior border of the thyroid cartilage, below the laryngeal prominence, you will come to its lower border. Immediately below this the **arch of the cricoid cartilage** (opposite C6) can be felt. Now continue to run your finger down the anterior midline of the neck to the **suprasternal notch** noting the cartilage rings in the wall of the trachea. About 1 cm below the arch of the cricoid (at the level of the second to fourth tracheal rings) you may be able to feel the **isthmus of the thyroid gland** crossing the front of the trachea. The relationships of the larynx and trachea are particularly important to any one who has charge of unconscious (e.g. anaesthetized) patients because of the occasional need to carry out the life-saving operation of tracheostomy (see p. 204).

The main lobes of the thyroid gland lie deep to the infrahyoid muscles with their upper poles reaching to the level of the middle of the thyroid cartilage and their lower poles to a level just above the sternal ends of the clavicles. The gland is, however, variable in both its size and position (sometimes not being located in the neck at all, see page 49). It may become greatly enlarged in pathological states, a condition known as goitre.

In thin subjects the hyoid bone (opposite C4) is palpable a short distance above the laryngeal prominence. Note that the **greater cornua** extend posteriorly as far as the anterior border of the sternocleidomastoid muscle. Above the hyoid bone are the **inferior**

border of the body and angle of the mandible. The **submandibular lymph nodes** lie just under cover of the posterior part of the inferior border while in an equivalent position behind the mental protuberance are the **submental nodes**. They may be enlarged in infections of their areas of drainage (which include most of the oral structures).

Now turn your attention to the face and braincase. Note the upper and lower **eyelids**, the **palpebral fissures** (the gaps between the lids) and the **eyelashes**. Near the medial end of each eyelid is a small prominence, the **lacrimal papilla**, on the summit of which can be seen the opening, or **punctum**, of a **lacrimal canaliculus** through which tears drain from the eye. At the medial angle, or **medial canthus**, of the eye, the eyelids are separated by a small space called the **lacrimal lake**. Its floor is formed by a pinkish fold of skin, the **lacrimal caruncle**.

In members of the mongoloid ethnic group the medial canthus of the eye is covered by a small fold of skin called the **epicanthal fold**.

Examine the lips noting their free **red borders** and the presence of a broad groove, the **philtrum**, running down the midline of the upper lip.

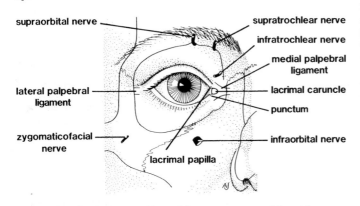

Fig. 4.36. Surface markings of the structures around the orbit.

The upper part or bridge of the external nose has a rigid skeleton provided by the bony part of the nasal septum and the nasal bones. Its lower part is more flexible because both the septum and side walls (the **alae of the nostrils**) in this region have a cartilaginous skeleton.

The external ear, also called the **pinna or auricle**, surrounds the opening of the **external acoustic meatus**. This is some 2–3 cm long and terminates medially at the tympanic membrane. The lateral part of the meatus has a cartilaginous wall and the medial part a bony wall. A small flap of skin and cartilage, the **tragus**, partially covers the opening of the meatus. Each of the many folds of the auricle is named but these names are of no significance to the dental student.

The **zygomatic arch** can be palpated from the lateral wall of the orbit to the anterior border of the tragus. The superficial surface of the arch is subcutaneous throughout its length. From the lower border of the arch arises the masseter muscle which can be felt as a fleshy mass extending downwards to the angle of the mandible. The muscle can be made to stand out by clenching the jaws. The temporal fascia is attached to the upper border of the arch. The fascia extends upwards and posteriorly to the **superior temporal line** which may be palpable as a faint ridge arching round on the side of the braincase. When the jaws are clenched the **temporalis muscle** can be felt contracting beneath the temporal fascia.

A considerable amount of fat is often present in the cheek in front of the masseter muscle. It is especially well developed in infants where it is called the **suckling pad.**

Beneath the posterior part of the zygomatic arch just in front of the tragus, the **head of the mandible** can be felt. When the mandible is depressed the head slides forwards and downwards on the **articular tubercle.**

The **anterior rim of the orbital cavity** can be palpated around its entire extent. About 2–3 cm from the midline of the face the superior border of the orbit is indented by the **supraorbital notch** (or foramen), for the transmission of the correspondingly named nerve and vessels. The superciliary arches (eyebrow ridges) are easily recognizable immediately above the superior orbital borders.

The **infraorbital foramen** lies about ½ cm below the inferior orbital border on a line drawn from the supraorbital notch to the interval between the first and second premolar teeth. The **mental foramen** lies on a downward continuation of this line about 1 cm above the inferior border of the mandible.

The **parotid gland** occupies the wedge-shaped space between the ramus of the mandible in front and the mastoid process and the attached sternocleidomastoid muscle behind. Its approximate extent is shown in Fig. 4.35. The course of the **parotid duct** is indicated by the central section of a line drawn from the lower margin of the tragus to a point midway between the lower border of the external nose and the red border of the upper lip. The duct opens into the vestibule of the mouth opposite the crown of the second upper molar tooth.

Five branches of the **facial nerve** leave the anterior border of the parotid gland and radiate outwards to the temporal, zygomatic, buccal, and mandibular parts of the face and to the upper part of the neck.

The **scalp** is the hair-bearing area extending over the vault of the skull from the nape of the neck to the forehead and downwards on each side into the temple. It contains a dense sheet of deep fascia, the epicranial aponeurosis, to each corner of which is attached a muscle belly, the aponeurosis and four muscle bellies together making up the **occipitofrontalis muscle**. As a result many people can move the scalp backwards and forwards to some extent although the principal function of occipitofrontalis is to raise the eyebrows and wrinkle the forehead.

A number of arteries can be seen or felt in the head and neck and the course of a number of others represented by lines drawn with reference to surface landmarks. The course of the **common carotid artery** can be indicated by a line drawn from the sternoclavicular joint to a point 1 cm below the greater cornu of the hyoid bone. Deep to this point the artery bifurcates. Throughout its course in the neck it lies in the **carotid sheath** deep to the sternocleidomastoid muscle. The **external carotid artery** continues upwards from the bifurcation of the common carotid artery along a line passing immediately behind the angle and then the neck of the mandible. It enters the parotid gland where it ends by dividing into **maxillary** and **superficial temporal arteries**. The **internal carotid artery** runs on a deeper plane than the external carotid artery continuing upwards in the carotid sheath along a line drawn from the bifurcation of the common carotid artery through the head of the mandible.

The **facial artery** arises from the external carotid artery a little above the level of the hyoid bone. It becomes superficial as it crosses the inferior border of the mandible to enter the face. It makes this crossing at the anterior border of the masseter muscle (this can be made more readily palpable by clenching the jaws) where its pulsations can be felt. From here it pursues a tortuous course towards the medial canthus of the eye, passing about 1 cm from the angle of the mouth. The accompanying vein is less tortuous.

The pulsations of the **superficial temporal artery** can be felt above and behind the head of the mandible immediately in front of the external ear. Some distance above this point it divides into anterior and posterior branches which can sometimes be seen, especially in elderly bald men, following tortuous courses and branching within the subcutaneous tissue of the temple.

Small groups of lymph nodes are found at several sites within the head. These comprise: (i) the **parotid nodes** situated within and on the lateral surface of the gland, (ii) the **buccal group** located in the cheek close to the facial vein, (iii) a few **retroauricular nodes** lying superficial to the upper attachment of the sternocleidomastoid muscle, and (iv) the **occipital nodes** on the attachment of trapezius to the occipital region of the skull. The lymph from these nodes drains into the cervical nodes already described.

SCALP

Layers

The scalp consists of five layers. In order, from superficial to deep, these are: (i) **skin** (with numerous hair follicles), (ii) **dense subcutaneous tissue**, (iii) **occipitofrontalis muscle** and associated **epicranial aponeurosis** (the deep fascia of the scalp), (iv) **loose subaponeurotic layer** (v) **periosteum** (sometimes referred to as **pericranium** in this situation). Of these five layers only the third needs further description.

Occipitofrontalis muscle and epicranial aponeurosis

The occipitofrontalis muscle consists of two occipital and two frontal bellies connected over the cranial vault by the epicranial aponeurosis (Fig. 4.38). The occipital belly arises from the highest nuchal line on the ectocranial surface of the occipital region of the cranial vault. Its fibres run upwards and forwards to be inserted into the posterolateral border of the epicranial aponeurosis. In addition a few fibres are attached to the skin of the scalp. The frontal belly arises from the anterior lateral margin of the aponeurosis and is inserted into the skin of the corresponding eyebrow and into the orbicularis oculi muscle. The epicranial aponeurosis is a sheet of strong connective tissue which covers the vertex of the skull between the occipital and frontal bellies. It is firmly attached to the skin of the scalp by the dense subcutaneous layer. Laterally it fades out above the ears.

The occipitofrontalis muscle is derived from the mesoderm of the second pharyngeal arch and is supplied, therefore, by the facial nerve, the nerve of that arch (the occipital belly by the posterior auricular branch and the frontal belly by the superior zygomatic branch). The principal action of the occipital bellies is to fix the epicranial aponeurosis so allowing the frontal bellies to elevate the eyebrows.

Blood supply

The scalp is supplied with blood by the **occipital, posterior auricular, and superficial temporal branches** of the **external carotid arteries.** These branches, which run in the subcutaneous layer, have very

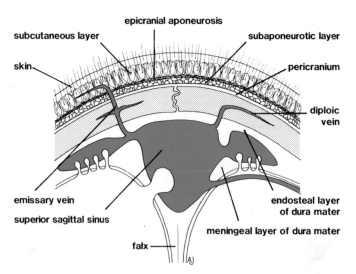

Fig. 4.37. Coronal section through the scalp over the cranial vault. A communication between the veins of the scalp and the intracranial venous sinuses is shown.

tortuous courses and anastomose freely with each other. The venous drainage follows the arterial supply. The veins of the scalp are in communication with the intracranial venous sinuses through a number of emissary veins. The most constant is the parietal emissary vein which passes through the parietal foramen to open into the superior sagittal sinus (Fig. 4.37).

Sensory innervation

The posterior part of the scalp receives its sensory nerve supply through the **greater occipital** and **third occipital nerves** (the posterior primary rami of the second and third cervical spinal nerves respectively). The region above and behind the ear is supplied by the **lesser occipital nerve** (from the cervical plexus) and the temple region by the **auriculotemporal nerve** (a branch of the mandibular division of the trigeminal nerve). The forehead and front of the scalp are innervated by the **supratrochlear** and **supraorbital nerves** (from the frontal branch of the ophthalmic division of the trigeminal nerve). Like the vessels the nerves run in the subcutaneous layer of the scalp.

Clinical aspects

The skin, subcutaneous tissue and epicranial aponeurosis are so firmly united that in scalping injuries they are always torn away as a single layer. The blood vessels, which lie in the subcutaneous tissue, do not contract and so tend to bleed profusely. Because of the rich anastomoses between the arteries flaps of scalp usually retain sufficient blood supply to prevent sloughing.

FACE

Superficial muscles

Like occipitofrontalis, the superficial muscles of the face are derived from the mesoderm of the second pharyngeal arch and receive their motor innervation from the facial nerve (their proprioceptive supply is believed to come from the trigeminal nerve through its connections with the terminal branches of the facial nerve). Many of these muscles take origin from the bones of the facial skeleton and are inserted into the dermis of the skin. Consequently there is no deep fascia in the face.

Although each of the many muscles making up this group has been individually described and named there is no practical reason for committing much of this detail to memory, especially as far as the smaller slips of muscle are concerned. It is of more value, and certainly much easier, to think of them as forming groups, each composed of constrictors and dilators, around each of the orifices of the face. The only important muscle which does not fit completely into such a scheme is buccinator, the muscle of the cheek.

The principal action of the superficial muscles of the face is to control the size of the orifices with which they are associated. In many mammals, and especially in man and other higher primates, they have the further important function of controlling facial expression and are often referred to in human anatomy as **muscles of facial expression**.

There are several small muscles associated with the external ears. These too are derived from the second pharyngeal arch and are innervated by the facial nerve. They are virtually functionless in man and are not described further.

Muscles of the lips

The sphincter of the lips is **orbicularis oris**. It consists of circular fibres surrounding the orifice of the mouth. Some of its fibres are contained entirely within the lips while others are contributed from the dilator muscles and especially from buccinator. The central fibres of buccinator decussate at the corner of the mouth so that those from above pass to the lower lip and vice versa. Several of the dilator muscles converge at the corner of the mouth and interlace with the fibres of buccinator and orbicularis oris. The knot of muscle so produced is termed the **modiolus**. Many of the fibres that are contained entirely within orbicularis oris pass obliquely through the thickness of the lips from the dermis of the skin on the outer labial surface to the mucous membrane on the inner aspect. Contraction of orbicularis oris compresses the lips against the teeth as well as closing the oral orifice.

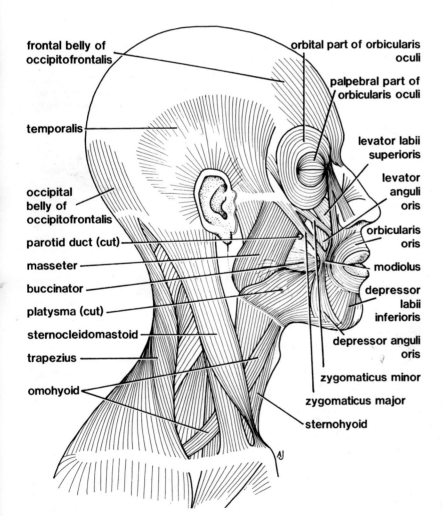

Fig. 4.38. The superficial muscles of the head and neck.

The major dilators of the mouth comprise the following. (i) **Levator labii superioris** arises from the bones of the inferior orbital rim above the infraorbital foramen and runs downwards to mingle with the fibres of orbicularis oris in the upper lip. (ii) **Levator anguli oris** takes origin from the canine fossa below the infraorbital foramen and is inserted into orbicularis oris lateral to levator labii superioris. (iii) **Zygomaticus major and minor** lie in a more superficial plane than the two preceding muscles, running from the zygomatic process of the maxilla and the zygomatic bone to the modiolus and upper lip. (iv) **Depressor labii inferioris** arises from the mandible anterior to the mental foramen and is inserted into the muscle and skin of the lower lip. (v) **Depressor anguli oris** arises from the mandible below depressor labii inferioris and runs superficial to that muscle to mingle with the modiolus.

A small slip of muscle, the **mentalis**, passes from the front of the mandible near to the midline to be inserted into the skin of the chin. It lies just to the side of the frenulum of the lower lip and is of some significance in that its contraction may dislodge a lower denture.

Also blending with orbicularis oris are some fibres of **platysma**.

Muscle of the cheek

Buccinator arises from the maxilla and mandible adjacent to the molar teeth and from the pterygomandibular raphe and pterygoid hamulus behind the last molar teeth. The lines of origin from the maxilla and mandible lie just above the reflections of the mucous membrane in the upper and lower buccal sulci. The position of these lines of attachment must be borne in mind when making dentures because if the edge of the denture impinges on the buccinator muscle it will be dislodged by movements of the cheek. The bulk of the buccinator muscle lies in the cheek but posteriorly the fibres arising from the pterygomandibular raphe cross behind the last molars and in front of the coronoid process of the mandible. At the raphe its fibres interdigitate with those of the superior constrictor muscle of the pharynx. From their origins the fibres run horizontally forwards, forming a sheet of muscle within the cheek, to mingle in the lips with orbicularis oris. The central fibres decussate at the modiolus but the upper and lower fibres continue into the corresponding lip without decussation.

Buccinator compresses the cheeks against the teeth and, with the cheeks first distended with air, is used in the acts of blowing and whistling.

Muscles of the eyelids

The sphincter of the eye is **orbicularis oculi.** It has two parts. The **palpebral part** is confined to the eyelids. Its fibres arch across the upper and lower lids, in front of the tarsal plates, passing between the medial and lateral palpebral ligaments (Figs. 4.36 and 4.60). The **orbital part** of the muscle is much larger and surrounds the palpebral part. Its fibres arise from the crest of the lacrimal bone, the frontal process of the maxilla and the neighbouring part of the frontal bone and run in concentric loops, many inserting into the skin of the eyebrow. The palpebral part of the muscle closes the eyes gently, as in blinking, whereas the orbital part is concerned with more forcible closure, as in 'screwing up' the eyes. Reflex closing of the eyes usually involves just the palpebral component.

The principal dilators of the palpebral fissure are **levator palpebrae superioris** (one of the muscles of the orbit, see page 166) and **occipitofrontalis.**

Muscles of the nostrils

There are weak compressors and dilators of the nostrils. The soft part of the nose can be raised to a limited extent by small levator muscles. These muscles are of little clinical consequence.

Parotid gland

This, the largest of the salivary glands, is mainly serous but contains a few scattered mucous acini. It lies below the external acoustic meatus wedged between the mandibular ramus in front and the mastoid process and sternocleidomastoid muscle behind. It has four surfaces. The small superior surface is related to the cartilaginous part of the external acoustic meatus and the posterior aspect of the capsule of the temporomandibular joint. A small part of the gland, termed the **glenoid lobe,** projects medially between the joint and the meatus. The anteromedial surface abuts on the posterior borders of the mandibular ramus and the attached masseter and medial pterygoid muscles. The posteromedial surface is related to the mastoid process and the upper part of the anterior border of sternocleidomastoid. The superficial surface is flattened and is covered by subcutaneous tissue and skin. The superficial part of the gland is extended to overlap the masseter in front and the sternocleidomastoid behind. The part overlying masseter may be separated from the remainder of the gland and is then termed the **accessory part** of the gland.

The gland lies within a well defined **parotid capsule** formed by diverging leaves of the deep cervical fascia.

Innervation

The parotid gland receives its parasympathetic supply through a complex pathway. The preganglionic fibres begin in the inferior salivatory nucleus in the medulla, leave the brainstem in the glosso-pharyngeal nerve and pass through its tympanic branch, the tympanic plexus, and the lesser petrosal nerve to the otic ganglion where they synapse with postganglionic fibres which pass to the gland in the auriculotemporal nerve.

The sympathetic supply to the gland is from the superior cervical ganglion of the sympathetic trunk. Postganglionic neurons travel from the ganglion to the gland in the plexus on the external carotid artery. The preganglionic neurons which relay in the ganglion begin in the upper thoracic segments of the spinal cord.

Stimulation of the parasympathetic innervation leads to the production of copious saliva rich in mucus and enzymes. Sympathetic stimulation, on the other hand, results in a reduced secretion of saliva which is low in organic content. The nature of the nerve endings in the gland is still debated. There is some evidence that both parasympathetic and sympathetic fibres end in direct contact with the myoepithelial cells. It is also possible that their effects are mediated by vasomotor changes.

Note that the facial nerve, which passes through the gland, does not supply it.

Parotid duct

The duct draining the gland begins by the confluence of tributaries within the anterior part of the gland. It emerges from the anterior border of the gland and runs forwards across masseter below the accessory part of the gland, if present. At the front edge of masseter it turns medially, pierces buccinator and opens on the oral surface of and cheek opposite the crown of the second upper molar (Figs 4.35 and 4.86, p. 188).

Structures within the gland

Three major non-glandular structures traverse the gland. From deep to superficial these are as follows (Figs 4.39, 4.40, and 4.72, p. 178).

1. The **external carotid artery** enters the gland through the lower part of its posteromedial surface. Within the gland the artery divides into its two terminal branches – the maxillary artery which leaves the gland through its anteromedial surface and the superficial temporal artery which leaves through the upper part of the superficial surface.

2. The **retromandibular vein** is formed, usually within the gland, by the union of maxillary and superficial temporal veins. It runs downwards lateral to the external carotid artery and in the lower part of the gland or after emerging therefrom splits into anterior and posterior divisions. The posterior division joins the posterior auricular vein to form the external jugular vein; the anterior division joins the facial vein.

3. The **facial nerve** enters the upper part of the posteromedial surface of the gland, runs forwards, superficial to the retromandibular vein, and divides into five branches (some may be multiple) which leave the anteromedial surface of the gland to supply the muscles of facial expression. Connections between these branches form a network called the parotid plexus.

The **auriculotemporal nerve**, as it passes behind the temporomandibular joint runs through the glenoid lobe of the parotid gland or within its covering fascia.

Blood supply and drainage

Blood reaches the gland through the external carotid artery and the branches given off within the gland. Venous drainage is to the external jugular vein. Lymph drains to the parotid nodes and thence to the deep cervical nodes.

Clinical aspects

Like other salivary glands the parotid gland may become inflamed. The commonest cause of this is mumps (epidemic parotitis), a viral infection which occurs most frequently in children. Acute and chronic parotitis may also result from infections ascending from the mouth through the parotid duct. When inflamed the gland is usually swollen and painful and, in chronic cases, the flow of saliva is reduced. A swollen gland may also be due to a stone (calculus) lodged in the duct. The significance of the parotid gland and its contents in inferior alveolar block local anaesthesia is described on page 177.

Benign and malignant tumours of the parotid gland are encountered. One of the commonest types of tumour is a pleomorphic adenoma, or mixed parotid tumour, which is locally invasive but does not usually metastasize. In operating to remove a tumour care must be taken to avoid damaging the facial nerve, although this may be un-avoidable with resulting paralysis of the facial muscles on that side. Facial paralysis may also result from an unoperated tumour invading the facial nerve.

Facial nerve

The facial nerve leaves the skull through the **stylomastoid foramen.** After giving the **posterior auricular branch** to the occipital belly of occipitofrontalis and auricular muscles, and a branch to the posterior belly of digastric and the stylohyoid muscle, the nerve enters the parotid gland and divides into five or more branches which are inter-connected to form the **parotid plexus.**

The five branches emerge from the anteromedial surface of the gland and then run forward across the face to supply the muscles of facial expression. They are: (i) the **temporal branch** which leaves the upper part of the parotid gland, crosses the zygomatic arch and supplies muscles of the external ear and part of frontalis; (ii) the **zygomatic branch** (often double) runs forwards to supply the remainder of frontalis, the two parts of orbicularis oculi and adjacent muscles; (iii) the **buccal branch** (again often double) to the buccinator, the upper half of the orbicularis oris and the dilator muscles inserting into the upper lip; (iv) the **mandibular branch** which emerges from the lower border of the gland, passes into the neck across the lower border of the angle of the mandible, runs forwards a short distance, and then crosses back into the face at the anterior border of the masseter muscle to supply the muscles of the lower lip; (v) the **cervical branch** which runs vertically downwards behind the angle of the mandible to supply platysma.

The first four of these branches of the facial nerve make numerous connections with cutaneous branches of the three divisions of the trigeminal nerve while the cervical branch communicates with the transverse cutaneous nerve (a branch of the cervical plexus). It is thought that proprioceptive fibres for the muscles of facial expression and platysma pass from the trigeminal and cervical spinal nerves to the facial branches in these connections.

As can be seen from Fig. 4.39 the branches of the facial nerve

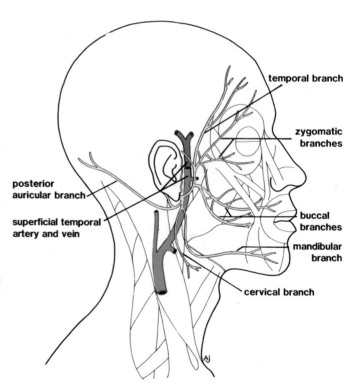

Fig. 4.39. The facial nerve in the face. The substance of the parotid gland has been removed to display the structures passing through it.

radiate outwards across the face and neck from the parotid gland. Incisions made in the face and neck should be in a direction parallel to these branches in order to reduce the likelihood of cutting them.

Blood supply

The face is supplied principally by the facial and superficial temporal arteries, both branches of the external carotid artery, while the forehead region is supplied by the supraorbital and supratrochlear branches of the ophthalmic artery. Blood also reaches the face through the infraorbital, masseteric, buccal, and mental arteries.

Facial artery

The facial artery, the most superior of the three branches which leave the anterior aspect of the external carotid artery in the neck, begins adjacent to the lateral wall of the pharynx. It passes upwards, deep to the posterior belly of the digastric muscle, and then arches over the superior aspect of the submandibular gland to run downwards again to the lower border of the mandible. It hooks around the latter at the anterior border of the masseter muscle piercing the deep fascia, and passes into the face. The artery then runs forwards and upwards following a tortuous course towards the inner angle of the eye. Its course is relatively superficial, passing deep to platysma and the two zygomaticus muscles but superficial to buccinator, levator anguli oris, and levator labii superioris. The artery is crossed by the branches of the facial nerve.

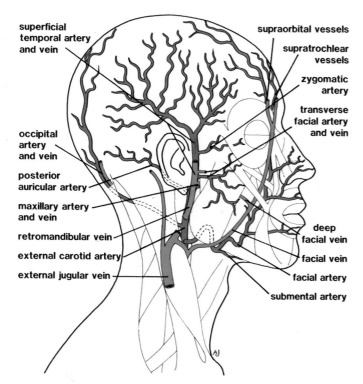

Fig. 4.40. The superficial arteries of the head. The parotid gland has been removed. Most of the veins accompanying the arteries have also been removed.

In the face the artery gives branches to the cheek, upper and lower lip and nose. There are numerous free anastomoses across the midline with corresponding vessels of the opposite side so that a severed artery in the face will bleed copiously from both cut ends. The pulse of the facial artery can be felt where the vessel crosses the lower border of the mandible just in front of the anterior border of the masseter muscle.

Superficial temporal artery

This is the smaller of the two terminal branches of the external carotid artery (the other being the maxillary artery). It begins in the parotid gland immediately behind the neck of the mandible, runs upwards across the posterior root of the zygomatic process of the temporal bone and then divides into anterior and posterior branches. It is crossed by the upper branches of the facial nerve within the parotid gland and accompanied in the scalp by the corresponding veins and the auriculotemporal nerve. Before dividing into its terminal branches the artery gives off several branches. These include: (i) the **transverse facial artery** which arises in the parotid gland and runs forwards across the masseter muscle supplying the gland and its duct and the masseter muscle; (ii) branches to the external ear; (iii) the **zygomatic artery** which runs along the upper border of the zygomatic arch towards the lateral angle of the eye supplying adjacent muscles; (iv) the **middle temporal artery** which arises above the zygomatic arch, pierces the temporal fascia and supplies, together with the deep temporal branch of the maxillary artery, the temporalis muscle. The terminal anterior and posterior branches supply the frontal and parietal regions of the scalp respectively.

Supraorbital and supratrochlear arteries

These arise from the ophthalmic artery within the orbit. They hook around the superior orbital rim, with the supraorbital artery (in the supraorbital notch or foramen) lying lateral to the supratrochlear branch. They ascend over the forehead, accompanied by correspondingly named veins and nerves (the latter being branches of the ophthalmic division of the trigeminal nerve), to supply the skin, muscle and pericranium of that region.

Facial veins

Most of the blood from the face returns by superficial channels. The forehead is drained by **supratrochlear** and **supraorbital veins** which pass downwards towards the inner angle of the eye where they fuse to form the **facial vein.** This vein runs downwards and backwards in company with, and just posterior to, the facial artery but following a less tortuous course. It receives tributaries corresponding to the branches of the facial artery. On the anterior part of the masseter muscle the facial vein crosses the lower border of the mandible, passes through the deep fascia and enters the neck. Here it is joined by the anterior division of the retromandibular vein and then drains into the internal jugular vein. A communication channel, the **deep facial vein,** connects the facial vein with the pterygoid plexus. It leaves the facial vein before the latter crosses on to the lateral surface of the masseter and runs deep to the muscle and to the mandibular ramus to reach the pterygoid plexus within the infratemporal fossa.

The **superficial temporal vein** is formed by numerous tributaries draining a wide area of the scalp. Just above the zygomatic arch it receives the **middle temporal vein** from the temporalis muscle and a little below this level the **transverse facial vein** from the side of the face. It then enters the parotid gland where it unites with the maxillary vein to form the **retromandibular vein.**

The retromandibular vein descends within the parotid gland, deep to the facial nerve but superficial to the external carotid artery. While still within the gland or after emerging from it the vein splits into anterior and posterior divisions. The anterior division passes forwards to join the facial vein as already described. The posterior division continues more directly downwards and is joined, either within or just outside the gland, by the **posterior auricular vein** to form the **external jugular vein.**

Cutaneous innervation

The skin of the face is supplied by the terminal branches of the three divisions of the trigeminal nerve.

Cutaneous branches of ophthalmic division

The area supplied by these branches includes the upper eyelid, the forehead region, and the external surface of the nose. There are five cutaneous branches of the ophthalmic division comprising: (i) the **lacrimal nerve** to the skin and conjunctiva of the lateral part of the upper eyelid; (ii) the **supraorbital nerve** to the lateral part of the forehead and frontal part of the scalp; (iii) the **supratrochlear nerve** to the medial part of the forehead; (iv) the **infratrochlear nerve** to the medial part of the upper eyelid; (v) the **external nasal nerve** to the skin of the nose.

Cutaneous branches of maxillary division

The large **infraorbital nerve,** the continuation of the main trunk of the maxillary nerve, emerges from the infraorbital foramen and breaks up into numerous branches which supply the lower eyelid, the upper lip and the upper part of the cheek as well as the adjacent mucous membrane of the mouth. The connections between the infraorbital nerve and the nearby branches of the facial nerve form the small **infraorbital plexus.**

The small **zygomaticofacial** and **zygomaticotemporal** nerves supply an area of skin lateral to that supplied by the infrabital nerve. The zygomaticofacial nerve emerges into the face through one or more foramina on the lateral surface of the zygomatic bone. The zygomaticotemporal nerve enters the temporal fossa through a foramen in the posterior surface of the zygomatic bone and then pierces the temporal fascia a short distance above the zygomatic arch to reach the face.

Cutaneous branches of mandibular division

The cutaneous branches of the mandibular division of the trigeminal nerve supply an extensive area including the chin, lower lip, much of the lower part of the cheek, the skin in front of the external ear, and the lower part of the temple.

The **auriculotemporal nerve** ascends from behind the neck of the mandible, over the posterior root of the zygomatic process of the temporal bone, to supply the temple, part of the skin lining the external acoustic meatus, the superficial aspect of the ear drum, and the upper part of the auricle.

The **buccal nerve** runs forwards from under cover of the mandibular ramus on to the buccinator muscle which it then pierces. It supplies the skin and the mucous membrane lining the cheek.

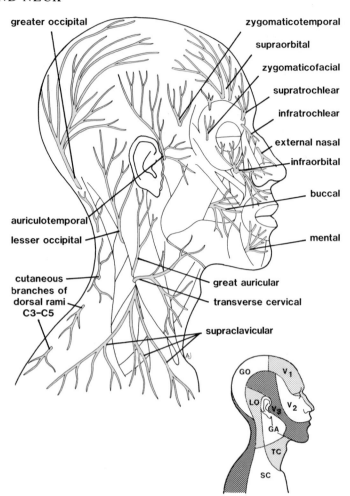

Fig. 4.41. The cutaneous innervation of the head and neck.

The **mental nerve** is the cutaneous branch of the inferior alveolar nerve. It emerges from the mandibular canal through the mental foramen and then breaks up into several branches which supply the skin and mucous membrane of the lower lip.

TEMPOROMANDIBULAR JOINT AND TEMPORALIS AND MASSETER MUSCLES

The temporomandibular joints are the only freely movable (synovial) articulations in the skull apart from the joints between the ossicles of the middle ear. A jaw joint located between the mandible and the squamous part of the temporal bone is peculiar to mammals. In all other vertebrates the jaw joint is between the articular, part of the lower jaw, and the quadrate, a bone of the upper jaw, but in mammals these two elements have become included in the tympanic cavity, as the malleus and incus respectively, and the original quadrate–articular jaw joint of lower vertebrates is represented by the joint between these two ossicles.

Movements of the jaw joints are brought about by numerous muscles, important amongst which are the muscles of mastication. Of these the temporalis and masseter are described in this section but the two pterygoid muscles are dealt with in the section on the infratemporal fossa. A full account of the functioning of the temporomandibular joint and of its associated musculature is given in the description of the mechanism of mastication in Chapter 4.9.

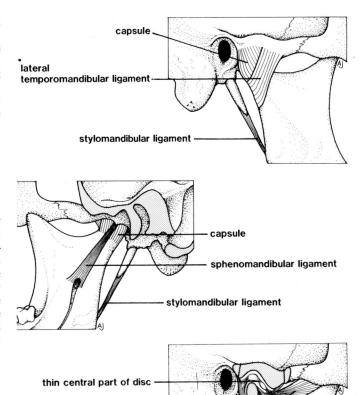

Temporomandibular joint

Articular surfaces

The temporomandibular joint is formed between the articular surfaces of the squamous part of the temporal bone and of the head (condyle) of the mandible. These surfaces are described in the appropriate sections of the chapter on skull (see pp. 122 and 129). The temporomandibular joint is atypical in that the articular surfaces are covered by white fibrocartilage (mostly collagen with only a few cartilage cells) not the more usual hyaline cartilage. Beneath the articular covering of the head of the mandible is a layer of hyaline cartilage (sometimes referred to as the **condylar cartilage**). It is an important growth site (p. 71), and is more readily apparent in the immature mandible.

Capsule and ligaments

The tough, fibrous capsule is attached above to the squamotympanic fissure and to the squamous bone around the margin of the upper articular surface, and below to the neck of the mandible a short distance below the limit of the lower articular surface. The capsule is slack between the articular disc and the squamous bone but much tighter between the disc and the neck of the mandible. The lateral pterygoid muscle is inserted, in part, into the anterior surface of the capsule.

The capsule is strengthened laterally by a thick band of fibrous tissue, the **lateral temporomandibular ligament**, extending downwards and backwards from the lateral pole of the articular tubercle, on the root of the zygomatic process of the temporal bone, to the lateral surface of the mandibular neck.

The **sphenomandibular** and **stylomandibular ligaments** are usually described as accessory ligaments of the temporomandibular joint. The former extends downwards and forwards from the spine of the sphenoid to the lingula of the mandible and lies some distance medial to the joint. The stylomandibular ligament lies behind the joint extending from the styloid process to the angle of the mandible.

Articular disc

The articular disc is a plate of fibrocartilage (mostly white fibrous tissue with relatively few cartilage cells) which in the majority of cases completely divides the joint cavity into an upper and lower compartment. Occasionally the disc is perforated and the two compartments are then in communication.

Laterally and medially the disc blends with the capsule of the joint. In front it is attached to the anterior border of the squamous articular surface as well as to the capsule. Posteriorly the disc is divided into

Fig. 4.42. Lateral (above) and medial (middle) views of the right temporomandibular joint. Below, the joint is shown in sagittal section.

two layers. The upper layer is attached to the anterior margin of the squamotympanic fissure while the lower layer is attached to the posterior surface of the neck of the mandible. The capsule on the posterior aspect of the joint is blended with these two layers. The tendon of the lateral pterygoid muscle is inserted into the anterior margin of the disc through its attachment to the capsule.

The upper surface of the disc is slightly concave anteriorly and markedly convex posteriorly. The under surface is concave over its whole extent. In both cases the surface is accommodated to the shape of the articular surface with which it is in contact.

The disc is not of uniform thickness. The central part is thinnest and is relatively avascular. It is here that occasional perforations may be found. The posterior part of the disc consists of a thick layer of loose vascular tissue and contains many blood vessels and sensory nerve endings. As just described this thickened part of the disc becomes divided into two layers which are attached separately to the squamous surface and head of the mandible. The front part of the disc is also thickened although not to the same degree as the posterior part.

Synovial membrane

As in other synovial joints all the non-load-bearing internal surfaces of the joint are covered with a layer of synovial membrane. These surfaces include the internal aspect of the capsule, the non-articular surfaces of the mandibular neck and, to a variable extent, the peripheral areas of the articular disc.

Nerve and blood supply

The joint is supplied with sensory fibres by branches of the **auriculo-temporal nerve** and the **nerve to masseter**, both branches of the mandibular division of the trigeminal nerve which also supplies the muscles acting upon the joint. The blood supply is through the **maxillary** and **superficial temporal arteries.**

Temporalis and masseter muscles

These two muscles, together with the medial and lateral pterygoid muscles, constitute the muscles of mastication. All are derived from the mesoderm of the first pharyngeal arch and are supplied, as would be expected, by the mandibular division of the trigeminal nerve.

Temporalis muscle and temporal fascia

The temporal fossa is roofed by the **temporal fascia.** This is a strong sheet of fibrous tissue attached above to the whole length of the superior temporal line. Below it splits into two laminae, the external one being attached to the lateral margin and the deep one to the medial margin of the upper border of the zygomatic arch. The superficial temporal blood vessels and the auriculotemporal nerve cross the fascia superficially; the zygomatic branch of the superficial temporal artery and a branch of the zygomaticotemporal nerve run between its two laminae just above the zygomatic arch.

The temporalis in subhuman primates (great apes and monkeys) is a large powerful muscle with well developed deep and superficial heads. The deep head arises from the side wall of the braincase and the superficial head from the internal surface of the temporal fascia. The fibres of the two heads converge, in a bipennate fashion, to attach to a strong central tendon which is inserted into the coronoid process of the mandible. By comparison the human temporalis muscle is much reduced in size but similar in arrangement. The bulk of the muscle arises from the external surface of the braincase from an area bounded by the inferior temporal line above and the infratemporal crest below and is equivalent to the deep head of the muscle in monkeys and apes. The fibres converge from this wide area of origin towards the coronoid process, passing deep to the zygomatic arch. The posterior fibres thus run downwards and forwards (the most posterior fibres run almost horizontally forwards), the middle fibres pass directly downwards, and the anterior fibres run downwards and slightly backwards. As they approach the coronoid process they attach to a well-developed tendon, equivalent to the central tendon of lower primates, which is inserted into the apex, anterior, and posterior borders and medial aspect of the coronoid process and, below the coronoid process, to the anterior border of the ramus as far as the retromolar fossa. The fibres arising low down on the braincase (i.e. close to the infratemporal crest) have a fleshy insertion into the medial surface of the coronoid process and ramus. The medial limit of this insertion is marked by the temporal crest. The superficial head of the human temporalis muscle is much smaller and

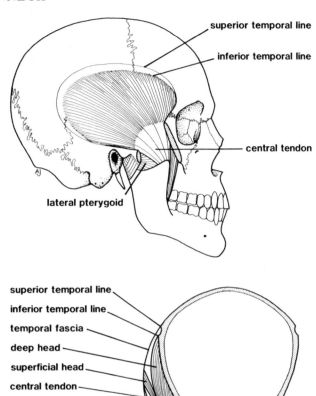

Fig. 4.43. The temporalis muscle. Above, lateral view; below in coronal section.

more variable than is that of lower primates. In most cases it consists of no more than a slip of muscle arising from the deep surface of the temporal fascia, usually opposite the coronoid process, and running downwards for a short distance before being inserted into the lateral surface of the temporalis tendon. Occasionally the superficial head is sufficiently well developed to form a thin layer of muscle covering most of the lateral aspect of the deep head. Again it arises from the temporal fascia and is inserted into the temporalis tendon. In a few cases no superficial head can be found at all and the space between the temporal fascia and the deep head contains merely loose connective tissue. Such variability is common in vestigial structures.

Temporalis is supplied by the deep temporal nerves from the anterior division of the mandibular nerve. Its action is to elevate the mandible. The posterior fibres, in addition, retract the mandible.

Masseter

The masseter muscle consists of three layers. The superficial layer, the largest component of the muscle, arises by a strong aponeurosis

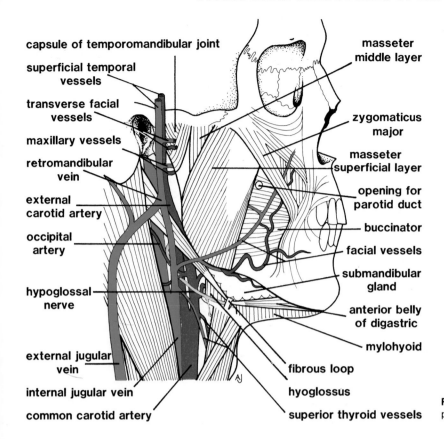

capsule of temporomandibular joint

superficial temporal vessels

transverse facial vessels

maxillary vessels

retromandibular vein

external carotid artery

occipital artery

hypoglossal nerve

external jugular vein

internal jugular vein

common carotid artery

masseter middle layer

zygomaticus major

masseter superficial layer

opening for parotid duct

buccinator

facial vessels

submandibular gland

anterior belly of digastric

mylohyoid

fibrous loop

hyoglossus

superior thyroid vessels

Fig. 4.44. The masseter muscle and related structures. The parotid gland has been removed.

from the anterior two-thirds of the lower border of the zygomatic arch. Its fibres pass downwards and backwards to be inserted into the lateral surface of the lower half of the ramus, including the angle of the mandible. The middle layer takes origin from the medial surface of the anterior two-thirds and the lower border of the posterior one-third of the arch. Its fibres run more directly downwards to be inserted into the lateral surface of the middle part of the ramus. The deep layer arises from the whole length of the medial surface of the zygomatic arch and its fibres pass downwards to attach to the upper part of the mandibular ramus. These three layers are quite distinct and separable posteriorly but anteriorly they fuse to form a single mass.

Within the muscle are several tendinous septa, some of which are attached to the zygomatic arch and which interdigitate with others attached to the lateral surface of the mandible. The muscle fibres run between these septa in a multipennate arrangement (p. 13).

The masseter muscle is innervated by the masseteric branch of the anterior division of the mandibular nerve. Having passed through the mandibular incisure the masseteric nerve enters the muscle from behind passing forwards and downwards in the space between the deep and middle layers. A branch of the transverse facial artery runs between the middle and superficial layers and provides the principal blood supply to the muscle.

The masseter muscle is a powerful elevator of the mandible. Its superficial fibres possess also a protruding action.

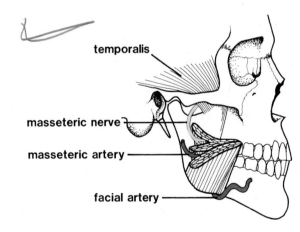

temporalis

masseteric nerve

masseteric artery

facial artery

Fig. 4.45. The three layers of the masseter muscle and its nerve and blood supply.

There is usually some intermingling of the most medial fibres of the deep layer of masseter with the most superficial fibres of temporalis. The description of these fibres as constituting a separate muscle, called **zygomaticomandibularis,** seems justified by the fact that such a muscle is well developed and quite distinct in many lower mammals.

CK

Fasciae

Superficial fascia

This is the subcutaneous layer of loose connective tissue. In some individuals it contains large amounts of fat although not usually as much as the equivalent layer in the trunk. It invests the platysma muscle.

Deep fascia

This name is employed to describe the condensations of connective tissue surrounding the deeper structures of the neck. In fact these layers are of varying thickness and practical importance. The following account is restricted to those layers that are sufficiently well defined to form separately identifiable membranes.

The **investing layer** of the deep cervical fascia is arranged like a cylinder around the neck, lying immediately deep to the superficial fascia and is clearly defined over much of its extent. Its inferior attachments are, on each side, to the spine and acromion of the scapula, to the clavicle and to the manubrium sterni. The superior attachments are more complicated. Posteriorly the upper attachment is to the external occipital protuberance, superior nuchal line, and mastoid process of the skull, the fascia splitting to enclose the attachments of the nuchal and sternocleidomastoid muscles. Between the mastoid process and the posterior border of the mandibular ramus the fascia splits into two layers which enclose the parotid gland so forming the **parotid capsule.** The deep layer of the capsule is attached to the base of the skull along the lower border of the tympanic plate.

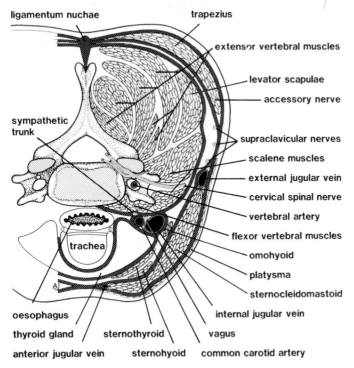

Fig. 4.46. Horizontal section of the neck at the level of the sixth cervical vertebra to show the arrangement of the deep fascia (dark cross-hatching).

A thickening of this deep layer, named the **stylomandibular ligament,** passes from the styloid process (which is ensheathed by the tympanic plate) to the angle of the mandible. The superficial layer of the parotid capsule passes forwards across the superficial surface of the parotid gland and onto the masseter muscle where it fades out. The upper border of this layer is attached from the mastoid process across the lower surface of the cartilaginous part of the external acoustic meatus to the lower border of the zygomatic arch.

Down the posterior midline of the neck the investing layer of the deep fascia fuses with the **ligamentum nuchae,** a strong fibrous band connecting the spines of the cervical vertebrae. Anteriorly, the investing layer is attached to the hyoid bone whence it passes upwards to attach to the lower border of the mandible. The investing layer splits to enclose trapezius and sternocleidomastoid muscles.

The remainder of the deep fascia consists of fibrous coverings ensheathing the structures lying within the investing layer. Although not strictly part of the superficial structures of the neck it is convenient to describe these sheaths here. The **prevertebral fascia** is a tough membrane covering the anterior aspect of the flexor muscles of the cervical spine. It extends from the base of the skull downwards to the body of the third thoracic vertebra. Laterally it passes in front of the lateral vertebral (scalene) muscles and becomes continuous with the thinner fascia enveloping the extensor vertebral muscles. The **carotid sheath** of each side consists of a tube of connective tissue surrounding the carotid artery (common carotid below the bifurcation, internal carotid above), internal jugular vein, and vagus nerve. It is better developed adjacent to the artery than over the vein. The sheath is attached above to the base of the skull around the opening of the carotid canal and is continued downwards along the common carotid artery to fuse with the connective tissue around the arch of the aorta. Embedded within the wall of the carotid sheath is the ansa cervicalis while immediately posterior to it is the cervical sympathetic trunk. The **pretracheal fascia** is a delicate covering around the thyroid gland. It is attached to the arch of the cricoid and is continued below into the superior mediastinum.

Clinical aspects

Between the various deep fasciae of the neck are tissue spaces. Together with corresponding spaces in the floor of the mouth with which they connect, these were of considerable clinical significance in the days before antibacterial drugs were available because of the tendency for pus and other pathological fluids to spread through the spaces rather than pierce the fasciae. In this way it was possible for infected material to track considerable distances from its point of origin and a knowledge of the fascial planes was clearly essential for correctly diagnosing and treating such conditions. The accumulation of large quantities of pus from dental foci is now an uncommon event, at least in developed countries, owing to the ready availability of early treatment and the widespread use of antibacterial drugs such as penicillin. Nevertheless a knowledge of the fascial planes in the neck and of the tissue spaces in the floor of the mouth (the latter are described on page 189) is still of occasional value to the practising dentist.

Muscle groups

The muscles of the neck fall into five main groups: (i) the **superficial muscles;** (ii) the **suprahyoid** and **infrahyoid muscles;** (iii) the **flexors of the cervical spine** (also termed **prevertebral** or **anterior vertebral** muscles); (iv) the **lateral vertebral muscles**; (v) the **extensors of the cervical spine** (consisting of the upper parts of the main extensors of the trunk and the small suboccipital muscles). Of these only the first two will be described in detail. A brief account will be given of the lateral vertebral muscles since they have important relationships in the root of the neck. The arrangement of the flexor and extensor groups has no relevance to the practice of dentistry and will not be described further.

Superficial muscles

Platysma

When well developed this is a broad sheet of muscle which arises from the fascia covering the large muscles on the front of the thorax. Its fibres sweep upwards and medially in the superficial fascia across the clavicle and into the side of the neck to be inserted into the lower border of the mandible and into the skin and muscle of the lower lip. It is innervated by the facial nerve (through its cervical branch). The action of platysma is to tighten the skin of the neck and to help depress the mandible and the angle of the mouth. It is variable in size and may be absent.

Sternocleidomastoid

Sternocleidomastoid is a strap-like muscle which passes obliquely upwards across the side of the neck (Fig. 4.38). Its origins are by a tendinous **sternal head** from the anterior surface of the manubrium sterni and by a fleshy **clavicular head** from the upper surface of the medial third of the clavicle. The two heads blend as they pass upwards and the muscle is inserted by tendon into the lateral aspect of the mastoid process and the lateral part of the superior nuchal line. The

muscle has a double innervation. It receives motor fibres from the accessory nerve (spinal root fibres) and proprioceptive fibres from the cervical plexus of nerves (principally from the second cervical spinal nerve). When the muscle contracts it approximates the mastoid process to the sternum. If one muscle is active the face is turned towards the opposite side and tilted upwards. Acting together the muscles of the two sides draw the head forwards.

Trapezius

This is a large flat muscle which is triangular in shape, the muscles of the two sides forming a trapezium from which the name is derived. Its origin is from the superior nuchal line, external occipital protuberance, ligamentum nuchae, the spinous process of the seventh cervical and the spinous processes and supraspinous ligaments of all the thoracic vertebrae. The fibres converge laterally from this extensive origin to be inserted into the lateral third of the clavicle and the acromion and spine of the scapula. The superior fibres (i.e. those in the neck) pass downwards and laterally from their origin to their insertion into the lateral third of the clavicle (Fig. 4.38). Like sternocleidomastoid the muscle has a double innervation receiving motor fibres from the spinal accessory nerve and proprioceptive fibres from the cervical plexus (C3, C4 spinal nerves). The muscle is concerned mainly with controlling the position of the scapula. With the scapula fixed the upper fibres can act to draw the head backwards and laterally.

Suprahyoid muscles

This group includes the **mylohyoid, geniohyoid, stylohyoid,** and **digastric muscles.** It is convenient to delay description of the mylo-

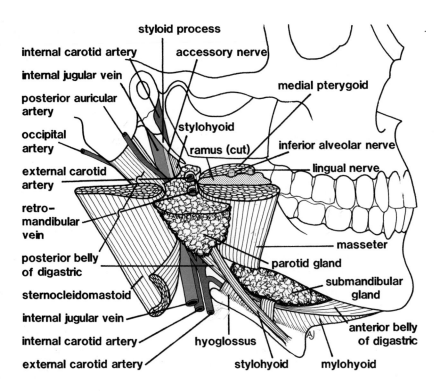

Fig. 4.47. The digastric muscle and its relationships.

hyoid and geniohyoid muscles until the section on the floor of the mouth (pp. 185–6) and of the stylohyoid muscle until the section on the styloid apparatus (p. 179).

Digastric

As its name suggests the digastric muscle has two bellies. The posterior belly arises from the mastoid notch of the temporal bone. It passes downwards and forwards towards the hyoid bone where it becomes continuous with the intermediate tendon. This passes through a perforation in the stylohyoid muscle, just above the latter's insertion into the hyoid bone, being held in place by a fibrous loop attached to the junction of the body and greater cornu. From the intermediate tendon the anterior belly passes upwards and forwards, below mylohyoid, to be attached to the digastric fossa on the lower border of the mandible. The posterior belly is derived from the second pharyngeal arch and is innervated by a branch of the facial nerve while the anterior belly is of first arch origin and is supplied by the trigeminal nerve through the mylohyoid branch of the inferior alveolar nerve (the latter being a branch of the mandibular division of the trigeminal). When the muscle contracts it depresses the mandible or elevates the hyoid.

Infrahyoid muscles

This group of paired strap-like muscles includes the **sternohyoid, sternothyroid, thyrohyoid,** and **omohyoid muscles.** They act to depress the hyoid bone or to fix it so that the suprahyoid muscles can act. They are supplied by branches of the ansa cervicalis apart from thyrohyoid which, together with geniohyoid, is innervated by fibres of the first cervical spinal nerve which run to their destination in the hypoglossal nerve.

The sternohyoid muscle arises from the medial end of the clavicle and adjacent manubrium sterni and is inserted into the lower border of the body of the hyoid bone. The sternothyroid muscle lies deep to sternohyoid running from the manubrium sterni to the oblique line on the lamina of the thyroid cartilage. The thyrohyoid muscle continues upwards from the oblique line to the lower border of the greater cornu and body of the hyoid bone. The omohyoid muscle

consists of two bellies. The inferior arises from the upper border of the scapula, passes forwards across the lower part of the neck and, deep to sternocleidomastoid, attaches to the intermediate tendon. The superior belly runs directly upwards from the tendon to attach to the body of the hyoid lateral to the insertion of sternohyoid. The intermediate tendon is held in place by a fibrous loop attached to the clavicle and first rib.

Lateral vertebral muscles

The three **scalene muscles (anterior, medius,** and **posterior)** take origin from the transverse processes of the cervical vertebrae and run downwards and outwards to the upper two ribs. They are supplied by the ventral rami of the cervical spinal nerves and act to elevate the ribs or bend the cervical spine laterally.

The subclavian vein crosses the first rib in front of the anterior scalene while the **subclavian artery** and the **brachial plexus** cross the first rib between the anterior and middle scalenes.

Triangles of neck

It was customary in the past to divide the neck into numerous triangles, related to the superficial muscles, in order to facilitate description. In fact this procedure merely added to the burden of memory. All that is worth remembering, from a practical viewpoint, is the general disposition of the **anterior** and **posterior triangles.** The latter lies between the trapezius and sternocleidomastoid muscles with a base formed by the middle third of the clavicle. The roof of the triangle is provided by the investing layer of the deep cervical fascia and the floor by the scalene muscles and, more posteriorly, by the muscles of the extensor group. The accessory nerve crosses the triangle almost vertically from the posterior border of sternocleidomastoid to the anterior border of trapezius. The four superficial branches of the cervical plexus emerge from the posterior triangle around the posterior edge of sternocleidomastoid.

The anterior triangle is bounded by the anterior border of the sternocleidomastoid on each side and by the lower border of the mandible above. Its apex lies at the manubrium sterni.

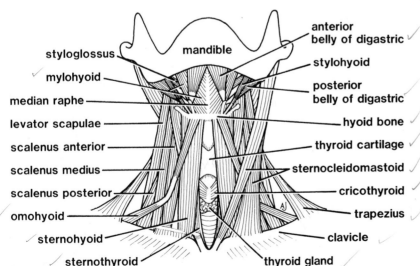

Fig. 4.48. The infrahyoid muscles. Sternocleidomastoid removed on left side of figure.

Cervical spinal nerves

There are eight cervical spinal nerves. Each of the upper seven nerves leaves the vertebral canal by passing above the vertebra of the same number (e.g. the first nerve emerges between the occipital bone and the atlas). The eighth emerges between the seventh cervical and the first thoracic vertebrae. Each nerve then divides into a dorsal and a ventral ramus. The dorsal ramus runs posteriorly to supply the extensor musculature of the vertebral column and, apart from that of the first cervical nerve, the skin over the back of the scalp and neck. The ventral ramus receives a grey ramus communicans from the corresponding ganglion of the sympathetic trunk, then enters into a plexus from which branches are distributed to skeletal muscle and skin.

The ventral rami of the upper four cervical spinal nerves join together to form the **cervical plexus.** The ventral rami of the remaining four cervical nerves and that of the first thoracic nerve join to form the **brachial plexus.** The latter is concerned with supplying the skin and muscles of the upper limb and is not described further.

Cervical plexus

The four ventral rami constituting the cervical plexus lie in series on the anterior surface of scalenus medius and are joined together consecutively by simple loops. The branches of the plexus can be divided into deep and superficial groups – the former supplying muscle and the latter being distributed to the skin of the front and sides of the neck and part of the side of the head.

Deep branches

The deep branches include the following.
1. A **communicating branch** from the first cervical nerve to the hypoglossal nerve. This carries motor fibres for the geniohyoid and thyrohyoid muscles which run to their destination in the hypoglossal nerve. It also carries fibres for the remaining infrahyoid muscles. The

latter fibres leave the hypoglossal nerve in its **descending branch** (also called the **superior root of the ansa cervicalis**) which passes along the front of the carotid sheath to join the descendens cervicalis and so form the **ansa cervicalis.**
2. **Muscular branches** pass from all four cervical nerves to the prevertebral muscles.
3. **Proprioceptive branches,** one from the second and third and another from the third and fourth cervical nerves, run to the sterno-cleidomastoid and trapezius muscles respectively.
4. The **descendens cervicalis** (or **inferior root of the ansa cervicalis**) from the second and third cervical nerves passes around the lateral surface of the internal jugular vein to join with the descending branch of the hypoglossal nerve and form the **ansa cervicalis** (Figs. 4.49 and 4.50). Branches of the latter supply the infrahyoid muscles except thyrohyoid.
5. The **phrenic nerve** is derived from the fourth cervical nerve with small additions from the third and fifth nerves. It runs vertically downwards over the anterior scalene muscle and then passes behind the subclavian vein to enter the mediastinum. Its further course is described in the section on thorax.

Superficial branches

The superficial branches of the cervical plexus hook around the posterior border of sternocleidomastoid and radiate outwards to supply skin over the sides and front of the neck, the front of the chest, a small area of scalp, the lower part of the auricle and an area of face just anterior to the auricle. They are four in number.
1. The **lesser occipital nerve** is derived from the second cervical nerve. It runs upwards along the posterior border of sternocleidomastoid to supply to skin of the scalp behind the auricle.
2. The **great auricular nerve,** having passed around the posterior border of sternocleidomastoid, runs upwards to supply the skin of the auricle and of the face over the parotid gland and angle of the mandible. It is derived from the second and third cervical nerves.
3. The **transverse cervical nerve** is also derived from the second and third nerves. It runs forwards to supply the skin of the side and front of the neck from symphysis menti to sternum.
4. The **supraclavicular nerves** are derived from the third and fourth cervical nerves. They pass downwards and fan out to supply skin over the chest and shoulder.

The dorsal rami

The dorsal ramus of the first cervical nerve supplies the muscles of the suboccipital region and usually has no cutaneous branch. The dorsal ramus of the second cervical nerve gives rise to a large cutaneous branch, the **greater occipital nerve,** which supplies the posterior aspect of the scalp as far as the vertex. The dorsal rami of the remaining cervical nerves have small cutaneous branches to the back of the neck.

Arteries in neck

Common carotid artery

The origin of the common carotid artery varies between the two sides of the body. On the right it begins behind the sternoclavicular joint at the bifurcation of the brachiocephalic trunk (Fig. 3.37). On the left it arises in the mediastinum directly from the arch of the aorta. On

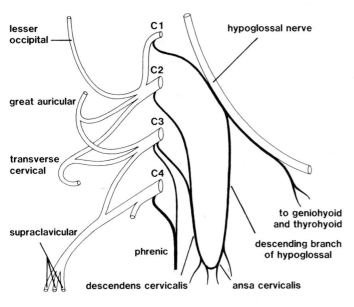

Fig. 4.49. The cervical plexus.

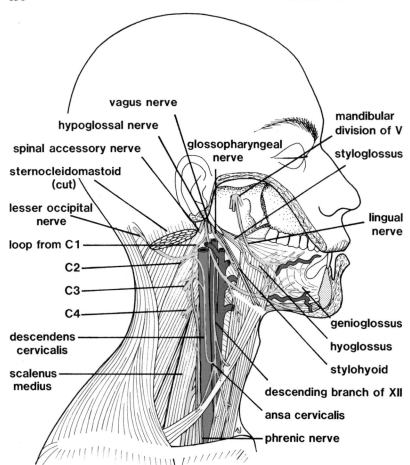

vagus nerve

hypoglossal nerve

spinal accessory nerve

sternocleidomastoid (cut)

lesser occipital nerve

loop from C1

C2

C3

C4

descendens cervicalis

scalenus medius

glossopharyngeal nerve

mandibular division of V

styloglossus

lingual nerve

genioglossus

hyoglossus

stylohyoid

descending branch of XII

ansa cervicalis

phrenic nerve

Fig. 4.50. The ansa cervicalis. The vagus and accessory nerves are cut shortly below their entrance into the neck.

either side the artery ascends, within the carotid sheath, to the level of the superior border of the thyroid lamina where it bifurcates into **internal** and **external** branches. It gives off no branches before the bifurcation. The terminal part of the artery and the first part of its internal branch are dilated to form the **carotid sinus.** Nerve endings in the wall of the sinus, the terminals of fibres in the carotid branch of the glossopharyngeal nerve, act as baroreceptors and are involved in the control of blood pressure.

Closely related to the carotid sinus is the **carotid body.** This structure is usually situated behind the sinus or between the internal and external carotid arteries and is only a few millimetres in width. It is innervated principally by the carotid branch of the glossopharyngeal nerve and functions as a chemoreceptor, responding to oxygen and carbon dioxide levels in the blood. Similar structures, the aortic bodies, are situated close to the arch of the aorta and are supplied by the vagus.

Internal carotid artery

The internal carotid artery continues upwards within the carotid sheath from its origin at the bifurcation of the common carotid. It lies at first superficial to the external carotid artery but as it ascends it comes to occupy a position behind and deep to that vessel. At the base of the skull it enters the carotid canal and so gains access to the

cranial cavity. The internal carotid artery has no branches within the neck. Its branches in the cranial cavity are described on page 137. The artery carries with it a network of nerves (the **internal carotid plexus**) from the superior cervical ganglion.

External carotid artery

The external carotid artery runs upwards in front of and eventually somewhat lateral to the internal carotid artery. It passes deep to the digastric and stylohyoid muscles and then pierces the parotid fascia to enter the gland where it ends by dividing into **maxillary** and **superficial temporal** branches. Before entering the gland it gives rise to the following six branches.

1. The **superior thyroid artery** arises from the front of the external carotid just below the level of the hyoid bone. It runs downwards to supply the gland and adjacent muscles. It gives off a **superior laryngeal branch** which accompanies the internal laryngeal nerve to the upper part of the larynx and adjacent part of the pharynx.

2. The **ascending pharyngeal artery** arises from the medial side of the external carotid artery close to its origin and ascends alongside the pharynx which it supplies. At the base of the skull it gives off a number of small meningeal branches which enter the cranial cavity through the foramen lacerum and the jugular foramen.

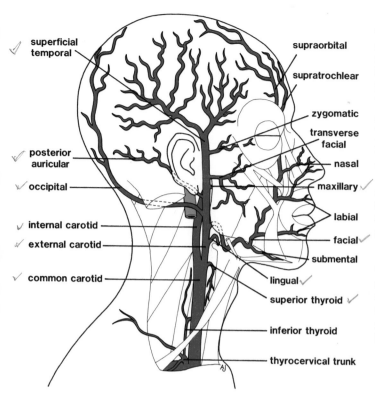

Fig. 4.51. The carotid arteries and their branches.

Thyrocervical and costocervical trunks

The **thyrocervical trunk** takes origin from the subclavian artery close to the medial border of the anterior scalene muscle. It divides into three branches. The **inferior thyroid artery** runs upwards to the lower border of the lobe of the thyroid gland (the relationships between its terminal branches and the recurrent laryngeal nerve are intimate but variable, see pages 160 and 163). As well as supplying the gland it gives branches to adjacent muscles, larynx (through its **inferior laryngeal branch**) and trachea. The **transverse cervical artery** runs posteriorly across the lower part of the neck to supply the muscles in the region of the posterior triangle. The **suprascapular artery** passes downwards to the region of the shoulder girdle.

The **costocervical trunk** arises from the subclavian artery behind the anterior scalene muscle. It divides into the **superior intercostal artery** to the upper intercostal spaces and the **deep cervical artery** which ascends between the extensor muscles of the neck which it supplies.

Vertebral artery

The vertebral artery of each side arises from near the root of the subclavian artery. It runs upwards through the foramina in the transverse processes of the upper six cervical vertebrae, passes behind the lateral mass of the atlas and enters the cranial cavity through the foramen magnum. Within the skull, at the lower border of the pons, it unites with the vessel of the opposite side to form the **basilar artery**.

3. The **lingual artery** leaves the anterior surface of the external carotid opposite the hyoid bone. It runs forwards, making a characteristic upward loop, and then passes deep to the hyoglossus muscle to enter the floor of the mouth.

4. The **facial artery** arises from the front of the external carotid artery a short distance above the lingual artery. It runs upwards in a deep groove on the posterior surface of the submandibular gland and deep to the ramus of the mandible, curves over the superior aspect of the gland and then runs downwards and forwards between the lateral surface of the gland and the medial surface of the mandible. It hooks around the inferior border of the mandible at the anterior edge of masseter to enter the face. In the neck it gives off an **ascending palatine branch** (Fig. 4.85, p. 187) which ascends alongside the pharynx to supply the soft palate, a **tonsillar branch** to the palatine tonsil and a **submental branch** which runs forwards on the superficial surface of the mylohyoid muscle to supply nearby muscles and skin.

5. The **occipital artery** leaves the back of the external carotid above the level of the hyoid bone. It runs medial to the digastric muscle and then in the occipital groove on the mastoid part of the temporal bone. On leaving the occipital groove it turns superficially to supply the posterior part of the scalp.

6. The **posterior auricular artery** arises from the posterior part of the external carotid above the digastric muscle. It ascends, between the parotid gland and styloid process, to supply the auricle and scalp behind the ear. At the stylomastoid foramen it gives off its **stylomastoid branch** which runs through the foramen to supply the tympanic cavity.

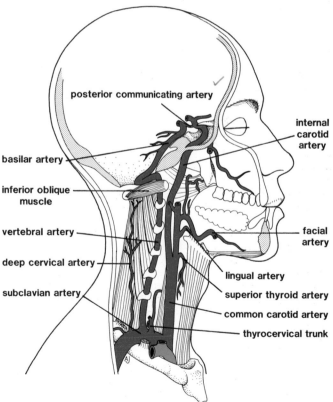

Fig. 4.52. The vertebral artery.

Veins in neck

Internal jugular vein

The internal jugular vein emerges from the jugular foramen to lie at first behind the internal carotid artery. Immediately below the cranial base it receives the inferior petrosal sinus. The vein passes downwards in the loose part of the carotid sheath coming to lie lateral to the internal carotid artery and, at a lower level, to the common carotid artery. Between the vein and the arteries is the vagus nerve. In the root of the neck the internal jugular vein joins the

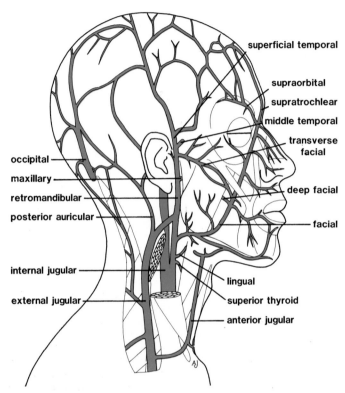

Fig. 4.53. The superficial veins of the head and neck.

External jugular vein

The external jugular vein is formed by the union of the posterior division of the retromandibular vein and the posterior auricular vein. It runs downwards superficial to the sternocleidomastoid muscle, pierces the deep cervical fascia above the middle of the clavicle, and ends in the subclavian vein. It receives a few small tributaries from adjacent structures.

Anterior jugular vein

An anterior jugular vein begins beneath the chin, on each side of the midline, and passes downwards to the suprasternal region where it pierces the deep fascia and empties into the external jugular vein.

Occipital vein

This large vein drains the occipital region of the scalp. It passes deep between the extensor muscles of the cervical vertebral column and usually opens into the vertebral vein.

Vertebral vein

The vertebral vein is formed in the region below the occipital bone by the union of numerous tributaries from the vertebral plexuses and from the deep musculature of the suboccipital region. It passes downwards in the foramina in the transverse processes of the upper six cervical vertebrae and ends by joining the brachiocephalic vein of the same side.

Cranial nerves in neck

The last four cranial nerves run for part of their course in the neck.

Glossopharyngeal

The glossopharyngeal nerve leaves the cranial cavity through the anterior compartment of the jugular foramen. It passes downwards and forwards between the internal and external carotid arteries, closely applied to the posterior border and lateral surface of the stylopharyngeus muscle, and enters the pharynx by passing between the adjoining borders of the superior and middle constrictor muscles. It then runs forwards deep to hyoglossus to supply the posterior part of the tongue.

In the jugular foramen the nerve bears a small **superior** and a larger **inferior ganglion** containing the cell bodies of the sensory neurons. The nerve is also functionally associated with the otic ganglion.

The branches of the glossopharyngeal nerve are as follows: (i) The **tympanic branch** leaves the inferior ganglion within the jugular foramen, passes through the canaliculus in the petrous part of the temporal bone to reach the tympanic cavity where it forms the **tympanic plexus** and supplies the lining mucous membrane; this branch also contains preganglionic parasympathetic fibres which continue from the tympanic plexus in the **lesser petrosal nerve** to relay in the otic ganglion with postganglionic neurons innervating the parotid gland. (ii) The **motor branch** innervates the stylopharyngeus muscle. (iii) **Pharyngeal branches** convey sensory and preganglionic parasympathetic fibres to the pharyngeal plexus. The sensory fibres pass through the plexus without interruption and supply the mucous membrane of the oropharynx. The preganglionic parasympathetic fibres synapse in the plexus with postganglionic fibres which supply the glands of this part of the pharynx. (iv) The

subclavian vein to form the **brachiocephalic vein**. The internal jugular is crossed superficially by the posterior belly of digastric, omohyoid, and sternocleidomastoid muscles, the posterior auricular and occipital arteries, and the accessory nerve and ansa cervicalis. In the lower part of its course it is covered by the infrahyoid muscles.

As well as the inferior petrosal sinus the internal jugular vein receives numerous tributaries. Their arrangement is subject to great individual variation but the more important tributaries usually include the following: (i) the facial vein (which has been joined by the anterior division of the retromandibular vein – page 147) (ii) veins draining the tongue (p. 189); (iii) the **pharyngeal veins** from the pharyngeal plexus (p. 177); (iv) the **superior thyroid vein** from the upper part of the gland; and (v) the **middle thyroid vein** from the lower part of the gland.

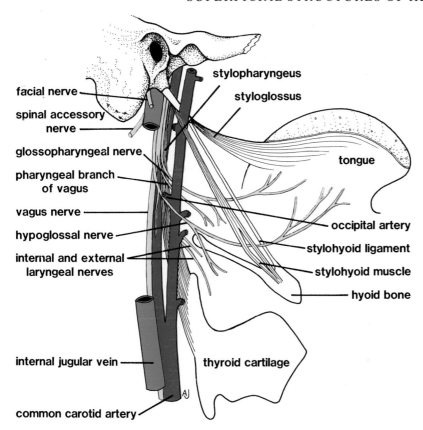

Fig. 4.54. The glossopharyngeal, vagus, accessory, and hypoglossal nerves in the neck.

carotid branch supplies the carotid sinus and body. (v) **Lingual branches** convey taste and general sensation from the posterior one-third of the tongue (including the vallate papillae).

Vagus

The vagus nerve leaves the cranial cavity through the middle compartment of the jugular foramen in company with the accessory nerve. In the foramen the nerve is swollen by the small **superior ganglion**. A short distance below the foramen it bears the larger **inferior ganglion**. The superior ganglion contains the cell bodies of the few somatic sensory (cutaneous) neurons which travel in the vagus (these are all distributed in its auricular branch), while the inferior ganglion contains the cell bodies of the taste and general visceral sensory neurons. Below the inferior ganglion the nerve is joined by the cranial root of the accessory nerve. It then continues vertically downwards within the carotid sheath running at first between the internal jugular vein and the internal carotid artery, then between the internal jugular vein and the common carotid artery.

In the root of the neck the relationships of the vagus differ between the two sides because of the asymmetry of the great vessels. On the right the vagus enters the thorax by passing in front of the right subclavian artery. On the left the vagus passes between the left common carotid and left subclavian arteries. The further course of the nerve is described in the chapter on mediastinum.

The branches of the vagus supplying structures in the head and neck include the following:

1. A **meningeal branch** leaves the superior ganglion to supply the dura mater of the posterior cranial fossa. As with the meningeal branch of the hypoglossal nerve, the constituent fibres are probably derived from the upper cervical spinal nerves.

2. The **auricular branch**, also from the superior ganglion, enters a small canal, the **mastoid canaliculus**, in the lateral wall of the jugular foramen and passes through the temporal bone to supply the skin of the auricle and of the external acoustic meatus and the outer surface of the tympanic membrane.

3. The **pharyngeal branch** emerges from the inferior ganglion, passes forwards between the internal and external carotid arteries, below and parallel to the glossopharyngeal nerve, to the middle constrictor where it joins with the pharyngeal branch of the glosso-pharyngeal nerve to form the pharyngeal plexus. Through this plexus, the vagus supplies motor fibres derived from the cranial accessory to the muscles of the pharynx and soft palate.

4. Several minute branches run from the inferior ganglion to the carotid body; alternatively the fibres making up these branches may run in the superior laryngeal branch.

5. The **superior laryngeal nerve** leaves the vagus below the pharyngeal branch. It descends on the side of the pharynx, deep to the internal carotid artery, and divides into **internal** and **external laryngeal branches**. The former passes down to pierce the postero-inferior part of the thyrohyoid membrane some distance above the superior laryngeal artery. It supplies the lining of the larynx down to the vocal folds and of the pharynx around the laryngeal inlet. The

external laryngeal nerve runs downwards on the inferior constrictor to supply the cricothyroid muscle.

6. The origin and course of the **recurrent laryngeal nerve** differ between the two sides. On the right the nerve leaves the vagus within the neck as the latter passes in front of the subclavian artery. It hooks under the artery and then ascends through the neck in the groove between the trachea and oesophagus. On the left side the recurrent laryngeal nerve arises from the vagus to the left of the arch of the aorta and within the thorax. It winds beneath the arch, posterior to the attachment of the ligamentum arteriosum, and then ascends on the right of the arch to reach the side of the trachea. As on the left side the nerve then continues upwards in the neck in the groove between the trachea and oesophagus. Near the lower pole of the lobe of the thyroid gland the recurrent laryngeal nerve is closely related to the terminal branches of the inferior thyroid artery, usually passing behind but not infrequently between or in front of these vessels. The nerve then runs close to the medial surface of the gland before passing deep to the lower border of the inferior constrictor, behind the cricothyroid articulation, to enter the larynx. It supplies all the muscles of the larynx, except cricothyroid, and the mucous membrane below the vocal folds. As it ascends in the neck it gives branches to the mucous membrane and muscular coats of the oesophagus and trachea. The relationships of the recurrent laryngeal nerve to the thyroid gland and its arteries are of special significance in surgery of the gland.

Within the neck the vagus also gives off **superior** and **inferior cardiac branches** which run downwards into the thorax to join the **cardiac plexuses**. They convey the parasympathetic innervation of the heart.

The vagus nerve within the head and neck supplies general visceral sensory fibres to the dura mater of the posterior cranial fossa and to the linings of the larynx, trachea, laryngopharynx and oesophagus, taste fibres to the epiglottis and vallecula, and somatic sensory fibres to the skin of the auricle, external acoustic meatus and outer surface of the tympanic membrane. The nerve also conveys parasympathetic fibres to glands in the pharynx and larynx and motor fibres (derived from the cranial accessory) to the muscles of the pharynx, soft palate, and larynx.

The bulk of the nerve is continued downwards into the thoracic and abdominal regions and is concerned with the parasympathetic and sensory supply of the viscera of the trunk.

Accessory

The **spinal** and **cranial roots of the accessory nerve** unite for a short distance within the jugular foramen through which they pass in close association with the vagus. The two roots then part company again.

The cranial root joins the vagus immediately below its inferior ganglion. The spinal root slopes downwards and backwards passing usually posterior but occasionally anterior to the internal jugular vein and then medial to the posterior belly of digastric to reach the upper part of the sternocleidomastoid muscle. It runs through the muscle, which it supples with motor fibres, crosses the posterior triangle and enters the trapezius muscle which it also supplies with motor fibres.

The cranial root, via the branches of the vagus, supplies the striped muscle of the pharynx, palate, and larynx.

Hypoglossal

The rootlets of the hypoglossal nerve are gathered together into two separate bundles which leave the cranial cavity through the hypoglossal canal. These then fuse to form a single nerve which is joined by a communicating branch from the first cervical spinal nerve (p. 155) and then runs downwards and laterally between the internal carotid artery and internal jugular vein and behind the glossopharyngeal and vagus nerves. Below the posterior belly of the digastric muscle, the hypoglossal nerve curves around the lateral aspect of the external carotid artery, passing under the origin of the occipital artery, deep to the digastric and stylohyoid muscles but superficial to the stylohyoid ligament. As it crosses the carotid sheath the nerve gives off its **descending branch** which joins with the descendens cervicalis to form the ansa cervicalis. It then runs forwards across the upward loop of the lingual nerve and on to the lateral surface of the hyoglossus muscle a little above the greater cornu of the hyoid bone. Its further course in the floor of the mouth is described on page 189.

The hypoglossal nerve supplies all the muscles of the tongue, except palatoglossus (in reality a muscle of the palate). The motor fibres which join it via the communicating branch from the first cervical spinal nerve are distributed through the ansa cervicalis to the sternohyoid, sternothyroid, and inferior belly of omohyoid and through branches to the thyrohyoid and geniohyoid muscles. A number of sensory fibres enter the hypoglossal nerve from connections with upper cervical spinal nerves. These pass in its small meningeal branch to the dura mater of the posterior fossa.

Cervical sympathetic trunk

The sympathetic trunk continues upwards from the thorax by crossing the neck of the first rib. It then ascends in the neck, lying between the prevertebral fascia and the carotid sheath, to end in front of the lateral mass of the atlas. It bears three swellings, the **superior, middle,** and **inferior cervical sympathetic** ganglia. Each of these has been formed during evolution by fusion of a number of separate cervical ganglia (there being originally one ganglion for each cervical spinal nerve).

The superior is the largest of the three ganglia. It lies in front of the transverse process of the axis. It is formed by fusion of the ganglia originally associated with the upper four cervical nerves. The middle ganglion is the smallest and represents the ganglia of the fifth and sixth cervical nerves. The inferior ganglion represents the ganglia of the remaining two cervical nerves. It is often fused with the first thoracic ganglion to form the **cervicothoracic (stellate) ganglion**. It lies close to the neck of the first rib. Continuing upwards from the superior ganglion is the **internal carotid nerve**. This runs behind the internal carotid artery, enters the carotid canal in the cranial base and ends by forming a plexus around the artery. From the plexus branches of communication are given to the oculomotor, trochlear, trigeminal, abducent, and glossopharyngeal nerves. It also gives branches to the ciliary and pterygopalatine ganglion (the latter through the deep petrosal nerve).

It will be clear from the description of the sympathetic trunk given on pages 251–2 that no white rami (i.e. no preganglionic fibres) pass from the cervical nerves to the cervical ganglia. All the preganglionic fibres involved in the sympathetic innervation of the head and neck enter the trunk in the upper thoracic segments and run upwards to end in one or other of the cervical ganglia. The postganglionic fibres pass to their destination in branches of the cervical ganglia which, like those of the ganglia in the remainder of the sympathetic trunk, can be divided into **somatic, visceral,** and **vascular** groups.

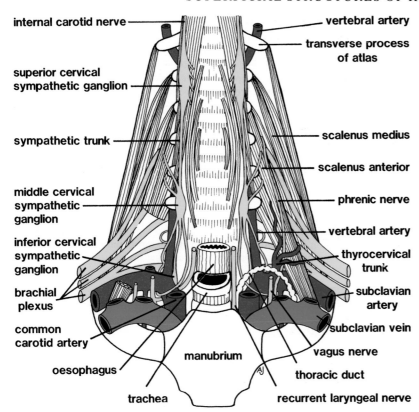

internal carotid nerve

superior cervical sympathetic ganglion

sympathetic trunk

middle cervical sympathetic ganglion

inferior cervical sympathetic ganglion

brachial plexus

common carotid artery

oesophagus

trachea

manubrium

vertebral artery

transverse process of atlas

scalenus medius

scalenus anterior

phrenic nerve

vertebral artery

thyrocervical trunk

subclavian artery

subclavian vein

vagus nerve

thoracic duct

recurrent laryngeal nerve

Fig. 4.55. The cervical sympathetic trunks.

The somatic branches comprise the **grey rami communicantes** to the cervical spinal nerves. As would be expected from the phylogenetic derivation of the ganglia, grey rami pass from the superior ganglion to the upper four cervical nerves, from the middle ganglion to the fifth and sixth cervical nerves and from the inferior ganglion to the seventh and eighth cervical nerves. The grey rami contain postganglionic fibres which run in the spinal nerves to supply blood vessels, sweat glands and arrector pili muscles in the skin.

A visceral branch passes from each ganglion to the cardiac plexus in the thorax. These cardiac branches contain postganglionic fibres which provide the sympathetic innervation of the heart. The superior ganglion also gives rise to **laryngopharyngeal visceral branches** which enter the pharyngeal plexus. The middle ganglion gives a visceral branch to the thyroid gland.

The vascular branches from the ganglia form networks which pass along neighbouring arteries to reach their destination. Those from the superior ganglion run with the common and external carotid arteries, and their branches, and so reach structures over a wide area of the head and neck. The vascular branches of the middle ganglion pass with the subclavian and inferior thyroid arteries to the larynx, trachea, and oesophagus. Those of the inferior ganglion accompany the vertebral artery and its branches.

LYMPH NODES OF HEAD AND NECK

All lymph from the head and neck eventually drains into the deep cervical lymph nodes which are situated beneath the sternocleido-

mastoid muscle from the base of the skull to the root of the neck. Lymph drains directly from some areas into these nodes while from other areas it passes first through one of the outlying groups of nodes.

Deep cervical nodes

These are conventionally divided into two groups. The **superior group** surrounds the upper part of the internal jugular vein. The **inferior group** lies close to the subclavian vessels. Two nodes are separately named: the **jugulodigastric node**, one of the superior group, is situated between the internal jugular vein and the digastric muscle; the **jugulo-omohyoid** node, one of the inferior group, lies close to the intermediate tendon of the omohyoid muscle. Both receive lymph from the tongue.

The deep cervical lymph nodes of each side drain into a **jugular trunk**.

Outlying groups of nodes

Submandibular nodes

This group lies on the surface of the superficial part of the submandibular gland beneath the investing layer of the deep cervical fascia and under cover of the inferior border of the mandible. It receives lymph from a wide area of the face and from the anterior part of the nasal cavity, teeth, floor of mouth, and anterior two-thirds of tongue, and drains into the deep cervical nodes, especially the jugulo-omohyoid node.

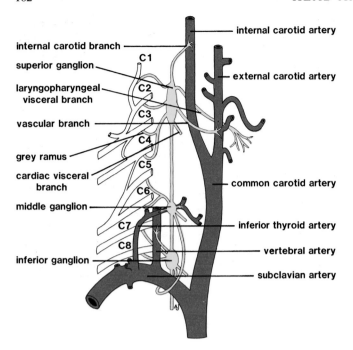

Fig. 4.56. Branches of the cervical sympathetic ganglia.

Parotid nodes

Lymph from the forehead, temple, eyelids, and external ear drains into the **superficial parotid nodes** situated on the lateral surface of the parotid gland. The **deep parotid nodes**, which are located within the gland, receive lymph from the eyelids and from the middle ear. The efferent vessels from the parotid nodes pass to the upper deep cervical group.

Buccal nodes

The vessels draining from the anterior part of the face into the submandibular nodes may have a few buccal nodes scattered along their course in the cheek.

Retroauricular nodes

This group lies superficial to the attachment of sternocleidomastoid to the mastoid process. It drains the scalp behind the external ear and empties into the upper deep cervical nodes.

Occipital nodes

These receive lymph from the posterior part of the scalp and empty into the lower deep cervical nodes. They lie at the apex of the posterior triangle.

Superficial and anterior cervical nodes

These two groups receive those lymph vessels from the superficial structures of the neck that do not empty directly into the deep cervical nodes. The superficial group is located around the external jugular vein on the lateral surface of the sternocleidomastoid muscle and the anterior group lies close to the anterior jugular veins. Their efferents pass to the deep cervical group.

Lymph from the deeper structures of the head and neck passes to groups of nodes around the pharynx, larynx, and trachea.

Submental nodes

These are situated on the superficial surface of the mylohyoid muscle behind the inferior border of the mandible in the region of the mental protuberance. They drain lymph from the tip of the tongue, floor of the mouth, the incisor teeth and associated alveolar process, and the central part of the lower lip. They empty into the submandibular group and the jugulo-omohyoid node.

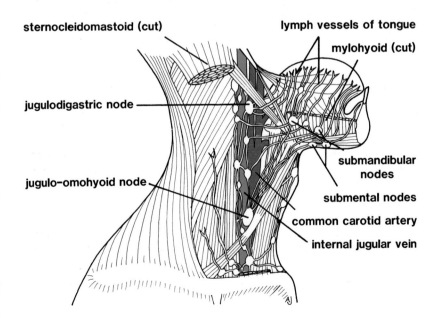

Fig. 4.57. The deep cervical lymph nodes.

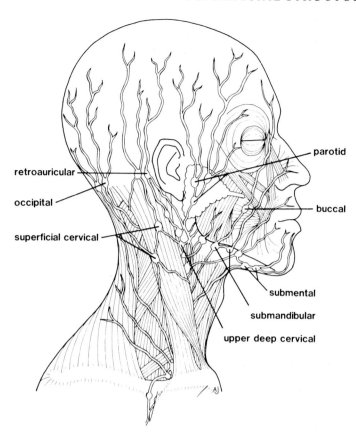

Fig. 4.58. The superficial lymph nodes of the head and neck.

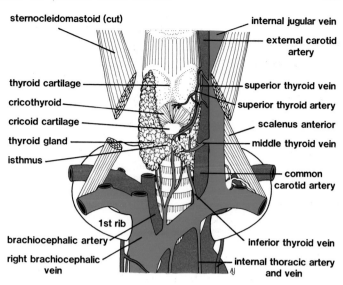

Fig. 4.59. Anterior view of the thyroid gland.

Clinical aspects

Although the lymph nodes of the head and neck are usually difficult to find during dissection, and may seem therefore to be rather unimpressive organs, they are in fact of the greatest clinical importance because they often become secondarily involved in infections and malignant disease of the organs they drain. Infections of the structures around the mouth, including the periapical tissues, are usually accompanied by tender enlargement of the submental or submandibular nodes. Occasionally one or more nodes in the deep cervical group may also be enlarged. Such inflamed nodes may subsequently become fibrotic in which case they remain palpable but not tender. Lymph nodes which are the site of malignant spread become enlarged and hard to the touch and in the early stages may be difficult to distinguish from fibrotic nodes. As the disease advances, however, the malignant cells tend to spread into neighbouring tissues and the nodes become fixed.

The lymph nodes of the head and neck may also become involved in generalized diseases of the lymphatic system such as Hodgkin's disease.

THYROID GLAND

The thyroid gland consists of two lobes united across the front of the trachea at the level of the second to fourth cartilaginous rings by a narrower portion called the **isthmus**. A small **pyramidal lobe** may project upwards from the isthmus, usually to the left of the midline. The gland is invested within the **pretracheal fascia** and lies deep to the sternothyroid and sternohyoid muscles. The four parathyroid glands are situated close to the thyroid gland, within the pretracheal fascia, one at the upper pole and one at the lower pole of each lobe.

The gland receives its blood supply from the superior and inferior thyroid arteries. The former pierces the pretracheal fascia as a single vessel but the latter divides into several branches which pass through the fascia independently. The recurrent laryngeal nerve usually passes behind but may pass between these branches before they enter the fascia. The venous return is through the superior, middle, and inferior thyroid veins (the first two are usually tributaries of the internal jugular vein and the last a tributary of the brachiocephalic vein).

Clinical aspects

Occasionally accessory thyroid glands are present. The sites at which these may occur are described with the embryology of the gland (p. 49). In rare cases all the glandular tissue may be located ectopically or the gland may fail totally to develop.

Enlargement of the thyroid gland, or goitre, is a relatively common condition. Simple, non-toxic goitre is a benign compensatory enlargement of the gland in response to low levels of iodine in the diet. Its principal manifestations are an unsightly lump in the neck and pressure effects on adjacent structures such as the trachea. Other forms of goitre are associated with either reduced or excessive secretion of thyroid hormone with the corresponding physiological effects. Carcinoma of the thyroid gland is rare. Ectopic glandular tissue is subject to the same diseases as are normally located glands.

Some forms of goitre are treated by thyroidectomy, care being taken not to remove parathyroid tissue or damage the recurrent laryngeal nerves.

CERVICAL VERTEBRAL COLUMN

This part of the vertebral column is composed of the seven cervical vertebrae and the intervening intervertebral discs. These have the same basic structure as the corresponding elements in the thoracic region of the vertebral column (pp. 79–80). A typical cervical vertebra has the following characteristics: (i) a small body; (ii) a large vertebral foramen; (iii) a bifid spinous process; (iv) a transverse process pierced by a **foramen transversarium** (Fig. 4.46). There are, of course, no facets for articulation with ribs.

The first, second, and seventh cervical vertebrae are modified. The first vertebra (**atlas**) has no body. It consists of two lateral masses connected by anterior and posterior arches. Each lateral mass bears a superior facet for articulation with the corresponding occipital condyle and an inferior facet for articulation with the superior articular process of the second vertebra. The second cervical vertebra (**axis**) has a strongly developed process, the dens or odontoid process, projecting upwards from its body. This process is, in fact, the centrum of the first vertebra which has fused with the body of the axis instead of being incorporated in the atlas. The front of the dens articulates with the back of the anterior arch of the atlas. The seventh cervical vertebra has a very long spinous process, hence its alternative name the **vertebra prominens**.

When articulated the cervical part of the vertebral column has a curvature which is convex forwards. This is a secondary curvature which appears in late fetal life and becomes accentuated in early childhood. The primary curvature of the vertebral column is concave forwards and this persists in the thoracic and pelvic regions. Although the degree of movement between adjacent vertebrae is small the cumulative effect is considerable giving the neck its characteristic flexibility. Nodding movements of the head take place principally at the joints between altas and occipital condyles and rotary movements at the joints between axis and atlas.

4

Orbit

Although the orbit is not intentionally involved in the practice of most aspects of dental surgery some knowledge of the anatomy of this region is required by the dental student because of its proximity to the upper jaw and because some of the nerves and vessels passing through it supply structures of dental importance. In addition infections of the oral region occasionally spread to the orbit and trauma to the face, including fractures of the upper facial skeleton, frequently involve this region.

In the account which follows the emphasis is on those aspects of orbital anatomy of vocational importance for the dental student. No description is given of the structure of the eyeball or of the mechanisms of vision.

Before reading this chapter make sure you are familiar with the anatomy of the bony orbit (pp. 115–16) and the surface anatomy of the orbital region (p. 142).

EYELIDS AND LACRIMAL APPARATUS

Eyelids

The eyelids are movable flaps which serve to protect the eye. The upper is the larger and more mobile with its own elevator muscle, the **levator palpebrae superioris.** Each eyelid consists of a **tarsal plate** covered by thin skin anteriorly and by **conjunctiva** posteriorly. In front of the tarsal plate are the fibres of the palpebral part of the orbicularis oculi muscle. Thin layers of loose connective tissue separate skin, muscle, and tarsal plate. The layer between the muscle and tarsal plate in the upper lid is continuous with the subaponeurotic layer of the scalp. Hence effusions of blood into the scalp can readily pass down into the upper lid.

The eyelashes are thick, curved hairs attached to the free margins of both eyelids from the **lateral angle (canthus)** to the lacrimal papilla. The **ciliary glands,** modified sweat glands of uncertain function, open close to the roots of the eyelashes. The margin of each eyelid, adjacent to the **medial canthus,** bears a small **lacrimal papilla** on the apex of which opens a **lacrimal canaliculus** through a small orifice or **punctum.**

Orbital septum and tarsi

The orbital septum is a thin connective tissue sheet attached to the margins of the bony orbit. It is deficient centrally at the palpebral fissure. It is greatly thickened above and below the palpebral fissure to form the superior and inferior tarsal plates. These are crescentic laminae of strong fibrous tissue which are shaped to fit the curvature of the eyeball. The upper tarsal plate is the larger of the two and receives the attachment of the levator palpebrae superioris muscle. The medial ends of the two plates are attached by the strong **medial palpebral ligament** to the lacrimal crest. A similar, but weaker, **lateral palpebral ligament** runs from the lateral ends of the plates to the zygomatic bone. The roots of the eyelashes are anchored in the tarsal plates.

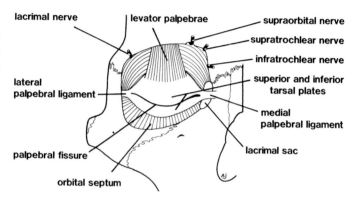

Fig. 4.60. Anterior view of the orbital septum and tarsal plates.

Tarsal (Meibomian) glands

These modified sebaceous glands are embedded in the deep surface of the tarsal plates and open by small ducts on to the free margin of the eyelids. They number about 30 in the upper lid and rather fewer in the lower lid. Their oily secretion spreads over the tear film (produced by the lacrimal gland) and delays its evaporation.

Conjunctiva

The conjunctiva is a transparent membrane consisting of a thin layer of fibrous tissue covered by stratified squamous epithelium. It covers the anterior aspect of the sclera of the eyeball and the inner surfaces of the eyelids. It is continuous with skin at the free margins of the lids and, at the sclerocorneal junction, with the corneal epithelium covering the transparent part of the eyeball. The line of reflection of the conjunctiva from the inner surface of the eyelid on to the sclera is known as the **conjunctival fornix.**

The conjunctiva of the sclera and upper eyelid is innervated by branches of the ophthalmic division of the trigeminal nerve and that of the lower lid by the infraorbital branch of the maxillary division. The blood supply of the conjunctiva is through branches of the ophthalmic artery.

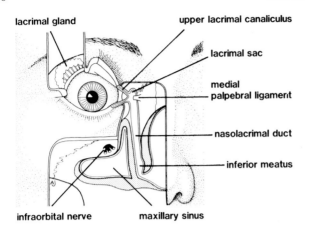

lacrimal gland

upper lacrimal canaliculus

lacrimal sac

medial
palpebral ligament

nasolacrimal duct

inferior meatus

infraorbital nerve   maxillary sinus

Fig. 4.61. The lacrimal apparatus.

Lacrimal apparatus and circulation of tears

Lacrimal gland

This serous gland consists of a large **orbital** and a smaller **palpebral** part. The orbital part, often described as being like an almond in size and shape, lies immediately adjacent to the periosteum of the lateral part of the roof of the orbit in a shallow fossa located just within the orbital margin. It is continuous with the palpebral part of the gland which lies in the lateral part of the upper eyelid deep to the orbital septum. The gland drains by a dozen or so small ducts which run from the palpebral part to open into the upper conjunctival fornix.

Lacrimal sac and nasolacrimal duct

The lacrimal sac is lodged within the lacrimal groove in the medial wall of the orbit. It receives the lacrimal canaliculi and is continuous below with the nasolacrimal duct. The latter runs downwards through the nasolacrimal canal to open into the inferior meatus of the nose. Both sac and duct have a fibrous wall and are lined by ciliated columnar epithelium.

Circulation of tears

The secretions of the lacrimal gland are released into the upper conjunctival fornix. From here the tears pass medially across the front of the eyeball to the lacrimal lake, their flow being aided by closing the eyelids. From the lake the tears pass through the lacrimal canaliculi to the lacrimal sac and thence through the nasolacrimal duct to the nasal cavity. Closing the eyelids helps to drain tears first by pressing the openings of the lacrimal canaliculi into the lake and secondly because the contraction of orbicularis oculi tends to dilate the lacrimal sac and so draw in the tears. From time to time the lids are closed reflexly (blinking) to draw tears across the eyes in response to dryness of the cornea.

CONTENTS OF ORBITS

The principal contents of the orbit are (i) the eyeball and optic nerve, (ii) the extraocular muscles which move the eyeball and upper eyelid, (iii) the vessels and nerves that supply these structures, and (iv) the vessels and nerves that pass through the orbit to reach structures in other regions.

The anteroposterior axis of the eyeball and the long axis of the bony orbit do not coincide. In the rest position the two eyeballs face forwards, usually with their long axes parallel to each other. The long axes of the bony orbits, by contrast, diverge anteriorly. It should be clear, therefore, that the optic nerve and the cone of rectus muscles, in passing from the apex of the orbit to the eyeball, will run forwards and laterally, not directly forwards (see Fig. 4.62). This point is important in understanding the relationships of the orbital structures and the functions of the extraocular muscles.

Extraocular muscles

The extraocular muscles include the elevator of the upper eyelid and six muscles that move the eyeball.

Levator palpebrae superioris

The elevator of the upper lid arises from the bone of the roof of the orbit close to its apex. It is a flat muscle which runs forwards beneath the orbital roof from which it is separated by the frontal nerve. Anteriorly the muscle broadens out and is attached to the tarsal plate and to the skin and conjunctiva of the upper eyelid. Most of the fibres of the muscle are of the striated variety and are innervated by the superior ramus of the oculomotor nerve. The part of the levator that is attached to the tarsal plate also contains some smooth muscle supplied by sympathetic fibres from the superior cervical ganglion. Interference with this sympathetic supply, such as may occur from compression of preganglionic neurons in the thoracic sympathetic trunk (by, for example, a tumour in the mediastinum) will lead to drooping of the upper eyelid or ptosis. This may be accompanied by constriction of the pupil caused by interruption of the sympathetic supply to the dilator pupillae muscle (see below and also Horner's syndrome on page 253).

The recti

The four recti arise from a **common tendinous ring** attached to the bone around the opening of the optic canal and the medial end of the superior orbital fissure at the apex of the orbit. From this ring the recti pass forwards as a cone of muscles, surrounding the optic nerve, to be inserted into the eyeball.

The **superior rectus** lies beneath levator palpebrae superioris. It is inserted into the upper surface of the sclera anterior to the coronal equator of the eyeball (the coronal equator is the circumference where a coronal plane, dividing the eyeball into anterior and posterior halves, meets the surface of the eyeball). Its action is therefore to elevate the cornea and, because of the lateral inclination of the muscle, to draw it medially. The **inferior rectus** has an equivalent insertion on the inferior surface of the eyeball and acts to depress the cornea and draw it medially. The **medial rectus** passes along the medial wall of the orbit and is inserted into the sclera on the medial surface of the eyeball, again anterior to the coronal equator. Its action is to draw the cornea medially. The **lateral rectus** is similarly arranged on the lateral side of the eyeball and draws the cornea laterally.

The superior rectus is innervated by the superior ramus and the inferior and medial recti by the inferior ramus of the oculomotor nerve. The lateral rectus is supplied by the abducent nerve.

Superior oblique

This muscle arises from the bone above and medial to the tendinous

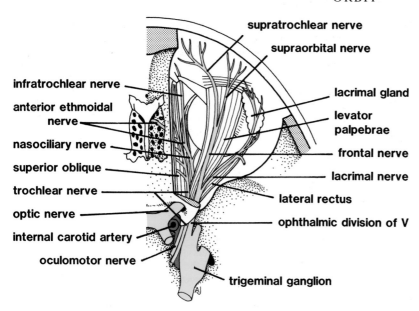

Fig. 4.62. Superior view of the contents of the right orbit. The orbital part of the frontal bone has been removed.

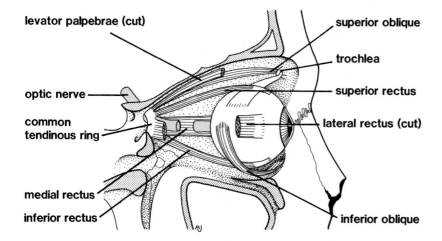

Fig. 4.63. Lateral view of the contents of the orbit.

ring. It passes forwards above the medial rectus and, towards the front of the orbit, becomes tendinous. The tendon passes through a loop of fibrous tissue, the **trochlea**, attached to the roof of the orbit immediately behind the superomedial angle of the orbital margin. At this point the tendon turns to run posteriorly and laterally across the upper surface of the eyeball, beneath the superior rectus, to be inserted into its upper surface behind the coronal equator. The action of the muscle is to pull the posterior part of the eyeball upwards and medially and so depress the cornea and turn it laterally. It is supplied by the trochlear nerve.

Inferior oblique

The inferior oblique muscle arises from the floor of the orbit lateral to the lacrimal groove. It is a narrow muscle which passes laterally and somewhat posteriorly beneath the eyeball, and also beneath the inferior rectus, to be inserted into the lateral surface of the eyeball behind the coronal equator. It elevates the cornea and draws it laterally. It is supplied by the inferior ramus of the oculomotor nerve.

Paralysis of one or more of the muscles moving the eyeball will alter its axis and so produce double vision, or diplopia, which will increase when an attempt is made to move the eyes in the direction of action of the paralysed muscle. Changes in the axis of the eyeball are called squints and the direction of the squint resulting from paralysis of one or other of the extraocular muscles can be worked out by considering the normal action of these muscles. Squints may also be congenital and in such cases diplopia is not a feature because the image from one eye is suppressed by the brain.

The vertical stability of the eyeball

The vertical position of the eyeball within the bony orbit is maintained by the sling-like **suspensory ligament**. This is attached, on either side of the eyeball, to the medial and lateral walls of the bony orbit, the points of attachment being near to the front edges of the walls and about midway between the roof and floor of the orbit. The ligament passes across the orbit beneath the eyeball where it is expanded to form a bed upon which the eyeball rests. Fractures involving the orbital walls below the attachments of the suspensory ligament will not affect the vertical stability of the eyeball but fractures above these attachments will result in dropping of the eyeball and hence in severe diplopia.

Nerves of the orbit

The nerves of the orbit comprise (i) the **optic nerve**, (ii) the **oculomotor, trochlear,** and **abducent nerves** to the extraocular muscles, (iii) the branches of the **ophthalmic division of the trigeminal nerve** which are sensory to structures within the orbit and to a wide area outside the orbit, (iv) the **ciliary ganglion** and associated branches which are concerned with the autonomic innervation of the eyeball, and (v) the **infraorbital** and **zygomatic branches of the maxillary division of the trigeminal nerve** which pass through the orbit without supplying its contents apart from fibres in the zygomatic nerve which pass to the lacrimal gland (see below and p. 179).

Optic nerve

The optic nerve, surrounded by its sheath formed from the three meningeal layers, enters the orbit through the optic canal, above and medial to the ophthalmic artery. It passes forwards and laterally within the cone of recti muscles to enter the eyeball medial to its posterior pole.

Nerves to the extraocular muscles

The **oculomotor nerve** divides into its **superior** and **inferior rami** whilst still within the lateral wall of the cavernous sinus. These enter the orbit by passing through the medial end of the superior orbital fissure within the common tendinous ring from which the recti muscles take origin. At their entrance to the orbit, therefore, the rami lie lateral to the optic nerve. The superior ramus crosses above the optic nerve to supply the overlying superior rectus and levator palpebrae superioris muscles. The inferior ramus divides immediately into three branches – one each to the medial rectus, inferior rectus, and inferior oblique muscles. The branch to the medial rectus passes below the optic nerve to reach its destination. The branch to the inferior oblique gives off a motor branch to the ciliary ganglion.

The **trochlear nerve** enters the orbit through the superior orbital fissure outside the tendinous ring. It then passes forwards above the origin of levator palpebrae superioris to reach the superior oblique muscle.

The **abducent nerve** enters the orbit by passing through the superior orbital fissure within the tendinous ring. It runs laterally and forwards to enter the lateral rectus muscle.

Branches of the ophthalmic division of the trigeminal nerve

This division of the trigeminal nerve splits into **lacrimal, frontal,** and **nasociliary** branches whilst still in the cavernous sinus. All three branches enter the orbit through the superior orbital fissure, the lacrimal and frontal outside and the nasociliary within the tendinous ring.

The **lacrimal nerve**, the smallest of the three branches, runs forwards along the lateral wall of the orbit above the lateral rectus muscle. It receives secretomotor fibres from the zygomatic nerve which are conveyed to the lacrimal gland. The lacrimal nerve pierces the orbital septum to supply the skin of the lateral part of the upper eyelid and much of the conjunctiva.

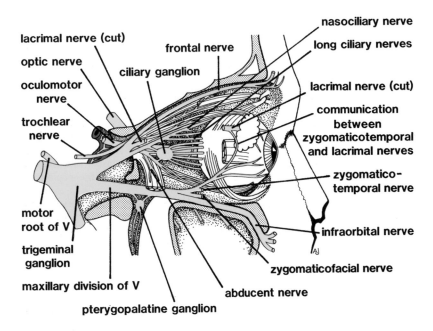

Fig. 4.64. Lateral view of the nerves of the orbit.

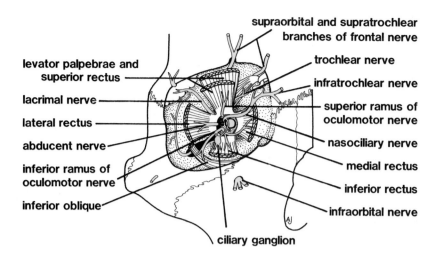

supraorbital and supratrochlear
branches of frontal nerve

trochlear nerve

infratrochlear nerve

superior ramus of
oculomotor nerve

nasociliary nerve

medial rectus

inferior rectus

infraorbital nerve

levator palpebrae and
superior rectus

lacrimal nerve

lateral rectus

abducent nerve

inferior ramus of
oculomotor nerve

inferior oblique

ciliary ganglion

Fig. 4.65. Anterior view of the nerves of the orbit.

The **frontal nerve** runs forwards between the levator palpebrae superioris and the roof of the orbit. A short distance before reaching the orbital margin it divides into a medial **supratrochlear** and a lateral **supraorbital** branch. These pierce the orbital septum and then occipitofrontalis to supply the skin of the forehead. The supraorbital nerve also gives branches to the mucous membrane of the frontal sinus.

The **nasociliary nerve** passes forwards within the cone of muscles, crosses above the optic nerve and then divides into its two terminal branches the **anterior ethmoidal** and the **infratrochlear**. Before bifurcating it gives off in proximal to distal sequence (i) the **sensory root of the ciliary ganglion**, (ii) the two **long ciliary nerves** carrying sensory fibres to the ciliary body and cornea and postganglionic sympathetic fibres (from the superior cervical ganglion; their route to the nasociliary nerve is uncertain) to the dilator pupillae muscle; these nerves enter the eyeball near the attachment of the optic nerve, and (iii) the **posterior ethmoidal nerve** which leaves the cone of muscles by passing beneath the superior oblique and then enters the posterior ethmoidal foramen in the medial wall of the orbit to supply the linings of the posterior ethmoidal air cells and the sphenoidal sinus. The anterior ethmoidal and infratrochlear branches also leave the cone of muscles by passing beneath the superior oblique. The anterior ethmoidal nerve enters the anterior ethmoidal foramen in the medial wall of the orbit, crosses beneath the roof of the ethmoidal labyrinth, where it supplies the lining of the anterior and middle ethmoidal air cells, to gain the supracribrous recess. It then passes through the nasal slit to supply an area of mucosa on the lateral wall and septum of the nasal cavity and continues, as the **external nasal nerve,** to innervate the skin over the nose. The infratrochlear nerve passes forwards below the trochlea to supply the lacrimal sac and adjacent conjunctiva and the skin of the upper lid and side of nose. Note that the branches of the ophthalmic division provide the sensory innervation of the upper lid; the lower lid is supplied with sensory fibres by the infraorbital branch of the maxillary division.

The ciliary ganglion

This is a small mass of nervous tissue lying on the lateral side of the optic nerve some distance behind the eyeball. It is a relay station for parasympathetic fibres. It receives three roots.

1. The **sensory root** is a branch of the nasociliary nerve; its fibres pass through the ganglion without interruption to supply the cornea and iris.

2. The **sympathetic root** is a branch of the sympathetic plexus on the internal carotid artery. It carries postganglionic vasoconstrictor fibres for the eyeball to the ganglion through which they pass without interruption. The cell bodies of these fibres are in the superior cervical ganglion of the sympathetic trunk. (Note that sympathetic fibres to dilator pupillae reach the eyeball in the long ciliary branches of the nasociliary nerve.)

3. The **motor root** is a branch of the nerve to inferior oblique, itself a branch of the oculomotor, and carries preganglionic parasympathetic fibres which synapse in the ganglion with postganglionic fibres to the sphincter pupillae and ciliary muscles.

The branches of the ciliary ganglion are the dozen or so **short ciliary nerves** which run to the back of the eyeball and pierce the sclera adjacent to the optic nerve. Each branch contains fibres from all three roots of the ganglion.

Orbital vessels

Ophthalmic artery

The ophthalmic artery branches from the internal carotid as the latter emerges from the cavernous sinus. It leaves the cranial cavity by passing through the optic canal where it lies lateral to and below the optic nerve. This relationship is preserved for a short distance within the orbit. The artery then crosses above the nerve to run forwards between the superior oblique and medial rectus muscles. The branches of the artery comprise the **central artery of the retina** (which runs to the retina within the optic nerve); the **lacrimal artery** to the lacrimal gland, eyelids, and conjunctiva; **muscular branches** to the extraocular muscles; **ciliary arteries** to the eyeball; **supraorbital, posterior ethmoidal, anterior ethmoidal,** and **supratrochlear** arteries (which accompany the nerves of the same name); and the **dorsal nasal artery** to the bridge of the nose.

Ophthalmic veins

Venous blood is drained from the orbit by the superior and inferior ophthalmic veins. Both pass through the superior orbital fissure to

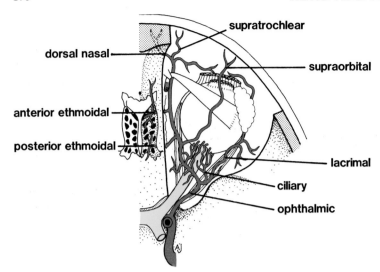

Fig. 4.66. Superior view of the ophthalmic artery and its branches.

open into the cavernous sinus. The superior vein has communications with the facial vein while the inferior vein frequently connects with the pterygoid plexus through the inferior orbital fissure.

Lymphatic drainage of orbit

Lymph drains from the orbit to the parotid group of nodes and thence to the deep cervical group.

5

Nasal cavity and paranasal sinuses

The nasal cavity in the living subject extends from the **external nostrils**, situated on the lower aspect of the external nose, to the **posterior nasal apertures** lying one each side of the posterior margin of the nasal septum. Through the posterior apertures it communicates with the nasopharynx. Because of the presence of the external nose the nasal cavity is larger from front to back in the living subject than it is in the dried skull.

Although extensive in its anteroposterior and vertical dimensions, the nasal cavity is narrow from side to side especially in its upper part where it lies between the two orbits. Below the orbits the nasal cavity lies between the right and left sides of the upper jaw. The roof of the nasal cavity is formed by the nasal bones, the cribriform plate of the ethmoid, and the body of the sphenoid. Inferiorly the nasal cavity is separated from the oral cavity by the palate. Deficiencies in the palate, either of a congenital or acquired nature, will thus place the two cavities in communication. The nasal cavity is completely divided into right and left compartments by the **nasal septum**.

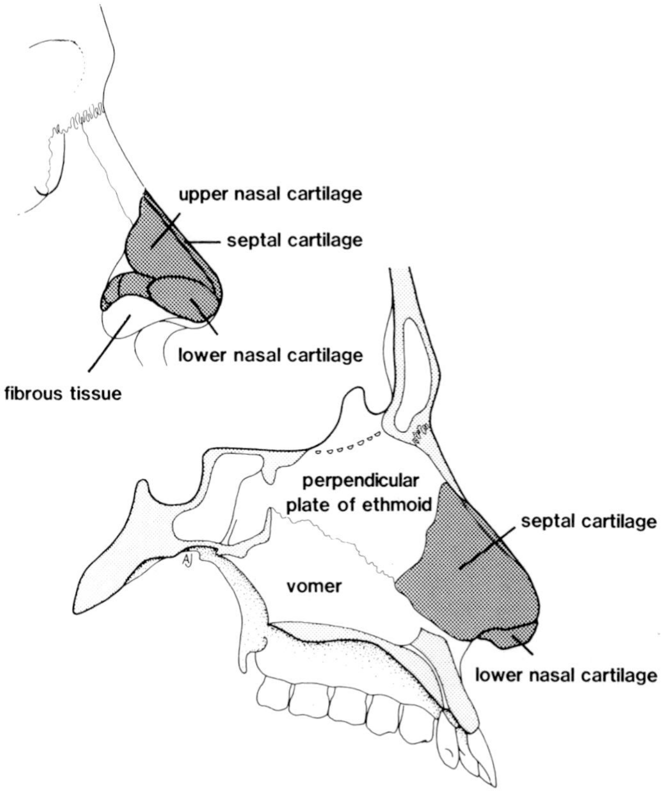

EXTERNAL NOSE

The skeleton of the external nose comprises the **nasal bones**, the **upper** and **lower nasal cartilages**, and the **cartilaginous part of the nasal septum** (or **septal cartilage**). The nasal bones and adjacent parts of the frontal processes of the maxillae form the bridge of the nose. The upper and lower nasal cartilages, together with a variable number of minor cartilages, form the skeleton of the lower, pliable part of the external nose. The septal cartilage is quadrilateral in shape. It is continuous posteriorly with the bony part of the nasal septum (i.e. with the anterior edge of the perpendicular plate of the ethmoid and the superior border of the vomer). In front of the bony septum it articulates above with the lower aspect of the internasal suture and below with the upper aspect of the median palatine suture. The various nasal cartilages represent unossified parts of the nasal capsule.

The lateral border of each external nostril is thickened and rounded, due to the presence of fibrofatty tissue, and is termed the **ala nasi**. Just inside the external nostrils the nasal cavity is dilated somewhat to form the **nasal vestibule**. This part of the nasal cavity is lined by skin with coarse hairs and sebaceous and sweat glands.

The skin covering the lower part of the external nose is adherent to the underlying structures and contains many large sebaceous glands. Its sensory innervation is by the infratrochlear, external nasal and infraorbital nerves and its arterial supply is through branches of the facial, ophthalmic, and infraorbital arteries. The venous drainage is into the facial and ophthalmic veins and the lymphatic drainage into the submandibular nodes.

Fig. 4.67. The nasal cartilages.

NASAL CAVITY PROPER

Most of the features of the nasal cavity have been described in the section dealing with this region in the dried skull (pp. 116–17). All that remains to be done is to describe the mucous membrane lining the cavity and its nerve and blood supply, and lymphatic drainage.

Nasal mucous membrane

Mucous membrane lines the whole of the nasal cavity apart from the vestibule. It is of two types, **olfactory** and **respiratory**.

Olfactory mucous membrane

Over the upper part of the septum and the roof and lateral walls of the nasal cavity down to and including the superior concha, the mucous membrane has an olfactory epithelium. This is rather thicker than the epithelium of the remainder of the nasal cavity and consists of receptor, supporting, and basal cells. The receptor cells are, in fact, primary sensory neurons (equivalent to the first-order neurons in other sensory pathways). From the basal aspect of these cells run unmyelinated axons which pass in the olfactory nerves, through the cribriform plate, to synapse with second-order neurons in the olfactory bulb.

The olfactory mucous membrane contains numerous serous glands.

Respiratory mucous membrane

The remainder of the nasal cavity, apart from the vestibule, is lined by mucosa with a respiratory (i.e. ciliated columnar or cuboidal) epithelium. Associated with this epithelium are numerous serous and mucous glands. Beneath the mucous membrane are extensive areas of vascular cavernous tissue. These are best developed over the conchae where their presence aids the warming of inspired air. In the meatus the mucous membrane tends to be thinner and less vascular and is adherent to the periosteum. The mucosa is thick over the bony part of the septum but over the cartilaginous part is thinner and is tightly bound down to the underlying perichondrium.

Nerve supply, blood supply, and lymphatic drainage of the nasal cavity

The innervation and arterial supply of the nasal cavity have a similar arrangement and can be conveniently described together.

The lateral wall

1. The **posterosuperior quadrant** is innervated by the lateral nasal branches of the pterygopalatine ganglion which enter the nasal cavity through the sphenopalatine foramen. The blood supply to this quadrant is via nasal branches of the sphenopalatine artery, a terminal branch of the maxillary artery which also enters the nasal cavity through the sphenopalatine foramen.

2. The **posteroinferior quadrant** is supplied by branches of the greater palatine nerve and artery (themselves branches of the pterygopalatine ganglion and maxillary artery, respectively). These pierce the perpendicular plate of the palatine bone to reach the nasal cavity.

3. The **anterosuperior quadrant** is supplied by the anterior ethmoidal nerve and artery (branches of the nasociliary nerve and ophthalmic artery) which enter the nasal cavity from the supracribrous recess through the nasal slit in the cribriform plate.

4. The **anteroinferior quadrant** is supplied by the anterior superior alveolar branches of the infraorbital nerve and artery.

The venous drainage of the posterior part of the lateral wall of the nasal cavity is to the pharyngeal and pterygoid plexuses while that of the anterior part is to the facial vein. The lymph drainage from the posterior part of the lateral wall is to the retropharyngeal lymph nodes and from the anterior part to the submandibular nodes.

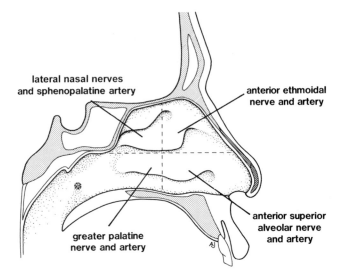

Fig. 4.68. The nerve and blood supply of the lateral wall of the nasal cavity.

The septum

Most of the septum is innervated by the medial nasal branches of the pterygopalatine ganglion and receives blood through the sphenopalatine branch of the maxillary artery. These structures, after gaining access to the nasal cavity through the sphenopalatine foramen, pass across the roof of the cavity to the upper border of the septum where they turn to run forwards and downwards in the mucous membrane towards the incisive fossa. The medial nasal nerves supply the roof of the nasal cavity and the mucous membrane over much of the septum. The nasopalatine nerve also supplies filaments to the septum but most of the nerve passes through the incisive fossa to supply the mucous membrane of the anterior part of the hard palate. The sphenopalatine artery finishes short of the incisive fossa, usually anastomosing with an ascending branch of the greater palatine artery which runs upwards through the fossa. A small area over the anterosuperior part of the septum is supplied by the anterior ethmoidal nerve and artery.

Venous blood from the posterior half of the septum flows into the pterygoid plexus and lymph into the retropharyngeal nodes. From the anterior half of the septum venous blood passes into the facial vein and lymph into the submandibular nodes.

The nerves supplying the lateral wall and septum of the nasal cavity contain sensory trigeminal fibres, mostly from the maxillary division, and postganglionic parasympathetic (secretomotor) fibres to the glands of the mucous membrane. The latter begin in the pterygopalatine ganglion where they are in synaptic connection with preganglionic fibres from the facial nerve (pp. 179–80).

PARANASAL SINUSES

A full account of the osteological features of the paranasal sinuses is given in the chapter on skull (see pp. 120–1).

The mucous membrane lining the sinuses is similar to that in the respiratory part of the nasal cavity. It is covered with cuboidal epithelium which is ciliated over much of its extent and especially near the openings of the sinuses into the nasal cavity. The movement of the cilia sweeps the mucus produced by the numerous mucous glands towards the openings and so aids drainage. The cilia are frequently reduced in number or lost altogether following chronic infection of the sinus thus reducing drainage and initiating a vicious circle in which continued infection is more likely. This is particularly likely to occur in the maxillary sinus where, because the opening is sited high up on the medial wall, drainage by gravity alone is impossible.

The mucous membrane lining the maxillary sinus is innervated by the infraorbital and superior alveolar nerves. Blood is supplied by the infraorbital, superior alveolar, and greater palatine arteries; the venous drainage is into the pterygoid plexus. Lymph drainage is to the submandibular nodes.

The lining of the frontal sinus is innervated by branches of the supraorbital nerve. Its blood supply is through the supraorbital and anterior ethmoidal arteries and the venous drainage is into the supraorbital and superior ophthalmic veins. Lymph drainage is into the submandibular nodes.

The sphenoidal sinus receives its nerve and blood supply through the posterior ethmoidal nerve and vessels. Lymph drainage is into the retropharyngeal nodes.

The ethmoidal sinuses are innervated by the anterior and posterior ethmoidal nerves and their blood supply and venous drainage are through the corresponding arteries and veins. Lymph from these sinuses passes into the submandibular and retropharyngeal nodes.

The secretomotor (parasympathetic) supply to the glands in the mucous membrane lining the maxillary sinus comes from the pterygopalatine ganglion via the infraorbital and superior alveolar nerves. The sphenoidal and ethmoidal sinuses are believed to receive their secretomotor supply through minute orbital branches of the pterygopalatine ganglion which enter the orbit through the inferior orbital fissure and then pass through the posterior ethmoidal foramen to reach the sinuses. The frontal sinus may also receive its secretomotor supply through orbital branches of the pterygopalatine ganglion.

6

Infratemporal and pterygopalatine fossae

A knowledge of the anatomy of the infratemporal and pterygopalatine fossae and their contents is essential for understanding the dental region. Many of the nerves and blood vessels supplying the structures of the mouth run through or close to these fossae. In addition the infratemporal fossa contains the pterygoid muscles which play an important part in movements of the mandible. The posterior boundary of the fossa is occupied by the styloid apparatus and carotid sheath and is closely related to the last four cranial nerves.

Before reading the following sections you should remind yourself of the osteological features of the infratemporal and pterygopalatine fossae which are fully described on pages 114 and 119–20.

INFRATEMPORAL FOSSA

Pterygoid muscles

The pterygoid muscles are two of the four muscles known collectively as the **muscles of mastication** (the remaining two are the masseter and temporalis which are described on pages 150–51). The muscles of mastication develop from the mesoderm of the first pharyngeal arch and are innervated, therefore, by the mandibular division of the trigeminal nerve.

Lateral pterygoid

This muscle arises by two heads. The upper head is attached to the infratemporal surface of the greater wing of the sphenoid, the lower head to the lateral surface of the lateral pterygoid plate. From these origins the fibres run backwards and laterally, converging as they do so, to be inserted by a short tendon into the pterygoid fovea on the anterior surface of the neck of the mandible and into the anterior aspect of the capsule, and hence into the disc of the temporomandibular joint. The muscle is innervated by a branch of the anterior trunk of the mandibular division of the trigeminal nerve. Its action is to pull the head of the mandible and the disc forwards. The part that it plays in translatory and opening movements of the mandible is described on pages 207–8.

The phylogenetic history of the muscle is of interest. It is believed that the corresponding muscle in the mammal-like reptiles was inserted into the prearticular, one of the bones of the lower jaw situated close to the quadrate–articular joint which formed the jaw articulation in these creatures as it does in all non-mammalian vertebrates. With the formation of the mammalian jaw joint between the squamous and dentary (mandible) and the inclusion of the quadrate and articular (the latter together with the prearticular) in

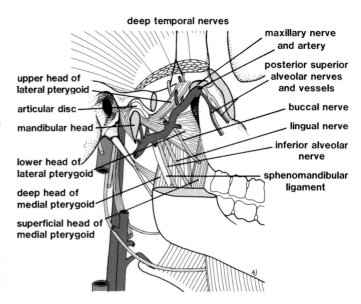

Fig. 4.69. Lateral view of the contents of the right infratemporal fossa. The ramus of the mandible has been removed at a level just above the mandibular foramen.

the middle-ear cavity, as the incus and malleus respectively, the lateral pterygoid gained a new insertion into the neck of the mandible and the front of the joint capsule. There is some evidence, mainly of an embryological nature, suggesting that the part of the lateral pterygoid that continued on to be inserted into the prearticular became trapped within the newly formed temporomandibular jaw joint where it is represented in modern mammals by the articular disc.

Medial pterygoid

The medial pterygoid also arises by two heads. Most of its fibres take origin from the medial surface of the lateral pterygoid plate but a small slip (the superficial head) arises from the maxillary tuberosity and neighbouring part of the palatine bone. The fibres pass downwards, backwards, and laterally to be inserted into the roughened area on the medial surface of the ramus and angle of the mandible. Like the masseter, the medial pterygoid muscle contains a number of tendinous septa which give it a multipennate arrangement

(p. 13). The gap between the muscle and the medial surface of the ramus above the insertion is called the **pterygomandibular space**. The muscle is innervated by a branch from the main trunk of the mandibular nerve. Its action is to pull the angle of the mandible upwards, forwards, and medially. Its role in mandibular movements is further discussed on pages 207–8.

Sphenomandibular ligament

This is a well-developed band of fibrous tissue which extends from the spine of the sphenoid to the lingula of the mandible and the adjacent margin of the mandibular foramen. As it passes downwards and forwards it is separated from the neck of the mandible by the maxillary vessels while more inferiorly (in the pterygomandibular space) it is separated from the ramus of the mandible by the inferior alveolar nerve and vessels. It is related medially to the pharyngeal wall above and to the medial pterygoid muscle below. The ligament is pierced near to its attachment to the lingula by the mylohyoid nerve and vessels.

Developmentally the sphenomandibular ligament is a remnant of the perichondrium surrounding the intermediate part of Meckel's cartilage.

Mandibular nerve

The mandibular branch of the trigeminal nerve arises from the lateral part of the trigeminal ganglion and almost immediately leaves the cranial cavity by passing through the foramen ovale into the infratemporal fossa. The trigeminal motor root runs beneath the ganglion and unites with the mandibular nerve within or just below the foramen ovale. As it emerges from the foramen the mandibular nerve lies between the upper head of the lateral pterygoid muscle and the tensor veli palatini. It is separated from the latter muscle by the **otic ganglion** from which it receives a few postganglionic parasympathetic fibres. After a brief course the nerve divides into **anterior** and **posterior** trunks (Figs 4.69 and 4.84).

Branches of the mandibular nerve before its division

A **meningeal branch (nervus spinosus)** runs back into the middle cranial fossa through the foramen spinosum (sometimes through the foramen ovale).

The **nerve to medial pterygoid** passes forwards to supply that muscle. It gives off a branch to the otic ganglion, the fibres of which pass through the ganglion without interruption and run in branches of the ganglion to supply tensor veli palatini and tensor tympani (the latter, a small middle-ear muscle inserted into the malleus, acts with stapedius to damp down oscillations of the ossicles in response to sounds of high intensity).

Branches from the anterior trunk

The anterior trunk is the smaller of the two and consists mainly of motor fibres. Its only sensory branch is the buccal nerve.

The **buccal nerve** runs at first laterally, to emerge between the two heads of the lateral pterygoid, and then continues downwards and forwards immediately deep to the temporalis muscle and onto the lateral surface of the buccinator. It gives branches to the skin of the cheek before piercing buccinator to supply the mucous membrane of the cheek, buccal sulcus, and lower alveolar process in the region of the lower molars and premolars. The buccal nerve also contains a few postganglionic parasympathetic fibres from the otic ganglion which are secretomotor to the small glands associated with the mucous membrane of the cheek.

The **masseteric nerve** passes laterally above the upper head of the lateral pterygoid and then through the mandibular incisure to reach the deep surface of the masseter. It gives a small branch to the temporomandibular joint.

The two **deep temporal nerves** also run above the lateral pterygoid muscle and then enter the deep surface of temporalis.

The **nerve to lateral pterygoid** has a short course to enter the deep surface of the muscle.

Branches from the posterior trunk

The larger posterior trunk is made up mainly of sensory fibres but receives a few motor fibres for the mylohyoid muscle and the anterior belly of the digastric. It divides into three large branches.

The **auriculotemporal nerve** arises by two roots which run posteriorly one either side of the middle meningeal artery. They unite behind the artery and the nerve then continues posteriorly, lying deep to the lateral pterygoid muscle and the neck of the mandible. It curves laterally around the posterior surface of the mandibular neck, passing through the glenoid lobe of the parotid gland or within its capsule, to emerge laterally from behind the temporomandibular joint to which it gives a small twig. It then ascends over the posterior root of the zygomatic process of the temporal bone, posterior to the superficial temporal vessels, and divides into **superficial temporal branches** which supply the skin of the temple. The nerve also gives branches to the external acoustic meatus and outer surface of the tympanic membrane, to the skin of the auricle and to the parotid gland. The branches to the parotid gland contain postganglionic parasympathetic (secretomotor) fibres which reach the auriculotemporal nerve in a communicating branch from the otic ganglion.

The **lingual nerve** runs downwards between the lateral pterygoid and tensor veli palatini muscles. Here it is joined at an acute angle by the **chorda tympani nerve**, a branch of the facial nerve given off in the tympanic cavity (Fig. 4.24 p. 130). The chorda tympani carries taste fibres for the anterior two-thirds of the tongue and preganglionic parasympathetic fibres for the salivary glands in the floor of the mouth. Emerging from beneath the lateral pterygoid muscle the lingual nerve curves downwards and forwards between the medial pterygoid muscle and the ramus of the mandible (i.e. in the pterygomandibular space) in front of the inferior alveolar nerve. It passes out of the pterygomandibular space br running forwards immediately adjacent to the medial surface of the mandible in the region of the third molar. In this situation it is covered by mucous membrane only and can, therefore, be palpated from within the mouth. It lies very close to the roots of the last molar and is at risk in operations upon this tooth. As the nerve runs against the surface of the mandible it has the mandibular attachment of the pterygomandibular raphe immediately above it and the corresponding attachment of the mylohyoid muscle immediately below.

Diverging medially from the mandible the nerve runs forwards across the floor of the mouth, supplying the mucous membrane as it does so, to the lateral surface of the hyoglossus muscle where it has connections with the **submandibular ganglion** (in which the preganglionic parasympathetic fibres brought to the lingual nerve in the chorda tympani synapse with postganglionic neurons innervating the submandibular and sublingual glands). It then divides into its terminal branches to supply the anterior two-thirds of the tongue with taste (chorda tympani fibres) and general sensation (trigeminal fibres). The course of the lingual nerve in the floor of the mouth and the connections of the submandibular ganglion are described in detail on pages 188–9.

The **inferior alveolar nerve** runs downwards deep to the lateral pterygoid muscle behind the lingual nerve. Emerging from beneath lateral pterygoid the nerve continues downwards between the ramus of the mandible and the sphenomandibular ligament into the pterygomandibular space. It enters the mandibular canal through the mandibular foramen and runs forwards to supply the lower teeth and, through its **mental branch**, the skin and mucous membrane of the lower lip. Just before the nerve enters the mandibular foramen it gives off its mylohyoid branch. This pierces the sphenomandibular ligament and runs downwards and forwards in a groove on the medial surface of the ramus to pass below the mylohyoid muscle which it supplies together with the anterior belly of the digastric. The mylohyoid nerve contains all the motor fibres of the posterior division of the mandibular nerve. The inferior alveolar nerve receives a few postganglionic fibres which have relayed in the otic ganglion and which pass in the mental branch to supply the small glands in the lower lip.

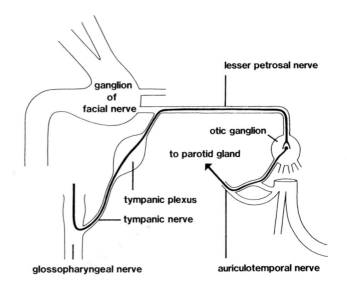

Fig. 4.70. The parasympathetic pathway to the parotid gland via the otic ganglion.

Otic ganglion

This ganglion is situated immediately below foramen ovale, between the main trunk of the mandibular nerve and tensor veli palatini, and close to the origin of the nerve to medial pterygoid. It receives preganglionic parasympathetic fibres from the inferior salivatory nucleus via the glossopharyngeal nerve and its lesser petrosal branch. These fibres synapse with postganglionic fibres which pass by a communicating branch to the auriculotemporal nerve and thence to the parotid gland to which they are secretomotor. A few postganglionic fibres pass to the main trunk of the mandibular nerve to be distributed through the inferior alveolar and buccal nerves to the mucous glands in the lower lip and cheek.

The ganglion receives a sympathetic root from the plexus on the middle meningeal artery. This contains postganglionic fibres from the superior cervical ganglion. These pass through the ganglion without relay and then run with the parasympathetic fibres to the parotid gland where they innervate the blood vessels.

The ganglion also receives a branch from the nerve to medial pterygoid. The fibres in this branch run through the ganglion without interruption and pass in its motor branches to supply the tensor veli palatini and tensor tympani.

Maxillary artery

One of the terminal branches of the external carotid artery, the maxillary artery begins in the parotid gland posterior to the neck of the mandible. It enters the infratemporal fossa by curving forwards deep to the mandibular neck. It then crosses the lower head of the lateral pterygoid, usually lying superficial but occasionally deep to that belly, to enter the pterygopalatine fossa through the pterygo-maxillary fissure. It is customary, and convenient for remembering the branches, to divide the artery into three parts – before, on, and beyond the lower head of the lateral pterygoid (Figs 4.69 and 4.76).

Branches of the first part

The first two branches arise from the maxillary artery while it is still in the parotid gland and supply structures of the ear. The **deep auricular artery** supplies the lining of the external acoustic meatus and the **anterior tympanic artery** passes through the petrotympanic fissure to supply part of the lining of the tympanic cavity.

The **middle meningeal artery** provides the principal source of blood to the meninges. It ascends deep to lateral pterygoid, passes between the two roots of the auriculotemporal nerve, and enters the cranial cavity through the foramen spinosum.

The **accessory meningeal artery** ascends in front of the middle meningeal artery to enter the skull through the foramen ovale. It gives branches to neighbouring muscles before entering the foramen.

The **inferior alveolar artery** runs downwards posterior, and in close relationship, to the nerve of the same name. Before entering the mandibular foramen it gives off its mylohyoid branch which pierces the sphenomandibular ligament and passes to the superficial aspect of the mylohyoid muscle in company with the corresponding nerve. The inferior alveolar artery runs forwards in the mandibular canal to supply the bone of the lower jaw, the inferior dentition and, through its **mental branch**, the lower lip.

Branches of the second part

The second part of the artery gives two **deep temporal branches** to the temporalis muscle, **pterygoid branches** to the pterygoid muscles, the **masseteric branch** which passes through the mandibular incisure to the masseter muscle, and the **buccal branch** which accompanies the buccal nerve to supply the structures of the cheek. A small **lingual branch** may similarly accompany the lingual nerve.

Branches of the third part

These arise within the pterygopalatine fossa and are described on page 180.

Pterygoid plexus of veins

This venous plexus lies around and partly within the lateral pterygoid muscle. Its tributaries correspond to the branches of the three parts of the maxillary artery although the area drained is somewhat smaller than that supplied by the artery. Blood from the periphery of the latter area drains via other routes such as the facial veins. The pterygoid plexus also communicates with the facial vein through the **deep facial vein**, with the cavernous sinus by means of one or more emissary veins passing through the foramen ovale (or the emissary sphenoidal foramen if present) and with the inferior ophthalmic vein through the inferior orbital fissure. It drains through the short but wide **maxillary vein** which runs between the neck of the mandible and the sphenomandibular ligament to

The pterygomandibular space and the anatomy of inferior alveolar block

The bone of the body of the adult mandible is so dense that it acts as an effective barrier to the passage of local anaesthetic solution. In order to anaesthetize the lower teeth it is necessary, therefore, to reach the main trunk of the inferior alveolar nerve before it enters the mandibular canal. The only practical place in which this can be done is in the pterygomandibular space. The resulting anaesthesia is called an **inferior alveolar (or inferior dental) block**. In order that such a block may be administered efficiently and safely a precise knowledge of the anatomy of the pterygomandibular space is essential.

The best way to appreciate (and to remember) the arrangement, contents, and relationships of the pterygomandibular space is by

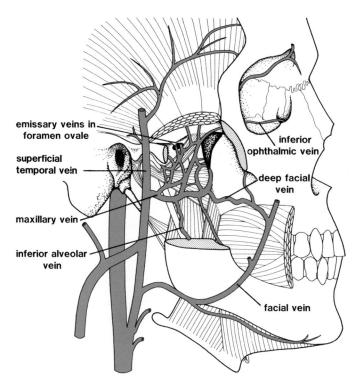

Fig. 4.71. The pterygoid plexus of veins.

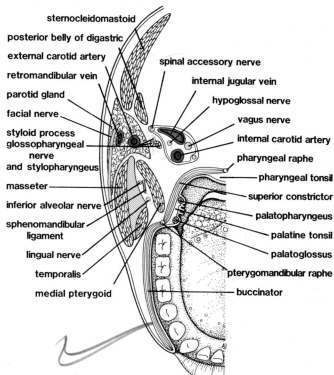

Fig. 4.72. Horizontal section through the pterygomandibular space at a level above the mandibular foramen.

unite with the superficial temporal vein and so form the **retromandibular vein**.

The plexus may be difficult to find in the cadaver where it is empty of blood but in the living subject it is frequently a prominent structure. Its importance in dentistry lies in the fact that it may be punctured by a needle delivering local anaesthetic solution to the posterior superior alveolar nerves, an event which may be followed by copious bleeding into the surrounding tissues. Blood may pass forwards through the inferior orbital fissure into the orbit with production of a 'black eye'. Through its communications the plexus forms a potential route whereby infection may spread from its area of drainage (including the jaws and, through the deep facial vein, the face) to the cavernous sinus (see Fig. 4.71).

studying a horizontal section through the infratemporal fossa located a short distance above the mandibular foramen. Such a section, in a slightly idealized form, is shown in Fig. 4.72. As can be seen the pterygomandibular space at this level is a narrow gap between the bulky medial pterygoid muscle and the ramus of the mandible. The medial surface of the ramus is not flat but presents anteriorly a ridge (the temporal crest) behind which is a shallow concavity. The lingual nerve is situated well forward in the space, approximately opposite the temporal crest, while the inferior alveolar neurovascular bundle, together with the closely associated sphenomandibular ligament lies further back within the concavity of the ramus. The temporalis

...d into the anterior border of the coronoid process ...rea of bone between this border and the temporal ...mainder of the pterygomandibular space is filled with ...ive tissue.

...rior boundary of the pterygomandibular space is formed by the anteromedial surface of the parotid gland. Within the gland are the facial nerve, retromandibular vein, and external carotid artery, in that order from superficial to deep. The gland is enclosed within the parotid capsule. Although tough and relatively impervious to fluid, the capsule is easily penetrated by the sharp tip of a syringe needle.

Access to the pterygomandibular space from within the mouth is gained by inserting the needle through the buccinator and the covering mucous membrane just lateral to the pterygomandibular raphe and then advancing it into the anterior opening of the space between the temporal crest and the front edge of the medial pterygoid muscle.

The various clinical techniques that are used to achieve inferior alveolar block share the same principal aims, namely: (i) to gain access to the pterygomandibular space without passing the needle into the insertion of temporalis or into the medial pterygoid, (ii) to advance the needle at a level such that the local anaesthetic solution is deposited around the inferior alveolar nerve just before it enters the mandibular foramen, (iii) to advance the needle far enough into the space so that it reaches the inferior alveolar nerve, and (iv) since lingual anaesthesia is often also required, to inject a few drops of solution around the lingual nerve as the needle is either advanced or withdrawn.

It is particularly important to ensure that the needle is advanced the correct distance into the pterygomandibular space. If it does not enter far enough satsifactory anaesthesia of the inferior alveolar nerve may not be achieved. If advanced too far there is a possibility that the tip of the needle will pierce the parotid capsule. Local anaesthetic solution will then enter the parotid gland through which it will spread rapidly to reach the branches of the facial nerve. A degree of facial paralysis will ensue which, though temporary, is uncomfortable for the patient and embarrassing to the operator. This can be avoided if it is remembered that the mandibular foramen is located approximately halfway between the anterior and posterior borders of the ramus, both of which can be readily palpated through the skin. In some patients, however, a lobule of the parotid gland projects forwards into the pterygomandibular space and in these cases it may be difficult to avoid local anaesthetic solution entering the gland.

Styloid apparatus

The styloid process is a curved bony spine, of variable length, which projects downwards and somewhat forwards from the inferior surface of the temporal bone and lateral to the internal carotid artery. Its upper part (the base) is fused with the tympanic plate. Its lower part gives attachment to two ligaments and three muscles.

Stylohyoid ligament

The styloid process ossifies in the dorsal part of the cartilage of the second pharyngeal arch. The lesser cornu and upper part of the body of the hyoid bone ossify in the ventral part of this cartilage. The intervening part atrophies but its perichondrium persists as the stylohyoid ligament, a well defined cord of fibrous tissue which runs from

the tip of the styloid process to the apex of the lesser cornu of the hyoid bone.

Stylomandibular ligament

This ligament is merely a thickening of the deep layer of the parotid capsule. It passes from the base of the styloid process and adjacent part of the tympanic plate to the angle of the mandible.

Stylopharyngeus muscle

The stylopharyngeus muscle arises from the medial surface of the styloid process. It runs almost vertically downwards, passes between the internal and external carotid arteries, crosses the lower border of the superior constrictor muscle and then continues downwards inside the middle constrictor, beneath the pharyngeal mucous membrane, to be inserted into the posterior border of the thyroid cartilage and

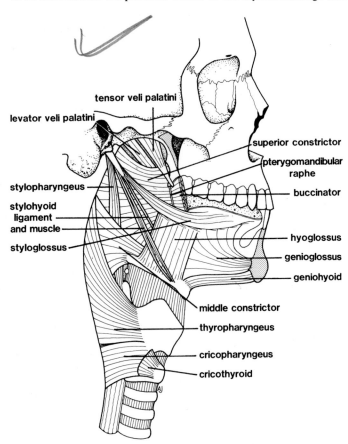

the side wall of the pharynx. The glossopharyngeal nerve curves around and supplies the muscle as it passes between the two carotid arteries.

The muscle is an elevator of the pharynx and larynx. As is obvious from its innervation the muscle is derived from the third pharyngeal arch, being in fact the only muscle so derived.

Fig. 4.73. The styloid apparatus and the muscles of the pharynx and the floor of the mouth.

Styloglossus muscle

This muscle takes origin from the anterior aspect of the lower part of the styloid process and of the neighbouring part of the stylohyoid ligament. It is fully described with the extrinsic muscles of the tongue on page 192.

Stylohyoid muscle

The stylohyoid muscle arises from the posterior surface of the styloid process. It runs downwards and forwards crossing superficial to the external carotid artery before the latter structure enters the parotid gland. A short distance above the hyoid bone the muscle divides into two slips which pass one either side of the intermediate tendon of the digastric muscle to be inserted into the base of the greater cornu of the hyoid bone. The muscle is derived from the second pharyngeal arch and is innervated, therefore, by the facial nerve. Its action is to elevate the hyoid.

All three styloid muscles are involved in swallowing (see p. 211).

PTERYGOPALATINE FOSSA

The pterygopalatine fossa contains the maxillary nerve, the pterygopalatine ganglion and the third part of the maxillary artery and its branches. It is intimately concerned, therefore, with the nerve and blood supply of the upper jaw.

Maxillary nerve and pterygopalatine ganglion

Maxillary nerve

The maxillary division of the trigeminal nerve enters the pterygopalatine fossa through the foramen rotundum. It runs forwards and somewhat laterally across the fossa and enters the orbit through the inferior orbital fissure. It then crosses the floor of the orbit, where it is known as the **infraorbital nerve,** to supply the skin of the face. The infraorbital nerve is described on page 148.

Within the fossa the maxillary nerve is attached to the **pterygopalatine ganglion** by two **ganglionic branches.** More anteriorly the **posterior superior alveolar nerves** are given off. Usually two or three in number, these pass downwards and laterally through the pterygomaxillary fissure into the infratemporal fossa. Here they run on the posterior surface of the maxilla and divide into numerous small branches which enter the maxilla through the posterior alveolar foramina and supply the upper molar teeth, the mucous membrane on the buccal surface of the associated alveolar process and the lining of the maxillary sinus. Anaesthesia of the upper molar teeth and associated buccal mucosa can be achieved by a **posterior superior alveolar block** in which local anaesthetic solution is injected adjacent to the nerves as they enter the maxilla.

As the maxillary nerve is about to enter the inferior orbital fissure it gives rise to the **zygomatic nerve.** This runs forwards through the fissure and along the lateral wall of the orbit where it divides into **zygomaticotemporal** and **zygomaticofacial branches.** These nerves leave the orbit through canals in the zygomatic bone, the zygomaticotemporal branch passing into the temporal fossa to supply the skin of the temple, and the zygomaticofacial nerve emerging more anteriorly to supply skin over the prominence of the cheek. The zygomatic nerve also contains postganglionic parasympathetic fibres from the pterygopalatine ganglion. Within the orbit these pass in a communicating branch from the zygomaticotemporal nerve to the lacrimal nerve and so reach the lacrimal gland.

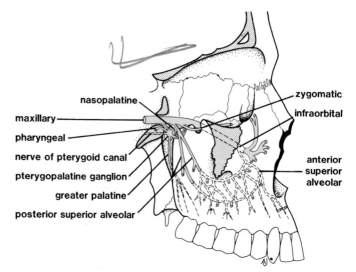

Fig. 4.74. The maxillary nerve in the pterygopalatine fossa. In the majority of individuals a middle superior alveolar nerve is also present, but variably located (Fig. 4.88A).

Pterygopalatine ganglion

This is located deep within the pterygopalatine fossa close to the sphenopalatine foramen. It is a relay station for parasympathetic secretomotor fibres derived from the facial nerve and destined for the lacrimal gland and the glands of the mucous membranes of the nose, nasopharynx, paranasal sinuses, palate, and upper lip. Most of the fibres in the branches of the ganglion, however, are of the sensory variety being derived from the maxillary nerve through the ganglionic branches of the latter. These fibres pass through the ganglion without interruption.

Preganglionic parasympathetic fibres from the superior salivatory nucleus reach the ganglion through the greater petrosal branch of the facial nerve. This branch fuses with the deep petrosal nerve from the carotid sympathetic plexus to form the **nerve of the pterygoid canal** which enters the pterygopalatine fossa through that canal and unites with the posterior aspect of the ganglion. The preganglionic fibres synapse in the ganglion with postganglionic neurons. The latter are distributed to the glands associated with the mucous membrane of the nose, nasopharynx, and palate through the nasal, pharyngeal, and palatine branches respectively of the ganglion and to the lacrimal gland through a complicated pathway comprising the ganglionic branches of the maxillary nerve, the maxillary nerve itself, its zygomatic and zygomaticotemporal branches, the communicating branch to the lacrimal nerve and then via the latter nerve to the gland. Postganglionic fibres pass to the small glands in the upper lip, upper part of the cheek, and mucous membrane of the maxillary sinus through the maxillary nerve and its infraorbital continuation. Postganglionic fibres to the linings of the sphenoidal, ethmoidal, and frontal sinuses run in the small orbital branches of the pterygopalatine ganglion.

The deep petrosal nerve contains postganglionic sympathetic fibres from the superior cervical ganglion. These are mostly vasoconstrictor in function and pass through the ganglion without interruption to be distributed in its branches.

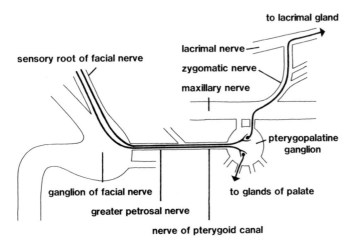

Fig. 4.75. The parasympathetic pathways through the pterygopalatine ganglion.

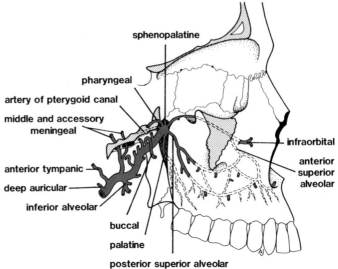

Fig. 4.76. The maxillary artery and its branches.

The principal branches of the pterygopalatine ganglion comprise the following.

1. The **greater palatine nerve** leaves the inferior aspect of the ganglion and descends through the greater palatine canal to emerge through the foramen of the same name on to the oral surface of the hard palate. It then runs forwards in a groove located approximately halfway between the midline of the palate and the palatal surface of the posterior teeth to supply the mucous membrane, and associated glands, of the palate as far forwards as the lateral incisor region. Within the greater palatine canal the nerve gives rise to nasal branches which pierce the perpendicular plate of the palatine bone to supply the mucous membrane of the posteroinferior quadrant of the lateral wall of the nose.

2. The **lesser palatine branches** also descend in the greater palatine canal but emerge on to the oral surface of the bony palate through the lesser palatine foramina. They supply the mucous membrane of the soft palate and of an area around the palatine tonsil. The taste fibres from this region are believed to pass back to the pterygopalatine ganglion (through which they pass without interruption) and then travel in the nerve of the pterygoid canal and in the greater petrosal nerve to the facial nerve.

3. The **nasal nerves** enter the nasal cavity through the sphenopalatine foramen. The **lateral branches** supply the mucous membrane of the posterosuperior quadrant of the lateral nasal wall. The **medial branches** supply the roof and most of the septum.

4. The **nasopalatine nerve** runs with the medial nasal branches to the septum. It then turns to run downwards and forwards on the vomer to reach the incisive fossa through which it passes on to the oral surface of the hard palate. It supplies a small part of the septum and the incisor region of the hard palate.

5. The **pharyngeal nerve** leaves the posterior aspect of the pterygo- palatine ganglion and passes through the palatovaginal canal to be distributed to the mucous membrane of the nasopharynx.

Maxillary artery

The maxillary artery enters the pterygopalatine fossa through the pterygomaxillary fissure. It passes across the fossa and then through the inferior orbital fissure to enter the orbit, where it is known as the infraorbital artery.

The third part of the maxillary artery (i.e. that part of the vessel within the pterygopalatine fossa) gives off **palatine, nasal,** and **pharyngeal branches** which accompany the corresponding branches of the pterygopalatine ganglion. It also gives rise to the **artery of the pterygoid canal** which runs posteriorly through the canal to supply the nasopharynx and tympanic cavity. As the maxillary artery enters the pterygopalatine fossa it gives off the **posterior superior alveolar branch** which runs with the corresponding branches of the maxillary nerve to supply the upper posterior teeth and adjacent structures. The posterior superior alveolar artery may give rise to a sizeable buccogingival branch which runs forwards on the posterior and then anterior surface of the maxilla, below the zygomatic process, to reach the infraorbital region where it may anastomose with the infraorbital artery. It is usually accompanied by a vein which is a tributary of the facial vein. The artery and vein lie immediately adjacent to periosteum, and may be at risk of being punctured in injections to obtain anaesthesia of the maxillary teeth.

The veins accompanying these branches of the maxillary artery emerge from the pterygopalatine fossa through the pterygomaxillary fissure and drain into the pterygoid plexus.

7

Oral cavity and related structures

As conventionally defined the oral cavity consists of an outer part, the **vestibule,** situated between the lips and cheeks externally and the teeth and alveolar processes internally, and a large inner part, the **oral cavity proper** located internal to the dental arcades. The various features to be seen inside the oral cavity are of the greatest importance to the dental student. The best way to examine the interior of the mouth is with the subject seated in a dental chair and with the aid of a powerful chairside light and a dental mirror. In the absence of these facilities you will be able to see most of the important features by examining the inside of your own mouth in a well-lit bathroom mirror.

The account which follows is for the adult mouth with a full complement of secondary (permanent) teeth. The only major differences in the child, apart from size, are found in the dentition, where, depending on age, primary (deciduous) teeth, some combination of primary and secondary teeth or an incomplete secondary dentition are found. Teeth tend to be lost, from one cause or another, with age and many middle-aged people have an incomplete dentition. A considerable proportion of elderly subjects is completely edentulous. In such cases the alveolar processes of both jaws are resorbed to some degree. Resorption may be so great that virtually no alveolar ridge can be seen.

The mucous membrane of the oral cavity may be divided into three types, although this is an oversimplification since there are regional variations within each type.

1. The **lining mucosa** covering the soft palate, ventral surface of the tongue, floor of the mouth, alveolar processes excluding the gingivae, and the internal surfaces of the lips and cheeks is invested by non-keratinizing epithelium covering a loose lamina propria and submucosa containing some fat deposits and mucous glands.

2. The **masticatory mucosa** of the hard palate and gingivae is lined by a parakeratinized epithelium. Submucosa is absent in the gingivae and the palatine raphe but present over the rest of the palatal surface. In regions where there is no submucosa the lamina propria is firmly attached to the underlying periosteum by a meshwork of collagen fibres to form a composite structure called **mucoperiosteum.**

3. The **specialized mucosa** of the dorsal surface of the tongue is orthokeratinized over the anterior two-thirds and bears four types of papillae. The lamina propria is rich in collagen fibres binding it to the underlying muscle. In the posterior third of the tongue the epithelium is non-keratinized and covers numerous nodules of lymphoid tissue which make up the lingual tonsil. Beneath this the lamina propria and indistinct submucosal layer contain lymphoid tissue and mucous glands.

EXAMINATION OF THE LIVING MOUTH

Vestibule

With the mouth closed the vestibule is little more than a potential space since the lips and cheeks are normally closely applied to the external aspect of the teeth and gums. In the presence of a complete dentition and with the teeth occluded the only communications between the vestibule and oral cavity proper are the narrow spaces behind the last molars. If the upper and lower teeth are fixed together, as, for example, in the reduction of a mandibular fracture, oral feeding can be achieved by passing nutrients through these spaces using a vessel with a specially designed spout. Note that when the jaw muscles are relaxed in the resting position the upper and lower teeth are not in occlusion but are separated by a narrow gap (the **freeway space**) of some 2–3 mm.

The vestibule is limited above and below by the reflections of the mucous membrane from the alveolar processes on to the cheeks and lips. The gutters formed by these reflections are called, in clinical dentistry, the **sulci** (upper and lower **buccal sulci** in the region of the cheeks and upper and lower **labial sulci** in the region of the lips).

If you pull the upper and lower lips outwards you will be able to see a narrow fold of mucous membrane, the **frenulum,** connecting each lip to the corresponding gum in the median plane. The upper frenulum is usually larger than the lower but both are variable in their degree of development. With the lips still everted examine the upper and lower sulci in the premolar regions. Here the sulci are usually shallower than elsewhere because of the attachment of the fibres of levator anguli oris and depressor labii inferioris to the upper and lower jaw respectively. If you move the lips around you will see that the folds of mucous membrane over these muscle attachments (sometimes called the **buccal fraena**) are very mobile. In constructing a denture care has to be taken to ensure that its margins do not impinge on the frenula or muscle attachments otherwise movements of the lips and cheeks will dislodge it.

The lining mucosa of the lips and cheeks and the sulci has a smooth shiny appearance, is dark red in colour and is loosely attached to underlying structures. A short distance from its reflection on to the alveolar processes the mucous membrane changes to the masticatory variety which is tightly attached to the underlying periosteum to form a mucoperiosteum. As a result the mucous membrane of the gingivae is non-mobile and pinkish in colour. The presence of numerous bundles of fibrous tissue connecting the deep surface of this mucous membrane to the bone gives it a stippled (so called 'orange peel') appearance. The demarcation between the two types of mucous membrane is quite distinct and can be seen as a pair of scalloped lines running horizontally above and below the dentition, a short distance from the gingival margins. When injecting local anaesthetic solution it is important to insert the needle into the mobile part of the mucous membrane and not into the mucoperiosteum since, in the latter case, the periosteum will be stripped from the bone causing pain and discomfort.

The **parotid duct** opens into the vestibule opposite the crown of the

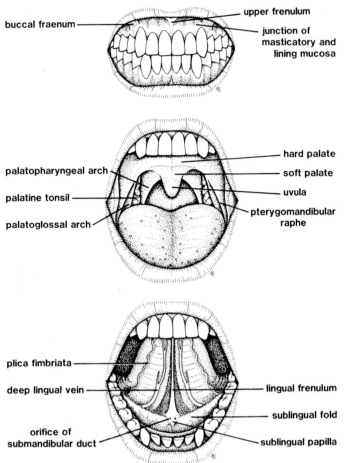

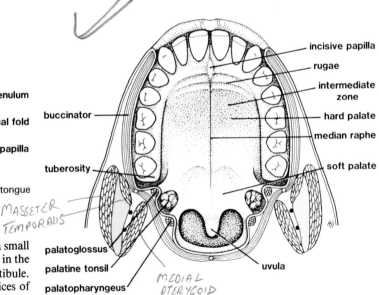

Fig. 4.77. Above, the vestibule; middle, the oral cavity proper with the tongue lowered; lower, the oral cavity proper with the tongue raised.

Fig. 4.78. Inferior view of the palate.

membrane covering the mylohyoid muscles. The posterior limit of the oral cavity lies at the **oropharyngeal isthmus.** This is bounded on each side by a fold of mucous membrane, the **palatoglossal arch,** (or **anterior pillar** of the **fauces**) running from the side of the palate to the side of the tongue. Behind the oropharyngeal isthmus is the oral part of the pharynx.

Palate

The palate can be divided into two parts of different structure and function. Anteriorly is the **hard palate,** which forms the partition between the nasal and oral cavities. The **soft palate** is attached to the posterior border of the hard palate and projects posteriorly into the pharynx, separating its nasal and oral parts. The 'skeleton' of the soft palate is formed by the fibrous palatine aponeurosis to which are attached numerous muscles. The soft palate is thus highly mobile and its movements are important in preventing food and drink entering the nasopharynx and nose during the act of swallowing.

The submucous layer of the hard palate varies in thickness from one region of the palate to another and is absent altogether in some areas. This variation produces the following zones which are easily recognizable in the living mouth (Fig. 4.78).

upper second molar tooth. The site of the orifice is marked by a small papilla. Numerous **buccal** and **labial mucous glands** are present in the mucous membrane of the lips and cheeks and open into the vestibule. These glands are sufficiently large to be palpated but the orifices of their ducts are too small to see. Four or five larger mucous glands are located external to the buccinator muscle around the parotid duct. These are the **molar glands.** Their ducts pierce buccinator to open into the vestibule close to the opening of the parotid duct.

Occlusion of the duct of one of the buccal or labial glands, as a result, for example, of minor trauma to the inside of the cheeks or lips, leads to retention of secretion within the gland. Such a swollen gland is termed a buccal or labial cyst.

Oral cavity proper

With the mouth widely open you will be able to see that the roof of the oral cavity proper is formed by the palate and that the floor is largely obscured by the highly mobile tongue. If the tongue is now raised you will see the floor of the mouth formed by the mucous

1. In the **gingival region,** adjacent to the teeth, and in the median **palatine raphe** the submucous layer is absent and the lamina propria of the mucous membrane and the periosteum are united to form a mucoperiosteum. In these regions the mucosa is pink in colour and tightly adherent to the underlying bone. The bone beneath the raphe is often raised to form a pronounced ridge, the **palatine torus.**

The palatine raphe ends anteriorly at a small elevation, the **incisive papilla,** overlying the incisive fossa.

2. Between the raphe and the gingival region on each side is an **intermediate zone** in which the submucosa is relatively well developed. Despite the presence of this layer the mucous membrane is still tightly

bound down to the bone by bands of tough fibrous tissue passing from the periosteum to the lamina propria. In the anterior part of the intermediate zone the spaces between these bands are filled with adipose tissue and the mucous membrane is thick and pale in colour and presents a number of transverse corrugations called the **palatine rugae.** These provide a rough surface against which the upper surface of the tongue can press in speech and in the preparation of food for swallowing. Failure to copy the rugae on the palate of a denture is often followed by complaints that speech has become difficult and food tasteless. Further posteriorly the mucous membrane of the intermediate zone is thinner and red in colour. Here the spaces between the fibrous bands are filled with numerous mucous glands.

The anterior (oral) surface of the soft palate at rest is concave and bears a low median raphe. Projecting downwards from its free (inferior) margin is a small conical process, the **uvula.**

It is important to be able to locate the junction of the hard and soft palate. This may be visible as a faint transverse groove in the mucous membrane covering the oral surface of the palate. If not, it can be palpated but the procedure is uncomfortable and liable to cause gagging. A more convenient procedure is to ask the subject to say 'aah' when the soft palate will be seen to vibrate. The boundary line between the vibrating and non-vibrating parts of the palate is called the **vibrating line** and lies a short distance behind the junction of hard and soft palates. The posterior edge of the palatal part of a full upper denture is positioned between the junction and the vibrating line, in the narrow non-mobile part of the soft palate. If it is placed in front of the junction it will ride on an area where the submucosa is thin or absent and will consequently lack peripheral seal and cause discomfort; if behind the vibrating line it will be dislodged by movements of the soft palate and may cause nausea.

Behind the last molar tooth the upper alveolar process ends in a rounded prominence, the **maxillary tuberosity.** If pressure is applied to the soft palate a short distance behind the tuberosity you will be able to feel the **pterygoid hamulus.** Between the tuberosity and the hamulus is the **hamular notch**. The posterior edge of an upper denture is continued laterally through the hamular notch which, since it is covered by compressible tissue, gives a better peripheral seal than either the tuberosity or the hamulus.

Tongue

The mucous membrane covering the tongue has a number of marked regional variations. The dorsum is divided by the V-shaped **sulcus terminalis** (the point of the V is directed posteriorly) into anterior two-thirds and posterior one-third which differ in epithelial specializations, development, and nerve supply.

The anterior two-thirds of the dorsal surface are covered by mucous membrane tightly bound down to the underlying muscle and bearing stratified squamous epithelium formed into numerous papillae over the irregularities in the underlying lamina propria. The papillae take several forms.

1. The **filiform papillae** are the most numerous. They are 2–3 mm long and arranged in rows parallel to the arms of the sulcus terminalis. The connective tissue of these papillae is set with secondary papillae with pointed ends. The epithelium covering these secondary papillae also forms pointed processes, so that the whole structure resembles a minute fir tree. The outer layer of epithelium is continuously shed. In illness this shedding may be delayed and the accumulated tissue mixed with bacteria, is seen as a grey coating (fur) on the tongue.

2. The **fungiform papillae** are less numerous. They have a slightly

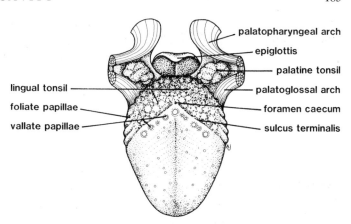

Fig. 4.79. The dorsal surface of the tongue.

constricted stalk and a hemispherical upper part which appears on the tongue as a bright red spot due to its rich blood supply. They are most easily seen towards the sides and the tip of the tongue. Taste buds are present on many fungiform papillae.

3. The **vallate papillae** are about twelve in number and are the largest of the lingual papillae. They are situated parallel and immediately anterior to the sulcus terminalis. They are recessed into the mucous membrane and surrounded by a deep circular furrow. The surface of each papilla bears a large number of taste buds. Serous glands (of Von Ebner) open into the bottom of the furrow and help to rinse the area around the papilla.

Other taste buds are found on the palatoglossal arches, the soft palate, the posterior surface of the epiglottis and the posterior wall of the pharynx as far down as the inferior margin of the cricoid cartilage. Taste buds distinguish only four sensations, sweet, bitter, acid, and salt. The distribution of taste sensation may be mapped out experimentally using swabs dipped in suitable chemicals.

The apex of the sulcus terminalis is marked by a shallow median pit, the **foramen caecum** marking the embryological origin of the thyroid gland and the upper end of the transient thyroglossal duct.

Filiform and fungiform papillae are absent from the posterior third of the tongue but the covering mucous membrane is raised into numerous low elevations by the presence of nodules of lymphoid tissue in the submucous layer. These are known collectively as the **lingual tonsil.**

On the posterior part of the lateral margins of the tongue are several vertical folds termed **foliate papillae**. These are rudimentary in man but well developed in other mammals.

If the tongue is now raised you will see that its under surface is smooth and is covered by a thin mucous membrane of the lining variety which is deep red in colour and firmly attached to the connective tissue ensheathing the lingual muscles. A median fold of mucous membrane, the **lingual frenulum,** connects the inferior surface of the tongue to the floor of the mouth. On each side of the frenulum is a fringed fold of mucous membrane called the **plica fimbriata.** Between the frenulum and the plica, the **deep lingual vein** can be seen through the thin mucous membrane. The presence of a short frenulum may lead to the condition of 'tongue-tie' in which speech is defective.

Associated with the mucous membrane of the tongue are numerous

lingual glands. Over the posterior one-third of the dorsum these are mainly mucus-secreting; over the anterior two-thirds serous glands are found opening into the neighbourhood of the taste buds, especially in the sulci of the vallate papillae. A few mucous glands are present on the under surface of the tongue near its tip.

Floor of the mouth

The floor of the mouth is lined with a smooth thin mucous membrane bearing a stratified squamous epithelium similar to that found on the under surface of the tongue.

Either side of the attachment of the lingual frenulum to the floor of the mouth is a small elevation, the **sublingual papilla.** On the surface of the papilla you may be able to see the orifice of the submandibular duct. Extending posterolaterally from the papilla is a ridge, the **sublingual fold,** produced by the underlying sublingual gland. The gland opens on to the crest of the fold by several tiny ducts which are too small to see with the naked eye.

Oropharyngeal isthmus and neighbouring region

The **palatoglossal arches** can be seen most clearly if the tongue is depressed and the soft palate raised (the latter by saying 'aah'). They are produced by the underlying palatoglossal muscles which run, one on each side, from the lateral part of the soft palate to the posterior part of the tongue. If the tongue is protruded you will see that the arches are pulled forwards. A short distance behind the palatoglossal arches is a second pair of folds, the **palatopharyngeal arches** (or **posterior pillars of the fauces**). These overlie the palatopharyngeal muscles which arise from each side of the soft palate and descend in the lateral walls of the pharynx. Beneath the mucous membrane between the palatoglossal and palatopharyngeal arches is the **palatine tonsil,** a mass of lymphoid tissue occupying the gap between the palatoglossal and palatopharyngeal muscles. Penetrating into the upper part of the tonsil is the deep **intratonsillar cleft.** Below this are the openings of the tonsillar crypts. The size of the palatine tonsil is extremely variable and much of its substance may have been removed by the not uncommon operation of tonsillectomy.

With the mouth wide open palpate the mucous membrane in front of and lateral to the palatoglossal arch. You will be able to feel the sharp front edge of the ramus of the mandible. This can be traced down towards the last lower molar tooth. Between the palpating finger and the ramus is the layer of mucous membrane and the underlying buccinator muscle. Medial to the ramus the mucous membrane is

furrowed by a shallow groove which begins just behind the last lower molar tooth and runs upwards and medially. This marks the position of the **pterygomandibular raphe** which runs from the body of the mandible just behind the last tooth to the pterygoid hamulus. Attached to its lateral aspect is the buccinator muscle and to its medial aspect the superior constrictor. A needle inserted through the mucous membrane just lateral to the raphe will pierce the buccinator muscle, pass medial to the ramus and enter the pterygomandibular space. This, in essence, is the route followed in making an inferior alveolar block (see pp. 177–8).

Lying immediately beneath the mucous membrane below the inferior attachment of the pterygomandibular raphe and adjacent to the bone on the medial surface of the body of the mandible below the last molar tooth is the **lingual nerve** curving forwards, downwards, and medially from the infratemporal fossa to the floor of the mouth. It is usually possible to feel the nerve between finger and bone in this position. Behind the last molar tooth is the small **retromolar pad** of soft tissue.

STRUCTURES BOUNDING THE ORAL CAVITY

Lips and cheeks

The lips are fleshy folds consisting of skin superficially and mucous membrane internally, with the orbicularis muscle, loose connective tissue, and the labial nerves and blood vessels contained between them. The mucus-secreting labial glands are situated internal to orbicularis oris. Similarly the cheeks have an external layer of skin, an internal layer of mucous membrane and a middle layer of muscle, principally buccinator, and connective tissue with the contained nerves and blood vessels. The buccal glands are internal to the buccinator.

The lips and cheeks are supplied with blood through the mental artery and the labial and buccal branches of the facial artery and their venous drainage is through tributaries of the facial vein. The sensory innervation of the skin and mucous membrane of the upper lip is from the infraorbital nerve, of the lower lip from the mental nerve and of the cheek from the buccal nerve. Secretomotor fibres to the

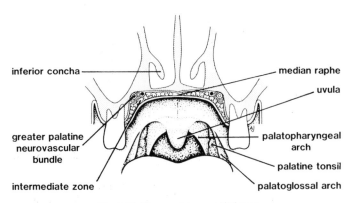

Fig. 4.80. The oropharyngeal isthmus.

inferior concha — — median raphe
— uvula
greater palatine neurovascular bundle — — palatopharyngeal arch
— palatine tonsil
intermediate zone — — palatoglossal arch

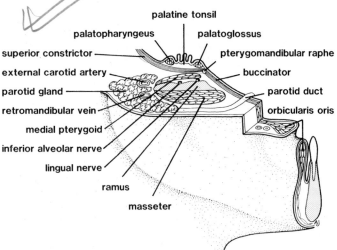

Fig. 4.81. The structure of the lips and cheeks.

palatine tonsil
palatopharyngeus — — palatoglossus
superior constrictor — — pterygomandibular raphe
external carotid artery — — buccinator
parotid gland — — parotid duct
retromandibular vein — — orbicularis oris
medial pterygoid
inferior alveolar nerve
lingual nerve
ramus
masseter

glands in the upper lip and upper cheek pass from the pterygopalatine ganglion in the maxillary nerve and its infraorbital continuation; similar fibres to the glands in the lower lip and lower cheek pass from the otic ganglion in the mandibular nerve and its inferior alveolar and buccal branches. The muscles, like the remainder of the muscles of facial expression, are supplied by the facial nerve. Lymph drainage is to the submandibular nodes apart from the central region of the lower lip which drains to the submental nodes.

Hard palate

The skeleton of the hard palate is provided by the palatine processes of the maxillae and the horizontal processes of the palatine bones. Its oral surface is covered by mucous membrane lined by stratified squamous epithelium. The regional variations in the mucous membrane are described on pages 182–3.

From the region of the greater palatine foramen forwards to the canine tooth the palatine mucosa receives its sensory innervation from the **greater palatine nerve.** After emerging from the greater palatine foramen the nerve runs forwards along a curved line situated approximately halfway between the palatal gingival margin and the midline of the palate. It lies close to the bone, often in a distinct groove, in the submucous layer of the intermediate zone. The greater palatine nerve also carries parasympathetic postganglionic fibres from the pterygopalatine ganglion to the palatine glands. The mucous membrane in the incisor region of the hard palate is innervated by the **nasopalatine nerve** which emerges on to the hard palate through the incisive fossa. The fact that the nerves supplying the palate run in a region where the submucous layer is present allows small quantities of local anaesthetic solution to be injected alongside the nerves without too much discomfort.

The blood supply of the whole of the hard palate is provided by the **greater palatine artery.** This vessel emerges from the greater

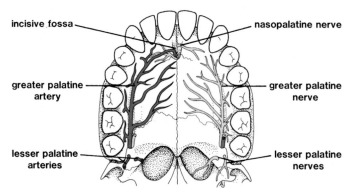

Fig. 4.82. The nerve (to right) and blood (to left) supply of the palate.

palatine foramen and passes forwards, lateral to the correspondingly named nerve, in the submucosa in the intermediate zone of the palate. It continues forwards into the incisor region and passes through the incisive fossa to supply a small area of mucous membrane within the nasal cavity.

Blood drains from the hard palate through veins that accompany the artery and terminate in the pterygoid plexus. The lymph drainage is to the deep cervical nodes.

Congenital clefts of the palate are amongst the commonest disorders of development. They are described on pages 51–2.

Floor of the mouth

The key to understanding the floor of the mouth is the disposition of the mylohyoid, geniohyoid, and hyoglossus muscles.

Mylohyoid muscle

The mylohyoid muscles of the two sides form a mobile diaphragm flooring the oral cavity. Below this diaphragm is the neck. Each muscle is a thin sheet which arises from the whole length of the mylohyoid line on the medial aspect of the mandible. It has a posterior free edge. The posterior fibres run medially and downwards to be inserted into the anterior surface of the body of the hyoid bone. The more anterior fibres pass similarly in a medial and downwards direction to meet the corresponding fibres of the opposite side at a median raphe which runs from the internal surface of the symphysis menti to the front of the hyoid bone. The muscle is innervated by the mylohyoid branch of the inferior alveolar nerve and its action is to elevate the floor of the mouth and hyoid or, with the latter fixed, to depress the mandible.

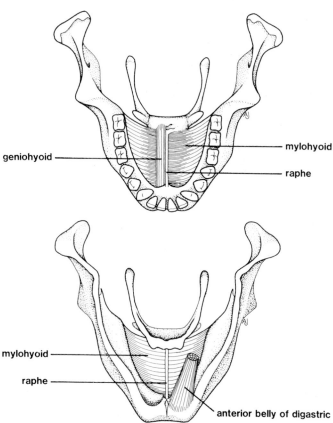

Fig. 4.83. Superior (above) and inferior (below) views of the mylohyoid muscles. The geniohyoid muscle and the anterior belly of the digastric are shown in place on the right side only of the specimen.

Geniohyoid muscle

This is a narrow band of muscle fibres which arises from the inferior mental spine and runs backwards and downwards to be inserted into the anterior surface of the hyoid bone. It lies on the medial part of the upper surface of the mylohyoid muscle in contact with its fellow of the opposite side. Immediately above it is the genioglossus muscle. Geniohyoid is supplied by a branch of the hypoglossal nerve but the fibres are derived from the first cervical spinal nerve. Its action is to elevate and draw forwards the hyoid bone or conversely to depress the mandible.

Hyoglossus muscle

Although hyoglossus is an extrinsic muscle of the tongue it is more convenient to describe it here than with the other muscles of that group because a knowledge of its relationships is necessary for understanding the course of several important structures in the floor of the mouth. It is a quadrilateral sheet of muscle which arises from the upper surface of the whole length of the greater cornu and of the lateral part of the body of the hyoid bone. Its fibres ascend vertically in a parasagittal plane to be inserted into the side of the tongue where they interdigitate with the fibres of the styloglossus muscle.

The lateral (superficial) surface of the muscle is related to the **lingual nerve**, the **deep lobe of the submandibular gland** and the **submandibular duct**, the **hypoglossal nerve**, and the **deep lingual vein**.

Having gained access to the mouth, the lingual nerve curves forwards, downwards, and medially across the intermuscular space between mylohyoid and hyoglossus to reach the lateral surface of the latter. Here it continues forwards and has the **submandibular ganglion** suspended from it by two or three ganglionic branches. The lingual nerve lies at first superior to the submandibular duct, but at the anterior border of hyoglossus it passes beneath the duct, crossing from the lateral to the medial side of that structure as it does so.

The deep lobe of the submandibular gland lies against the posterior part of the lateral surface of the hyoglossus from which it is separated by the hypoglossal nerve and deep lingual vein. The submandibular duct leaves the deep lobe of the gland and passes forwards on the lateral surface of the hyoglossus, with the relationships to the lingual nerve just described, to open into the oral cavity at the sublingual papilla at the side of the frenulum of the tongue.

The hypoglossal nerve runs forwards on the lateral surface of hyoglossus a short distance above the greater cornu of the hyoid. At the anterior margin of the muscle it divides into several branches which run into the musculature of the tongue. In its course across hyoglossus the hypoglossal nerve is accompanied by the deep lingual vein.

Also related to the posterior part of the lateral surface of the hyoglossus are the stylohyoid muscle and the intermediate tendon of the digastric.

The medial surface of the hyoglossus is related to the **glossopharyngeal nerve**, **stylohyoid ligament**, and **lingual artery**. The glossopharyngeal nerve travels deep to the upper part of hyoglossus to supply the mucous membrane of the posterior one-third of the tongue. The stylohyoid ligament runs deep to the posterior part of hyoglossus to attach to the lesser cornu of the hyoid bone. The lingual artery passes medial to the lower part of the posterior border of hyoglossus, runs forwards above the greater cornu of the hyoid

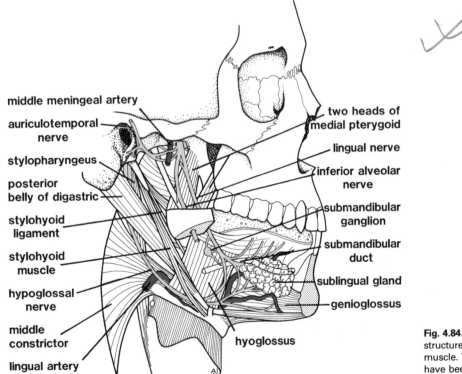

middle meningeal artery
auriculotemporal nerve
stylopharyngeus
posterior belly of digastric
stylohyoid ligament
stylohyoid muscle
hypoglossal nerve
middle constrictor
lingual artery

two heads of medial pterygoid
lingual nerve
inferior alveolar nerve
submandibular ganglion
submandibular duct
sublingual gland
genioglossus
hyoglossus

Fig. 4.84. Lateral view of the floor of the mouth to show the structures related to the lateral surface of the hyoglossus muscle. The mylohyoid muscle and submandibular gland have been removed.

and then turns upwards at the anterior border of the muscle to pass on to the lower surface of the tongue. Also related to the medial surface of hyoglossus is the genioglossus muscle.

Like other muscles of the tongue (except palatoglossus), hyoglossus is innervated by the hypoglossal nerve. Its action is to depress the tongue.

Salivary glands in the floor of the mouth

The sublingual gland lies wholly in the floor of the mouth whereas the submandibular gland lies partly in the floor of the mouth and partly in the neck. Both glands are predominantly mucus secreting in man.

Submandibular gland

The submandibular gland consists of a **superficial lobe,** situated in the neck lateral (i.e. superficial) to the mylohyoid muscle, and a **deep lobe,** lying in the floor of the mouth between mylohyoid and hyoglossus. The two lobes are continuous with each other posteriorly around the free edge of mylohyoid.

The lateral surface of the superficial lobe is in contact with the medial surface of the mandible below the mylohyoid line, where its position is marked by the submandibular fossa. The facial artery, after curving over the posterior belly of the digastric muscle, runs downwards between the lateral surface of the superficial lobe and the medial surface of the mandible, usually in a deep groove in the gland. At the lower border of the mandible the artery arches upwards into the face. The medial surface of the superficial lobe is related anteriorly to the inferior surface of the mylohyoid muscle and more posteriorly to the stylohyoid muscle and ligament. The inferior surface of the lobe is covered by the investing layer of the deep cervical fascia, as it passes from the hyoid bone to the lower border of the mandible, and is crossed by the facial vein.

The deep lobe is the smaller of the two. It lies in the narrow intermuscular gap between mylohyoid and hyoglossus, extending as far forwards as the posterior pole of the sublingual gland (approximately opposite the second molar tooth). It is related above to the lingual nerve and below to the hypoglossal nerve.

The **submandibular duct** begins in the superficial lobe. It traverses the gland, curving around the posterior margin of mylohyoid in the connection between the superficial and deep lobes, to emerge from the anterior surface of the latter. It then runs forwards, with its close relationship to the lingual nerve, first between mylohyoid and hyoglossus and subsequently between the sublingual gland and genioglossus to open into the oral cavity through a narrow orifice on the summit of the **sublingual papilla**.

Sublingual gland

This is the smallest of the three principal salivary glands. It is situated in front of the deep lobe of the submandibular gland, between the mylohyoid laterally and the genioglossus medially, extending from opposite the second molar tooth to the premolar region. Its superior surface is covered by the mucous membrane of the floor of the mouth which it raises to form the **sublingual fold**. Above the mylohyoid muscle the lateral surface of the gland comes into contact with the sublingual fossa on the medial surface of the body of the mandible. The medial surface of the gland is crossed by the lingual nerve and submandibular duct. The gland opens onto the surface of

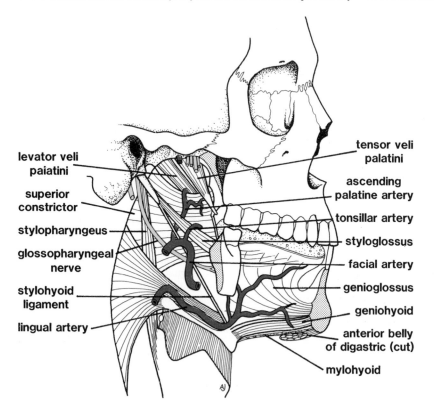

Fig. 4.85. Lateral view of the floor of the mouth with the hyoglossus muscle removed to show the structures related to the medial surface of that muscle.

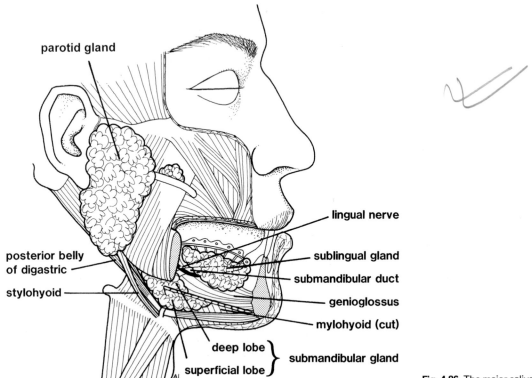

parotid gland

posterior belly
of digastric

stylohyoid

lingual nerve

sublingual gland

submandibular duct

genioglossus

mylohyoid (cut)

deep lobe }
superficial lobe } submandibular gland

Fig. 4.86. The major salivary glands.

the sublingual fold through a variable number (usually about 15) of small ducts.

The innervation of the submandibular and sublingual glands is through the submandibular ganglion and is described below.

The blood supply of the submandibular gland is through branches of the facial and lingual arteries. Its venous drainage is by accompanying veins. The blood supply and drainage of the sublingual gland is through the sublingual artery and vein.

Clinical aspects

Like the parotid gland the submandibular and sublingual glands may be involved in viral or bacterial infections and in stone formation. Stones are formed most frequently in the submandibular duct and gland and lead to enlargement and tenderness of the gland which are usually worse at mealtimes because of the increased secretion of saliva. Cysts may occur in the glands in the floor of the mouth sometimes as a result of chronic blockage of their ducts but more frequently of obscure aetiology. A swelling of this type is sometimes referred to as a ranula.

Nerves in the floor of mouth

Three important nerves – **lingual**, **glossopharyngeal**, and **hypoglossal** – pass through the floor of the mouth. The courses of these nerves before they enter the mouth are described respectively on pages 175, 158, and 160.

Lingual nerve

As the lingual nerve leaves the infratemporal fossa it contains sensory trigeminal fibres and also taste and preganglionic parasympathetic fibres which have reached it from the facial nerve in the chorda tympani. It gains access to the mouth by passing beneath the lower margin of the superior constrictor muscle close to the mandibular attachment of the pterygomandibular raphe, lying close to the medial surface of the mandible adjacent to the roots of the last molar tooth. It then runs forwards, downwards, and medially in a smooth curve across the gap between mylohyoid and hyoglossus to reach the lateral surface of the latter muscle (Fig. 4.84). Continuing forwards it reaches the front edge of hyoglossus where it crosses beneath the submandibular duct from its lateral to its medial side. Running now forwards and upwards it passes between the sublingual gland and genioglossus, with the duct beneath it, and divides into its terminal branches which supply general sensory and taste fibres to the anterior two-thirds of the tongue. The lingual nerve also supplies sensory fibres to the mucous membrane lining the floor of the mouth and the lingual surface of the mandibular alveolar process through branches given off as the nerve traverses the floor of the mouth.

The **submandibular ganglion** is suspended from the lingual nerve, as it crosses hyoglossus, by short anterior and posterior ganglionic branches. It is the major relay station for the parasympathetic supply to the glands in the floor of the mouth. The parasympathetic root of the ganglion is the posterior ganglionic branch from the lingual nerve. This conveys preganglionic parasympathetic fibres which

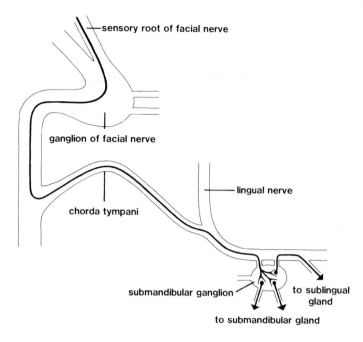

Fig. 4.87. The parasympathetic pathways through the submandibular ganglion.

begin in the superior salivatory nucleus in the brainstem and travel via the facial nerve, chorda tympani, and lingual nerve to the ganglion. The sympathetic root is a branch from the plexus on the facial artery. It contains postganglionic fibres which commence in the superior cervical ganglion. Most of the preganglionic parasympathetic fibres synapse in the ganglion with postganglionic fibres which pass to the submandibular gland through glandular branches of the ganglion and to the sublingual gland and the small glands of the floor of the mouth and tongue through the anterior ganglionic branch and the lingual nerve. A few of the preganglionic neurons to the submandibular gland synapse within the gland itself. The sympathetic fibres pass through the ganglion without interruption to run with the parasympathetic fibres to the glands. The role of the autonomic innervation in the control of glandular secretion is discussed on page 145.

Hypoglossal nerve

Having crossed the external and internal carotid arteries, the hypoglossal nerve enters the mouth by passing deep to the posterior border of mylohyoid (Fig. 4.84). It then runs forwards in the intermuscular space between that muscle and hyoglossus below the lingual nerve and a short distance above the greater cornu of the hyoid bone. As it crosses the lateral surface of hyoglossus it inclines upwards and passes deep to the stylohyoid muscle and the tendon of digastric. After leaving the lateral surface of hyoglossus the nerve continues forwards on genioglossus as far as the tip of the tongue. During its course in the floor of the mouth the hypoglossal nerve gives branches to the extrinsic (except palatoglossus) and intrinsic muscles of the tongue and has numerous connections with the lingual nerve.

Glossopharyngeal nerve

This nerve has a short course in the mouth (Fig. 4.85). It passes deep to the upper part of hyoglossus and supplies the mucous membrane of the posterior one-third of the tongue and the vallate papillae with general sensory, taste and secretomotor fibres.

Blood vessels in the floor of the mouth

Lingual artery

The lingual artery provides the main blood supply to the floor of the mouth and to the tongue. It leaves the anterior surface of the external carotid opposite the tip of the greater cornu of the hyoid. The first part of its course is in the neck (Fig. 4.85). Here the artery forms a characteristic loop, running at first upwards and then descending again to the level of the hyoid. It is related medially to the middle constrictor and has skin, platysma, and deep fascia laterally. It is crossed superficially by the hypoglossal nerve. The artery then enters the floor of the mouth by running deep to hyoglossus. Its medial relationships in this part of its course are, in posterior to anterior sequence, the middle constrictor, stylohyoid ligament and genioglossus. At the anterior border of hyoglossus the artery gives off its **sublingual branch** which runs forwards between mylohyoid and genioglossus to supply the sublingual gland and the muscles of the floor of the mouth. The main trunk, now known as the **deep lingual artery**, turns upwards and then runs forwards just beneath the mucous membrane on the inferior surface of the tongue close to the frenulum. It is accompanied in this part of its course by the lingual nerve and deep lingual vein. The artery gives off numerous branches which pass upwards to supply the substance of the tongue.

Venous channels

The veins of the floor of the mouth comprise two main channels. The **deep lingual vein** begins near the tip of the tongue. It accompanies the lingual artery on the inferior surface of the tongue but at the anterior border of hyoglossus, where it receives the sublingual vein from the sublingual gland and the floor of the mouth, it parts company with the artery to run lateral to the muscle close to the hypoglossal nerve. The vein ends by draining into the facial, lingual, or internal jugular vein. The dorsal lingual veins join to form the **lingual vein** which runs with the lingual artery deep to hyoglossus and opens into the internal jugular vein posterior to the greater cornu of the hyoid bone.

Tissue spaces in the floor of the mouth

A dental abscess from an infected lower tooth may erode the cortex of the body of the mandible allowing the escape of pus into the adjacent soft tissues. If this occurs in a lateral direction the abscess will usually point into the buccal sulcus. If the erosion takes place medially pus may enter the floor of the mouth or the neck, depending upon whether the cortex is eroded above or below the attachment of the mylohyoid muscle to the medial surface of the mandibular body (Fig. 4.89). Because this attachment slopes downwards as it passes forwards, an abscess from the posterior teeth is more likely to open below mylohyoid and one from the anterior teeth above mylohyoid. The tissue space above mylohyoid is bounded below by the muscle, above by the mucous membrane lining the floor of the mouth and laterally and anteriorly by the body of the mandible. Posteriorly it communicates freely with the tissue spaces in the neck. The genioglossus and geniohyoid muscles form a midline partition which acts as an effective barrier to the spread of infection from one side of the space to the other. The tissue space below the mylohyoid muscle is bounded inferiorly by the investing layer of the deep cervical fascia and laterally and anteriorly by the mandibular body. This space too communicates posteriorly with the tissue spaces in the neck.

Nerve supply, blood supply, and lymphatic drainage of the teeth and supporting structures

The upper teeth, their supporting structures (i.e. the bone of the alveolar process and the periodontal ligaments), and the mucous membrane covering the alveolar process are supplied by branches of the maxillary nerve and artery. The lower teeth and supporting structures and the mucous membrane of the lower alveolar process receive their blood supply mainly from the maxillary artery but their innervation is by branches of the mandibular nerve.

Upper dentition

The **maxillary nerve,** having crossed the pterygopalatine fossa, enters the orbit by passing through the inferior orbital fissure and is then called the **infraorbital nerve** (Figs 4.74 and 4.88A). It runs forwards in the floor of the orbit, lying first in the infraorbital groove and then in the infraorbital canal, and emerges into the face through the infraorbital foramen. In the majority of individuals, the upper teeth are supplied by **posterior, middle,** and **anterior superior alveolar nerves.** In the remaining cases, the middle superior alveolar nerve is absent.

The posterior superior alveolar nerves (usually two or three in number) leave the maxillary nerve while it is still in the pterygopalatine fossa. They pass downards and laterally through the pterygomaxillary fissure to reach the posterior surface of the maxilla. Here they divide into numerous small branches which enter the maxilla through the posterior alveolar foramina, and then run downwards and forwards, the lower branches passing in bony canals in the posterior part of the maxilla and the upper branches passing in the posterolateral wall of the maxillary sinus immediately beneath the lining mucous membrane which they supply. Towards the front of the infraorbital canal, the anterior superior alveolar nerve leaves the infraorbital nerve and enters the fine **sinuous canal** which passes downwards in the maxilla, close to the anterior wall of the maxillary sinus and the lower margin of the nasal aperture, towards the incisor teeth. The nerve gives a small nasal branch to the mucous membrane of the antero-inferior quadrant of the lateral wall of the nasal cavity.

The middle superior alveolar nerve, when present, most frequently arises as a branch of the infraorbital nerve. It may leave the infraorbital nerve anywhere along its course between the inferior orbital fissure and the anterior superior alveolar branch. It runs downwards and forwards, immediately beneath the mucous membrane lining the posterior, lateral or anterior wall (depending upon its point of origin from the infraorbital nerve) of the maxillary sinus. In a few individuals, the middle superior alveolar nerve arises directly from the maxillary nerve in the pterygopalatine fossa and enters the maxilla through a small foramen located a short distance lateral to or below the commencement of the infraorbital groove. Another variation is for the middle superior alveolar nerve to arise as a branch of the anterior superior alveolar nerve.

Within the maxilla the superior alveolar nerves divide into numerous fine branches which join together to form the **superior alveolar plexus** located within the alveolar process a short distance above the apices of the roots of the upper teeth. Branches of the plexus supply the upper teeth, the bone of the alveolar process, the periodontal ligaments and the mucous membrane on the buccal aspect of the alveolar process. The part of the plexus formed by the posterior superior alveolar nerves supplies the molar and premolar regions while that formed by the anterior superior alveolar nerve supplies the canine and incisor regions. When the middle superior alveolar nerve is present it innervates, through the plexus, the premolar teeth and also supplies fibres to the first molar (which then has a double innervation).

As the **maxillary artery** enters the pterygomaxillary fissure it gives off a **posterior superior alveolar branch** which passes downwards on the posterior surface of the maxilla and divides into several branches. Some of these branches accompany the posterior superior alveolar nerves into the maxilla where they supply the bone, the molar and premolar teeth and the lining of the maxillary sinus. The remaining branches continue downwards and forwards on the external surface of the maxilla to supply the mucous membrane on the buccal surface of the upper alveolar process (see also p. 180).

Anterior superior alveolar branches arise from the infraorbital artery as it traverses the infraorbital canal. These accompany the corresponding nerve to supply the anterior teeth and supporting structures.

As already described (p. 185) the mucous membrane covering the palatal aspect of the upper alveolar process is innervated by the **greater palatine** and **nasopalatine nerves** and is supplied with blood through the **greater palatine artery**.

The venous drainage of the upper dentition and associated structures is by alveolar and palatine veins which run with the similarly named arteries and nerves and drain into the pterygoid plexus. The lymph from these structures drains mainly into the submandibular nodes and upper deep cervical nodes.

Lower dentition

The lower teeth, alveolar process, and periodontal ligaments are innervated by the **inferior alveolar nerve.** This branch of the posterior trunk of the mandibular nerve enters the mandible through the mandibular foramen. It runs forwards in the mandibular canal below the roots of the posterior teeth to the mental foramen through which the main trunk of the nerve emerges, as the **mental nerve,** to supply the skin and mucous membrane of the lower lip and the skin of the chin. Just before the main trunk passes through the mental foramen it gives off an incisive branch which continues forwards within the mandible to supply the canine and incisor teeth.

The arrangement of the nerve within the mandible is subject to considerable individual variation (Fig. 4.88B). In the majority of cases it runs forwards as a single trunk immediately below the apices of the roots of the molar teeth (occasionally the apices actually project into the mandibular canal). The branches to the posterior teeth are then short and direct. Less commonly the main trunk of the nerve is situated more inferiorly in the body of the mandible, close to its lower border and some distance below the roots of the teeth. In these cases the dental branches are much longer and slope obliquely upwards and forwards to unite and form an alveolar plexus from which the molar and premolar teeth are supplied. In yet other cases the inferior alveolar nerve, soon after entering the mandible, gives

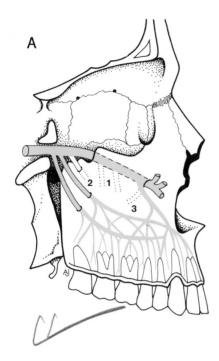

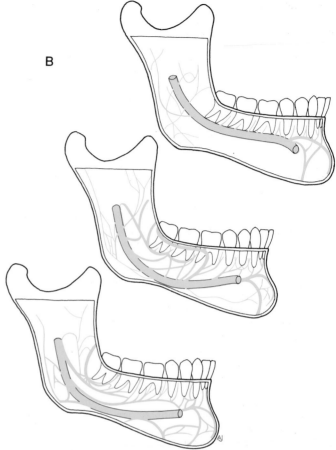

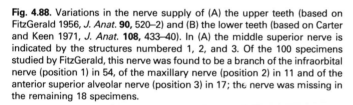

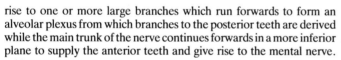

Fig. 4.88. Variations in the nerve supply of (A) the upper teeth (based on FitzGerald 1956, *J. Anat.* **90,** 520–2) and (B) the lower teeth (based on Carter and Keen 1971, *J. Anat.* **108,** 433–40). In (A) the middle superior nerve is indicated by the structures numbered 1, 2, and 3. Of the 100 specimens studied by FitzGerald, this nerve was found to be a branch of the infraorbital nerve (position 1) in 54, of the maxillary nerve (position 2) in 11 and of the anterior superior alveolar nerve (position 3) in 17; the nerve was missing in the remaining 18 specimens.

rise to one or more large branches which run forwards to form an alveolar plexus from which branches to the posterior teeth are derived while the main trunk of the nerve continues forwards in a more inferior plane to supply the anterior teeth and give rise to the mental nerve.

Neurovascular bundles have been demonstrated entering the mandible through foramina situated in the areas of insertion of the muscles of mastication, especially those of the lateral pterygoid and temporalis. These ramify within the bone to form a fine network located in the ramus and in the body of the mandible lateral to the roots of the molar teeth. Numerous connections are made between the nerves in this network and the inferior alveolar nerve and its dental branches. It is possible therefore that some of the sensory innervation of the posterior teeth is derived from the nerves supplying the muscles of mastication. Further forwards similar connecting branches between the mylohyoid nerve and dental branches to the anterior teeth have been demonstrated passing through foramina on the medial surface of the mandible opposite the premolar teeth. The presence of these various connections may well provide the explanation for the not uncommon observation that some patients continue to feel pain (so called 'escape pain') in the lower teeth after the main trunk of the inferior alveolar nerve has been blocked by the injection of local anaesthetic solution at the mandibular foramen.

The inferior alveolar nerve is accompanied by the **inferior alveolar artery**, a branch of the first part of the maxillary artery. The artery gives rise to branches which accompany, and receive the same names as, the branches of the nerve.

The mucous membrane on the lingual surface of the mandibular alveolar process is innervated by the **lingual nerve** and receives its blood supply from the **lingual artery**.

Venous drainage from the lower dentition and associated structures, like that from the upper dentition, is into the pterygoid plexus through vessels which accompany the arteries. Lymph drains to the submental and submandibular nodes and thence to the deep cervical nodes.

Tongue

The tongue is a highly mobile, muscular organ which plays a major part in the mechanisms of swallowing and speech. It is attached, at its root, to the hyoid bone, itself highly mobile, and its free surfaces are covered by mucous membrane showing the regional specializations described on page 183. The complex developmental history of the tongue described in Chapter 2.3 is reflected in its multiple nerve supply.

The bulk of the tongue is made up of striated muscle. This can be

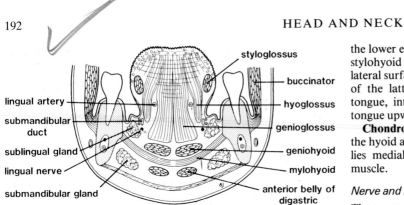

Fig. 4.89. Coronal section through the tongue and the floor of the mouth.

divided into two components – the **intrinsic muscles**, contained entirely within the tongue and responsible for altering its shape, and the **extrinsic muscles** which have attachments outside the tongue and act principally to change its position.

Intrinsic muscles

The tongue is divided into right and left halves by a median fibrous septum. On each side of this septum the intrinsic muscles are arranged in four groups.

1. The **superior longitudinal fibres** lie in a band immediately beneath the mucous membrane of the dorsum of the tongue. They are attached to the mucous membrane over the posterior part of the tongue and run forwards to attach to the mucous membrane at its edges and tip. When these fibres contract they shorten the tongue and turn its tip and edges upwards (so making the dorsum concave).

2. The **inferior longitudinal fibres** are situated lateral to genioglossus in the lower part of the tongue. They also act to shorten the tongue but turn its tip and edges downwards (so making the dorsum convex).

3. The **transverse fibres** arise from the median septum and pass laterally to be inserted into the mucous membrane at the sides of the tongue. The action of these fibres is to narrow and elongate the tongue.

4. The **vertical fibres** run from the dorsum of the tongue to the mucous membrane on its ventral surface and act to flatten and broaden the tongue.

Extrinsic muscles

These include **hyoglossus, chondroglossus, genioglossus, styloglossus,** and **palatoglossus.** Hyoglossus has been described in the section dealing with the floor of the mouth (p. 186). Palatoglossus on the basis of its development, nerve supply, and actions is better considered as a muscle of the soft palate and is dealt with in that section (p. 198).

Genioglossus (Fig. 4.85) arises from the upper mental spine of the mandible. It lies adjacent to the median plane in contact with its fellow of the opposite side and immediately above geniohyoid which arises from the lower mental spine. Its fibres run posteriorly radiating outwards as they do so to intermingle with the intrinsic fibres along the whole length of the ventral surface of the tongue from root to tip. Genioglossus draws the tongue forwards and pulls down the central part of the dorsum making it concave from side to side.

Styloglossus (Fig. 4.73) takes its origin from the anterior surface of the lower end of the styloid process and the neighbouring part of the stylohyoid ligament. It passes downwards and forwards across the lateral surface of the superior constrictor muscle. At the lower border of the latter muscle styloglossus is inserted into the side of the tongue, interdigitating with the fibres of hyoglossus. It draws the tongue upwards and backwards.

Chondroglossus is a slip of muscle arising from the lesser cornu of the hyoid and ascending to blend with the intrinsic lingual muscles. It lies medial to hyoglossus and is often described as part of that muscle.

Nerve and blood supply

The mucous membrane of the posterior one-third of the dorsum of the tongue is supplied with both taste and general sensibility by the glossopharyngeal nerve. This nerve also supplies taste fibres to the vallate papillae on the anterior two-thirds of the tongue. The remainder of the anterior two-thirds receives taste fibres from the facial nerve, via the chorda tympani and lingual nerve, while general sensibility for the anterior two-thirds is conveyed by trigeminal fibres in the lingual nerve. A small area of the posterior one-third, immediately in front of the epiglottis, is supplied by the internal laryngeal branch of the vagus. The fact that the vallate papillae are supplied by the glossopharyngeal nerve (the nerve of the third arch) despite being located anterior to the sulcus terminalis is attributable to forward migration of tissue across the boundary between the third arch and first arch territories during development.

Both the intrinsic and extrinsic muscles of the tongue, apart from palatoglossus, are derived from occipital myotomes and are innervated, therefore, by the hypoglossal nerve. Palatoglossus is a pharyngeal arch derivative and is supplied through the cranial part of the accessory nerve.

The main source of blood to the tongue is the lingual branch of the external carotid artery. Small lingual branches are also given off the ascending palatine and ascending pharyngeal arteries. There may also be a small lingual branch from the second part of the maxillary artery. The venous drainage is via the lingual and deep lingual veins.

Lymph drainage (Fig. 4.57)

The lymph drainage of the tongue is complex but must be thoroughly understood because of the tendency for malignant lingual neoplasms to spread through this route. Carcinoma of the tongue may first be detected by the presence of metastases in the draining lymph nodes, especially if the primary lesion is in the posterior one-third of the tongue where it may not be apparent to the patient.

There is a plexus of lymphatic vessels in the mucous membrane and another in the musculature of the tongue. The two are continuous. Drainage from the tongue anterior to the vallate papillae is into **marginal** and **central vessels**, that from behind the papillae is into **dorsal vessels**. The marginal vessels receive lymph from the tip of the tongue. They descend under the mucous membrane on the inferior surface of the tongue and pierce mylohyoid to drain mostly into the submental nodes and thence into the jugulo-omohyoid node. Some of the marginal vessels end in the submandibular nodes which themselves drain into the deep cervical nodes, principally the jugulo-omohyoid. Vessels arising on one side of the tongue may cross on its undersurface to end in nodes of the opposite side. The central vessels receive lymph from the remainder of the tongue anterior to the vallate papillae. They descend between the two genioglossi close to the median plane. Some pass posteriorly to the jugulo-omohyoid and jugulodigastric nodes while others pierce mylohyoid to enter the submandibular nodes. Again there is some overlap between the two sides. The dorsal vessels drain bilaterally into the jugulodigastric nodes and, to a lesser extent, into the jugulo-omohyoid nodes.

SUMMARY OF SENSORY INNERVATION OF ORAL CAVITY

Because of its importance in the practice of dentistry the information about the sensory innervation of the structures of the oral cavity presented in the previous sections of this chapter is summarized below. You must know this.

1. The upper teeth and supporting structures and the lining of the maxillary sinus are supplied by the **anterior** and **posterior superior alveolar nerves** plus the **middle alveolar nerve** when present.

2. The lower teeth and supporting structures receive their sensory innervation through the **inferior alveolar nerve** and its **incisive branch**.

3. The mucous membrane on the buccal aspect of the upper alveolar process is innervated by the **superior alveolar nerves** with a contribution from the **buccal nerve** in the molar region.

4. The mucous membrane of the hard palate (including the palatal aspect of the upper alveolar process) is supplied by the **nasopalatine nerve** in the incisor region and by the **greater palatine nerve** posterior to this.

5. The mucous membrane on the buccal surface of the lower alveolar process is supplied by the **buccal nerve** in the molar and premolar region and by the **mental nerve** in the canine and incisor region.

6. The mucous membrane lining the lingual surface of the lower alveolar process and the floor of the mouth is innervated by the **lingual nerve**.

7. The mucous membrane of the cheek is innervated by the **buccal nerve**.

8. The upper lip receives its sensory supply from the **infraorbital nerve** while the lower lip is supplied by the **mental nerve**.

9. General sensation from the anterior two-thirds of the tongue is supplied by the **trigeminal fibres in the lingual nerve**. Taste from this part of the tongue is conveyed by **facial fibres** which reach the lingual nerve through the **chorda tympani**.

10. The posterior one-third of the tongue (including the vallate papillae) receives both taste and general sensation from the **glossopharyngeal nerve**.

SUMMARY OF LYMPH DRAINAGE OF ORAL CAVITY

Since both infections and malignant neoplasms tend to spread through the lymphatic system a knowledge of the lymph drainage of the structures of the oral cavity is essential for dental practitioners. Like most other attributes of living organisms the arrangement of the lymph channels and nodes is variable. The following summarizes the most usual arrangement.

1. Lymph from the teeth drains into the **submandibular, submental,** and **deep cervical nodes**.

2. The lymph vessels from the alveolar processes and from the mucous membrane lining their buccal surfaces end in the **submandibular nodes**.

3. Lymph vessels from the hard and soft palates and the palatal aspect of the upper alveolar process end in the **retropharyngeal** and **deep cervical nodes**.

4. Lymph from the structures of the floor of the mouth drains into the **submandibular** and **deep cervical nodes**. From a small area of the floor of the mouth behind the incisor teeth drainage is into the **submental nodes**.

5. Lymph from the tip of the tongue passes to the **submental** and **submandibular nodes** while that from the remainder of the tongue passes mainly to the **jugulo-omohyoid** and **jugulodigastric nodes**.

6. Lymph from the cheek, upper lip and lateral part of the lower lip drains into the **submandibular nodes**. Drainage from the central part of the lower lip is into the **submental nodes**. Note that a wedge of tissue including the central parts of the lower lip, floor of mouth, and tip of tongue drains into the **submental nodes**.

8

Pharynx, soft palate, and larynx

The pharynx is a fibromuscular tube continuous below with the oesophagus and incomplete anteriorly where it receives the posterior openings of the nasal and oral cavities. Below the oral opening is the entrance to the larynx. The pharynx thus serves as part of both the alimentary and respiratory pathways, the two pathways crossing in its lower third. This anatomical arrangement necessitates a precisely controlled swallowing mechanism to ensure that food and drink enter the oesophagus and not the larynx. The neural control of this mechanism is in abeyance in the unconscious patient.

In order to carry out its functions during swallowing the pharynx requires a considerable degree of mobility. This is provided by the pharyngeal wall being composed principally of muscle sheets and by its posterior surface being in contact with the smooth prevertebral fascia upon which it can slide.

The larynx is situated in the midline of the neck in front of the pharynx and is covered anteriorly by skin, fascia, and the infrahyoid muscles. It opens from the pharynx just behind and below the root of the tongue and is continuous inferiorly with the trachea. It has a sphincteric action, guarding the lower part of the respiratory tract, and is also the organ of phonation. The laryngeal wall contains several cartilages and numerous small muscles.

The soft palate is a mobile flap of tissue which is attached to the posterior edge of the hard palate and hangs down into the pharynx. It is raised during swallowing by the contraction of its musculature to close off the part of the pharynx lying behind the nasal cavity and so prevent the passage of food and drink into the upper respiratory tract.

PHARYNX

The pharynx is about 12 cm long, extending from the base of the skull to the lower border of the cricoid cartilage opposite the sixth cervical vertebra where it is continuous with the oesophagus. It is divided into three parts: the naso-, oro-, and laryngopharynx.

The **nasopharynx** lies behind the nasal cavity and above the soft palate. The posterior nasal apertures open into it anteriorly. Below it is continuous with the oropharynx through the **pharyngeal isthmus**, the part of the pharyngeal cavity situated behind the soft palate. The nasopharynx is part of the upper respiratory tract and does not normally give passage to food or drink.

The **auditory tube** opens on to the lateral wall of the nasopharynx a short distance behind the nasal aperture. This opening is bounded above and behind by the **tubal elevation** produced by the underlying medial end of the auditory tube. The **salpingopharyngeal fold** of mucous membrane, overlying the salpingopharyngeus muscle, descends from the posterior end of the tubal elevation. Associated with the mucous membrane around the opening of the auditory tube

are numerous mucous glands and nodules of lymphoid tissue (the latter are known collectively as the **tubal tonsil**). Posterior to the tubal elevation is a shallow depression called the **pharyngeal recess**.

The roof and posterior wall of the nasopharynx lie immediately adjacent to the body of the sphenoid and the basilar part of the occipital bone in the central part of the cranial base. A collection of lymphoid tissue, the **pharyngeal tonsil**, or **adenoid**, is located beneath the mucous membrane lining the upper part of the posterior wall. The tonsil may become enlarged (so called 'adenoids') in chronic infections of the upper respiratory tract. This may block the airway and lead to mouth-breathing.

The mucous membrane lining the nasopharynx is of the respiratory type, being covered by ciliated cuboidal epithelium, and receives its sensory and secretomotor nerve supply through a branch of the pterygopalatine ganglion. In both of these respects it resembles the mucous membrane lining the nose.

The **oropharynx** extends from the soft palate to the level of the epiglottis. The oral cavity opens into the oropharynx anteriorly through the **oropharyngeal isthmus** which is bounded on each side by a fold of mucous membrane, the **palatoglossal arch**, descending from the soft palate to the side of the tongue. The arch is produced by the underlying **palatoglossus muscle**. Between the epiglottis and the posterior surface of the tongue are two shallow pits, termed the **valleculae**. They are separated from each other by a median fold of mucous membrane, the **median glossoepiglottic fold**, and bounded laterally by the two **lateral glossoepiglottic folds**. The lateral wall of the oropharynx, behind the palatoglossal arch, presents a vertical ridge of mucous membrane, the **palatopharyngeal arch**, produced by the underlying **palatopharyngeus muscle**.

Between the palatoglossal and palatopharyngeal arches is a depression, the **tonsillar sinus**. The **palatine tonsil**, a mass of lymphoid tissue, is situated beneath the mucous membrane lining the sinus. The deep **intratonsillar cleft** extends from the pharynx into the upper part of the tonsil. Below the cleft the medial surface of the tonsil is marked by several small orifices leading into deep recesses, the **tonsillar crypts**, within the tonsil. Laterally the tonsil is enclosed by a fibrous capsule. The tonsil is very variable in size and is frequently the site of infection which causes it to become enlarged and painful (tonsillitis). Chronic infections may be treated by tonsillectomy.

The pharyngeal, tubal, palatine, and lingual tonsils form a ring of lymphoid tissue around the upper parts of the respiratory and alimentary passages.

The oropharynx, including the clefts and crypts of the palatine tonsils, is lined by stratified squamous epithelium. Its nerve supply is from the pharyngeal plexus.

The **laryngopharynx** extends from the epiglottis to the lower

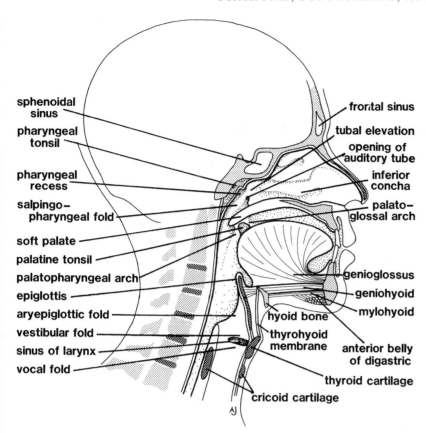

sphenoidal sinus
pharyngeal tonsil
pharyngeal recess
salpingo-pharyngeal fold
soft palate
palatine tonsil
palatopharyngeal arch
epiglottis
aryepiglottic fold
vestibular fold
sinus of larynx
vocal fold

frontal sinus
tubal elevation
opening of auditory tube
inferior concha
palato-glossal arch
genioglossus
geniohyoid
mylohyoid
hyoid bone
thyrohyoid membrane
anterior belly of digastric
thyroid cartilage
cricoid cartilage

Fig. 4.90. Sagittal section of the head and neck to show the pharynx and larynx.

border of the cricoid cartilage. Its anterior wall, below the epiglottis, is pierced by the **inlet of the larynx**. Either side of the inlet is a small recess termed the **piriform fossa**. The fossa is bounded medially by the **aryepiglottic** fold of mucous membrane which also forms the lateral boundary of the laryngeal inlet. The laryngopharynx is lined by stratified squamous epithelium and is innervated from the vagus through the internal and recurrent laryngeal branches.

On functional, developmental, and comparative anatomical grounds the nasopharynx would probably be better regarded as part of the nasal cavity. Unlike the oro- and laryngopharynx it is solely respiratory in function, is lined by respiratory mucosa which receives its sensory innervation from the trigeminal nerve, and has a permanently patent lumen.

Muscles

The principal components of the pharyngeal wall are the three paired **constrictor muscles**. These arise anteriorly from a variety of structures and sweep around the side of the pharynx to meet their fellows of the opposite side in the posterior pharyngeal wall at the median **pharyngeal ligament** and **raphe**. They are arranged in a superior–inferior sequence with the muscle below overlapping to some extent the muscle above.

Three other muscles are inserted into the pharyngeal wall. These are **stylopharyngeus**, **salpingopharyngeus**, and **palatopharyngeus**. Stylopharyngeus is described with the styloid apparatus (p. 178) and palatopharyngeus with the soft palate (p. 198).

Superior constrictor

This muscle arises from the lower two-thirds of the posterior border of the medial pterygoid plate (including the hamulus) and from the posterior end of the mylohyoid line on the medial surface of the mandible. Between the hamulus and the mandible the fibres arise from the **pterygomandibular raphe** where they interdigitate with fibres of the buccinator. A few fibres also arise from the side of the tongue.

From this multiple origin the muscle sweeps in a thin sheet around the side wall and into the posterior wall of the pharynx. The uppermost fibres are inserted into the pharyngeal tubercle on the basilar part of the occipital bone. Below this the fibres are inserted into the strong pharyngeal ligament which descends from the pharyngeal tubercle in the posterior midline as far as the lower limit of the nasopharynx. More inferiorly still the fibres are inserted into the expansile pharyngeal raphe.

Between the upper border of the muscle and the base of the skull is a gap through which the cartilaginous part of the auditory tube and the levator veli palatini muscle pass. The remainder of the gap is closed by the strong **pharyngobasilar fascia**.

Middle constrictor

The middle constrictor is attached anteriorly to the lower part of the stylohyoid ligament, the lesser cornu, and the upper border of the greater cornu of the hyoid bone. The fibres pass around the pharynx

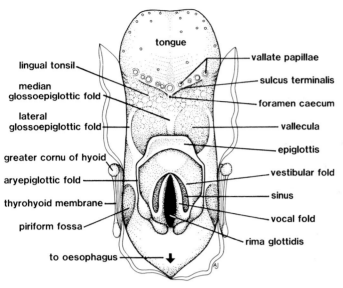

Fig. 4.91. The anterior wall of the oro- and laryngopharynx.

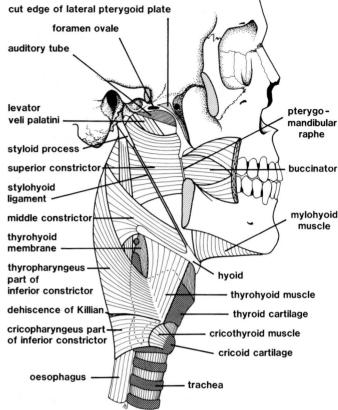

Fig. 4.92. Lateral view of the constrictor muscles of the pharynx. The antero-lateral surface of the auditory tube can be seen as the tube enters the interior of the pharynx by passing above the upper margin of the superior constrictor.

to interdigitate with the fibres of the opposite side at the pharyngeal raphe. The upper fibres diverge upwards, passing superficial to the lower part of the superior constrictor; the lower fibres run more horizontally passing deep to the upper part of the inferior constrictor.

Inferior constrictor

The inferior constrictor consists of two parts, the **thyropharyngeus** and **cricopharyngeus**. Thyropharyngeus arises from the oblique line on the lamina of the thyroid cartilage. The fibres run posteriorly and upwards to be inserted into the pharyngeal raphe, the uppermost fibres being situated superficial to the middle constrictor. Cricopharyngeus is attached anteriorly to the side of the arch of the cricoid cartilage. With its fellow of the opposite side it encircles the lowermost part of the pharynx in a thick band which is continuous inferiorly with the circular fibres of the upper part of the oesophagus. Between the thyroid and cricoid cartilages the fibres of the inferior constrictor arise from a tendinous band which crosses superficial to the cricothyroid muscle.

A weak area, called **Killian's dehiscence**, is present between thyropharyngeus and cricopharyngeus. The mucous membrane lining the pharynx may protrude through this weak area giving rise to a pharyngeal pouch.

Salpingopharyngeus

This muscle arises from the lower part of the cartilage of the auditory tube close to the opening of the latter into the nasopharynx (Fig. 4.96). It passes downwards beneath the pharyngeal mucous membrane, which is raised to form the **salpingopharyngeal fold,** and blends with the constrictor muscles.

The pharyngeal muscles, with the exception of stylopharyngeus, are innervated by fibres which leave the brainstem in the cranial accessory nerve. The pathway by which they reach the pharynx is described in the next section. Stylopharyngeus, the only muscle

derived from the third pharyngeal arch, is supplied by the glosso-pharyngeal nerve.

The action of the pharyngeal muscles is discussed with the mechanism of swallowing in Chapter 4.9.

Nerve supply

Lying in the connective tissue (sometimes, and inappropriately, referred to as buccopharyngeal fascia) on the superficial surface of the constrictor muscles, especially the middle constrictor, is the **pharyngeal plexus of nerves.** This is formed by union of the pharyngeal branches of the vagus and glossopharyngeal nerves and the laryngo-pharyngeal branch of the superior cervical sympathetic ganglion.

The glossopharyngeal supplies sensory fibres for the mucous membrane of the oropharynx and parasympathetic (secretomotor) fibres to the glands of this region. The latter are preganglionic fibres from the inferior salivatory nucleus which synapse in relay stations in the pharyngeal mucous membrane. The pharyngeal branch of the vagus carries motor fibres for the muscles of the pharynx (except stylo-pharyngeus) and soft palate (except the tensor). These fibres begin in the nucleus ambiguus, leave the brainstem in the cranial accessory nerve and pass to the vagus in the union of the two nerves in the

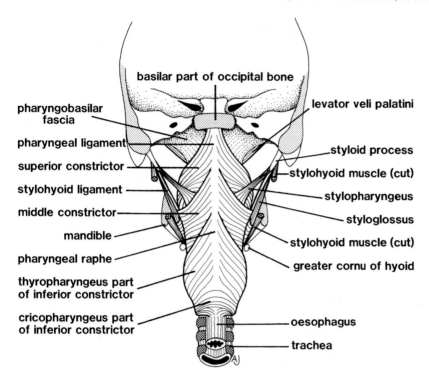

Fig. 4.93. Posterior view of the constrictor muscles of the pharynx.

jugular foramen. The sympathetic fibres which reach the plexus from the superior cervical ganglion are vasoconstrictor.

The mucous membrane of the naso- and laryngopharynx is not innervated by the pharyngeal plexus. The nasopharynx is supplied with general sensory (trigeminal) and postganglionic parasympathetic (originally facial) fibres through the pharyngeal branch of the pterygopalatine ganglion. The laryngopharynx receives its sensory and parasympathetic innervation through the internal and recurrent laryngeal branches of the vagus. The internal laryngeal nerve also conveys taste fibres for the mucosa of the epiglottis and valleculae.

Blood supply and lymph drainage

The pharynx receives blood from the ascending pharyngeal branch of the external carotid artery, the ascending palatine and tonsillar branches of the facial artery, the greater palatine and pharyngeal branches of the maxillary artery, branches of the lingual artery, and from the superior and inferior laryngeal branches of the superior and inferior thyroid arteries respectively.

The veins draining the pharynx form a pharyngeal venous plexus on the superficial surface of the constrictor muscles. The plexus drains into the pterygoid plexus and into the internal jugular vein.

The lymphatic channels from the pharynx pass to the deep cervical nodes, either directly or through the retropharyngeal nodes.

Principal relationships of the pharynx

Posteriorly the pharynx is in contact with the prevertebral fascia. The small amount of loose connective tissue between the fascia and the

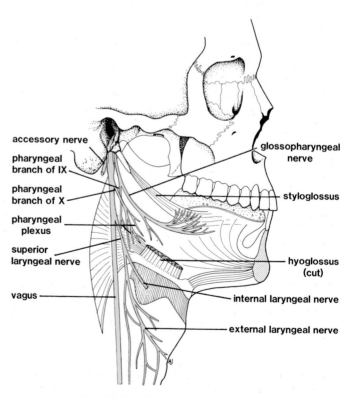

Fig. 4.94. The pharyngeal plexus of nerves.

pharyngeal wall, sometimes called the retropharyngeal space, provides a potential route for pathological fluids to spread from one side of the neck to the other. The anterior relationships of the pharynx are, from above downwards, the posterior nasal apertures, the soft palate, the oral cavity, the posterior surface of the tongue, the epiglottis, and the larynx. The floor of the piriform fossa, on each side of the laryngeal inlet, is related to the thyrohyoid membrane and the lamina of the thyroid cartilage. Laterally the pharynx is related to the carotid sheath, styloid apparatus, glossopharyngeal nerve, and the pharyngeal and superior laryngeal branches of the vagus.

SOFT PALATE

The soft palate is a mobile flap suspended from the posterior border of the hard palate. It projects downwards and backwards, separating the nasal and oral parts of the pharynx, and is continuous on each side with the lateral wall of the pharynx.

The soft palate consists in essence of an aponeurosis to which are attached several muscles, the whole enclosed in a fold of mucous membrane. Over most of its extent the mucous membrane is covered by stratified squamous epithelium but on the upper part of its posterior (or nasopharyngeal) surface the epithelium is ciliated cuboidal like that of the nasopharynx. Associated with the mucous membrane, especially on the anterior (or oral) surface, are numerous mucous glands.

Hanging from the lower free margin of the soft palate is a conical projection of variable length, the **uvula.** It contains a mass of mucous glands. Running downwards on to the side wall of the pharynx from the anterior surface of the soft palate are two folds of mucous membrane, the palatoglossal and palatopharyngeal arches. Between the palatoglossal arches of the two sides is the oropharyngeal isthmus through which the mouth communicates with the pharynx.

The principal function of the soft palate is to close off the nasopharynx from the oropharynx during swallowing.

Palatine aponeurosis

This is a thin but strong sheet of fibrous tissue attached to the posterior border and inferior surface (as far forwards as the palatine crest) of the bony palate. It is in reality the expanded tendons of the tensor veli palatini muscles. To it are attached all the other palatine muscles.

Palatine musculature

Tensor veli palatini

This thin, triangular muscle arises from the scaphoid fossa (located at the upper end of the posterior border of the medial pterygoid plate) and the lateral side of the cartilaginous part of the auditory tube. From this extensive origin the fibres descend and converge to form a tendon which pierces the origin of buccinator and turns medially around the pterygoid hamulus to gain access to the interior of the pharynx. The tendon then broadens out to form the palatine aponeurosis.

The muscle is supplied by the mandibular division of the trigeminal nerve through its branch to the medial pterygoid muscle and otic ganglion. Its action is to tense the palatine aponeurosis so that the other palatine muscles can act.

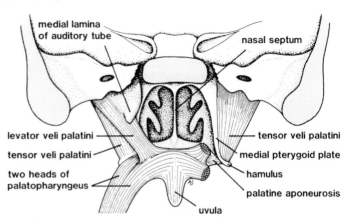

Fig. 4.95. Posterior view of the muscles of the soft palate. On the right the levator veli palatini and auditory tube have been removed.

Levator veli palatini

The levator of the palate arises from the inferior surface of the petrous temporal bone anterior and medial to the external opening of the carotid canal and from the medial lamina of the cartilaginous part of the auditory tube. It passes into the pharynx above the upper border of the superior constrictor and is inserted into the posterior surface of the palatine aponeurosis between the two heads of origin of palatopharyngeus. It is supplied from the pharyngeal plexus and acts, with the palatine aponeurosis tensed, to raise the soft palate.

Palatoglossus

This muscle arises from the anterior surface of the palatine aponeurosis and runs downwards beneath the mucous membrane of the oropharyngeal isthmus forming the palatoglossal arch. It is inserted into the side of the tongue. When the muscles of the two sides contract they pull up the posterior part of the tongue and approximate the palatoglossal arches so that the oropharyngeal isthmus is constricted. The motor nerve supply of the muscle is from the pharyngeal plexus.

Palatopharyngeus

Palatopharyngeus arises by two heads which are separated from each other by the insertion of levator veli palatini. The anterior head takes origin from the posterior border of the bony palate. The posterior head arises from the posterior surface of the palatine aponeurosis behind the attachment of the levator. The two heads pass laterally and then arch downwards over the lateral border of the aponeurosis and unite in the lateral wall of the oropharynx. The now single muscle continues downwards beneath the mucous membrane, raising the palatopharyngeal arch, to be inserted into the posterior border of the thyroid cartilage and into the inferior constrictor muscle.

The muscle is innervated from the pharyngeal plexus and acts to elevate the larynx and pharynx or conversely to depress the soft palate.

Palatopharyngeal sphincter

A separate group of palatopharyngeal fibres arises from the lateral end of the posterior border of the bony palate (in continuity with the anterior head) and runs horizontally backwards encircling, with the corresponding fibres of the opposite side, the pharynx within the superior constrictor. These fibres constitute the **palatopharyngeal sphincter,** or 'Passavant's muscle', and their presence raises an elevation, **'Passavant's ridge',** on the interior aspect of the pharyngeal wall. When the soft palate is elevated it meets the pharyngeal wall at this ridge. In cleft palate the palatopharyngeal sphincter is greatly hypertrophied and helps by its contraction to compensate, to some extent, for the deficiency in the soft palate. It is innervated by the pharyngeal plexus.

Nerve supply

Most of the mucous membrane of the soft palate is supplied with sensory fibres from the trigeminal nerve through the lesser palatine branches of the pterygopalatine ganglion. On the anterior surface there is a small area of overlap with the glossopharyngeal nerve.

All the muscles, except tensor veli palatini, are supplied through the pharyngeal plexus (cranial accessory fibres). The tensor is supplied by the mandibular nerve.

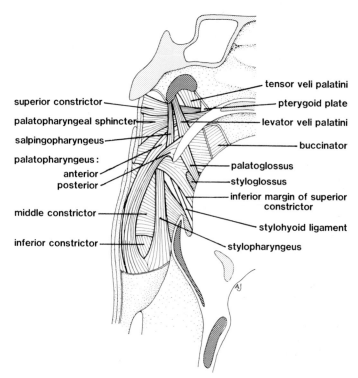

labels on figure:
superior constrictor
palatopharyngeal sphincter
salpingopharyngeus
palatopharyngeus:
  anterior
  posterior
middle constrictor
inferior constrictor
tensor veli palatini
pterygoid plate
levator veli palatini
buccinator
palatoglossus
styloglossus
inferior margin of superior constrictor
stylohyoid ligament
stylopharyngeus

Fig. 4.96. Internal view of the muscles of the pharynx and soft palate.

Blood supply and lymph drainage

The soft palate receives blood from the lesser palatine branches of the maxillary artery, the ascending palatine branch of the facial artery and palatine branches of the ascending pharyngeal artery. Venous blood drains into the pharyngeal and pterygoid plexuses.

Lymph drainage is into the retropharyngeal and upper deep cervical nodes.

Auditory tube

The **auditory tube** (also known as the **pharyngotympanic** or **Eustachian** tube) is the channel through which the tympanic cavity communicates with the nasopharynx. It serves to equalize the pressure on the two sides of the ear drum. It is about 35 mm in length of which the lateral one-third is bony and the medial two-thirds are cartilaginous. The diameter of the tube is greatest at the nasopharyngeal opening and least at the junction of bony and cartilaginous parts. In running from the tympanic cavity to the nasopharynx its general direction is downwards, forwards, and medially.

The bony part of the tube begins at the anterior wall of the tympanic cavity, within the petrous bone, and ends on the under surface of the cranial base in the angle between the squamous and petrous parts of the temporal bone just behind the spine of the sphenoid (see Fig. 4.23). Its lower opening has a roughened margin for attachment of the cartilaginous part of the tube.

The cartilaginous part of the tube is triangular in cross-section with anterolateral, posteromedial, and inferior walls. It is composed partly of fibrocartilage and partly of fibrous tissue. The cartilage consists of two laminae joined above. The larger medial lamina is situated in the posteromedial wall of the tube while the lateral lamina is in the anterolateral wall. The tube is completed below by a membrane of fibrous tissue which connects the free edges of the two laminae. At the opening of the tube into the nasopharynx the medial lamina is expanded beneath the pharyngeal mucous membrane to form the tubal elevation.

The tube is lined with mucous membrane bearing a ciliated columnar epithelium continuous with that lining both the tympanic cavity and the nasopharynx. It receives its sensory nerve supply from the tympanic plexus and from the pharyngeal branch of the pterygo-palatine ganglion. Its blood supply is from the ascending pharyngeal and middle meningeal arteries.

A knowledge of the relationships of the cartilaginous part of the auditory tube is helpful in understanding the anatomy of this rather complex region. This part of the tube is located in a groove which passes across the inferior surface of the cranial base along the line of the articulation between the greater wing of the sphenoid and the petrous part of the temporal bone. Anterolateral to the tube is the tensor veli palatini which separates the tube from the mandibular nerve and otic ganglion. Posteromedial to the tube is the levator veli palatini. Both muscles arise in part from the cartilage of the tube, attachments which explain the dilation of the auditory tube which occurs during swallowing. As it enters the nasopharynx the tube crosses above the superior margin of the superior constrictor and is in contact in front with the upper part of the posterior border of the medial pterygoid plate (the superior constrictor being attached to the lower two-thirds of this border). The space above the constrictor not occupied by the tube and levator veli palatini is closed by the pharyngobasilar fascia.

LARYNX

The larynx is a tube lined by mucous membrane and containing within its wall several cartilages and small muscles.

Cartilages

There are nine cartilages in the larynx. The cricoid, thyroid, and paired arytenoids, consist of hyaline cartilage and tend to ossify with age. The epiglottic and paired corniculate and cuneiform cartilages are composed of elastic fibrocartilage which does not ossify (or even mineralize).

Cricoid cartilage

Traditionally described as being shaped like a signet ring, this is the only complete ring of cartilage in the walls of the respiratory system. It consists of a quadrate **lamina** (equivalent to the part of a signet ring that bears the signature) situated posteriorly and a narrow **arch** anteriorly. On each side there are two articular facets which enter into synovial joints with other laryngeal cartilages. One facet is located on the lateral surface at the junction of arch and lamina and articulates with the inferior cornu of the thyroid cartilage; the second is situated on the superior border of the lamina close to its lateral corner and articulates with the base of the corresponding arytenoid cartilage. The posterior surface of the lamina bears a median ridge, on either side of which is a shallow depression for attachment of the posterior cricoarytenoid muscle. The cricothyroid and the crico-pharyngeus part of the inferior constrictor arise from the lateral surface of the arch. The internal surface of the cricoid is smooth and is lined with laryngeal mucous membrane.

Thyroid cartilage

This is the largest of the laryngeal cartilages. It consists of two **laminae** conjoined anteriorly. The two laminae make an angle with each other of about 90° in men and some 30° greater in women and form a projection in the midline of the neck known as the **laryngeal prominence**. The generally greater size of the larynx and the more acute angle between the thyroid laminae leads to the laryngeal prominence being accentuated in the male and hence to its more usual name of 'Adam's apple'. The prominence is greatest at the upper part of the laminae. Immediately above this point of greatest prominence the laminae are separated by the V-shaped **superior thyroid notch**.

Posteriorly the laminae diverge and have free superior, posterior and inferior borders, and internal and external surfaces. The thickened posterior border gives attachment to the stylopharyngeus and palato-pharyngeus muscles. It is continued upwards as the **superior cornu** and downwards as the **inferior cornu**, the latter articulating with the facet already described on the cricoid cartilage. The superior border is boldly convex and gives attachment to the thyrohyoid membrane. Just in front of the root of the superior cornu is the **superior tubercle**. The inferior border has a much straighter outline and bears, a short distance anterior to the inferior cornu, the **inferior tubercle**.

Running across the external surface of the lamina in a downwards and forwards direction from the superior to the inferior tubercle is the **oblique line**. It marks the attachment of the sternothyroid, thyro-hyoid, and inferior constrictor muscles. The internal surface of the lamina is smooth and featureless lying immediately beneath the fibroelastic membrane in the intact larynx and the floor of the piriform fossa.

Arytenoid cartilages

The two small arytenoid cartilages articulate, one on each side, with the facets on the superolateral corners of the cricoid lamina. Each is shaped like a three-sided pyramid, having a base, a posterior surface, a medial surface, an anterolateral surface, and an apex. The base is somewhat concave and provides the articulation with the cricoid lamina. The medial surface is smooth and is covered by the laryngeal mucous membrane. The anterolateral surface is convex. To its upper

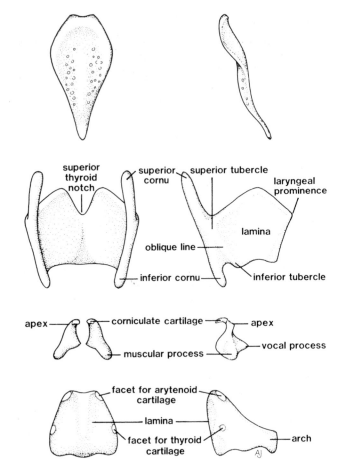

Fig. 4.97. The epiglottic, thyroid, arytenoid, and cricoid cartilages (in that order from above downwards). Posterior view to left, lateral view to right.

part is attached the vestibular ligament and to its lower part the lateral cricoarytenoid and vocalis muscles. The posterior surface gives attachment to the transverse arytenoid muscle. The lateral angle of the arytenoid is extended to form a rounded projection termed the **muscular process**. It gives attachment to the lateral and posterior cricoarytenoid muscles. The anterior angle forms a more pointed projection called the **vocal process**. Here is attached the vocal ligament. The apex curves backwards somewhat and articulates with the corniculate cartilage.

Epiglottic cartilage

This is a thin, curled leaf-shaped cartilage. It is attached below by its stalk to the inner aspect of the angle formed by the conjoined thyroid laminae, just below the thyroid notch. Its broad superior part projects upwards into the pharynx behind the hyoid bone and the posterior surface of the tongue and above the laryngeal inlet. The convex posterior surface of the cartilage is covered over its whole extent by mucous membrane and faces, in its upper part, into the laryngopharynx and, in its lower part, into the larynx above the vocal folds. Only the upper part of the anterior surface of the cartilage is

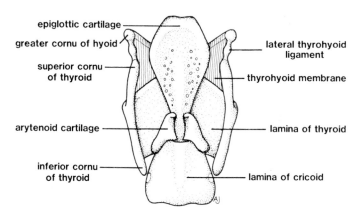

Fig. 4.98. Posterior view of the articulated cartilages of the larynx.

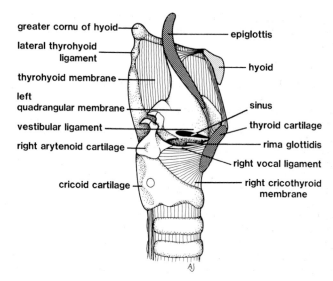

Fig. 4.99. Lateral view of right side of larynx to show the quadrangular and cricothyroid membranes. The right lamina of the thyroid cartilage and the right quadrangular membrane have been removed. Note that the *left* quadrangular but *right* cricothyroid membranes are shown.

free and is covered by mucous membrane reflected from the posterior surface of the tongue and from the lateral pharyngeal wall. This mucous membrane is raised into three folds – a median glossoepiglottic and two lateral glossoepiglottic folds – with the valleculae between them. The lower part of the anterior surface is situated behind the thyrohyoid membrane, from which it is separated by fatty tissue, and the hyoid bone, to which it is attached by the hyoepiglottic ligament.

Corniculate and cuneiform cartilages

A small cone of cartilage, the **corniculate cartilage**, articulates with the apex of each arytenoid cartilage, lying within the aryepiglottic fold of mucous membrane. Ventral to the corniculate cartilage, also in the aryepiglottic fold, is another small nodule called the **cuneiform cartilage**.

Ligaments and membranes

Thyrohyoid membrane and ligaments

The **thyrohyoid membrane** is a sheet of fibroelastic tissue attached below to the superior borders of the laminae and the anterior aspects of the superior cornua of the thyroid cartilage and above to the upper border of the posterior surface of the body and greater cornua of the hyoid bone. It is thickened in the midline, to form the **median thyrohyoid ligament**, and at its lateral margins, to form the two **lateral thyrohyoid ligaments**. It is separated from the posterior surface of the hyoid, below its attachment to the upper border of this surface, by a bursa. The thyrohyoid membrane is pierced on each side by the superior laryngeal vessels and internal laryngeal nerve.

Fibroelastic, quadrangular, and cricothyroid membranes

Beneath the mucous membrane of the larynx, separating it from the internal surface of the thyroid lamina and the thyrohyoid membrane there is, on each side, a broad sheet of mixed fibrous and elastic tissue termed the **fibroelastic membrane of the larynx**. It is divided into upper and lower parts by a horizontally placed interval.

The upper, less well-defined part, called the **quadrangular membrane**, extends from the anterior border of the arytenoid cartilage, between vocal process and apex, to the lateral border of the epiglottic cartilage. Its upper border is free and forms, with the

covering mucous membrane the **aryepiglottic fold**. Its lower border, also free, is somewhat thickened to form the **vestibular ligament**. The ligament raises a ridge, termed the **vestibular fold**, in the mucous membrane lining the larynx.

The lower part of the fibroelastic membrane is much better defined and is called the **cricothyroid membrane**. It is attached below to the upper border of the cricoid arch, behind to the vocal process of the arytenoid cartilage and in front to the lower border of the angle of the thyroid cartilage close to the midline. Its upper border is free and runs from the vocal process of the arytenoid forwards to the internal surface of the thyroid cartilage. It is termed the **vocal ligament** and forms, with its covering of mucous membrane, the **vocal fold**. The gap between the right and left vocal folds forms the anterior part of the **rima glottidis** (the posterior part of which lies between the arytenoid cartilages – see p. 203). The rima glottidis is the narrowest part of the lumen of the larynx. In the midline the cricothyroid membrane is thickened to form the **conus elasticus** connecting the upper border of the cricoid cartilage to the lower border of the thyroid cartilage.

Muscles

The muscles of the larynx comprise an extrinsic and an intrinsic group. The extrinsic group consists of muscles which arise outside the larynx and are inserted into the laryngeal cartilages. It includes stylopharyngeus, palatopharyngeus, sternothyroid, and thyrohyoid. Their action is to elevate or depress the larynx bodily during swallowing. Movements of the larynx are also brought about by the muscles acting on the hyoid. The functions of the extrinsic laryngeal and hyoid musculature are described further in the section on swallowing (p. 211).

The intrinsic group consists of muscles which are attached at both ends to the laryngeal cartilages. They are named according to the cartilages to which they are attached. With the exception of the transverse arytenoid each is paired.

The cricothyroid muscle is innervated by the external laryngeal branch of the superior laryngeal nerve. The remaining intrinsic muscles are supplied by the recurrent laryngeal nerves.

Cricothyroid

The cricothyroid arises from a small area on the anterolateral aspect of the cricoid arch. Its fibres fan out to be inserted into the anterior border of the inferior cornu and the adjacent lower border of the lamina of the thyroid cartilage. When the muscles of the two sides contract the angle of the thyroid cartilage is tilted downwards or conversely, with a fixed thyroid cartilage, the arch of the cricoid is tilted upwards, both movements taking place about a transverse axis passing through the articulations between the inferior cornua of the thyroid cartilage and the sides of the cricoid cartilage. The effect is to increase the distance between the angle of the thyroid cartilage and the arytenoid cartilage and so lengthen the vocal fold.

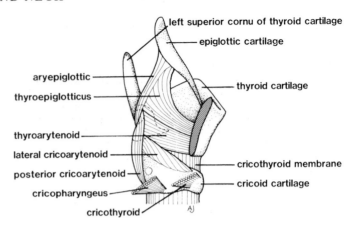

Fig. 4.101. Lateral view of the laryngeal muscles. The right lamina of the thyroid cartilage and the cricothyroid muscle have been removed.

This movement results in the rima glottidis opening into a diamond-shaped aperture. Contraction of the lower more vertically directed, fibres exerts a downward pull on the arytenoid which, because the base of this cartilage articulates with the sloping corner of the cricoid lamina, results in it moving laterally as well as downwards. In consequence the rima glottidis opens into a triangular aperture.

Lateral cricoarytenoid

This muscle arises from the superior border of the cricoid arch and passes upwards and backwards to be inserted into the muscular process of the arytenoid. By drawing the muscular process forwards the lateral cricoarytenoid rotates the arytenoid cartilage about its vertical axis so that the vocal process moves medially. The muscle is thus an opponent of the upper part of the posterior cricoarytenoid, acting with its fellow of the opposite side to approximate the vocal folds by rotation of the arytenoids.

Transverse arytenoid

This is an unpaired muscle which consists of transversely running fibres attached on each side to the muscular process and lateral border of the arytenoid cartilage. Its action is to draw the arytenoids together by pulling them upwards and medially along the sloping

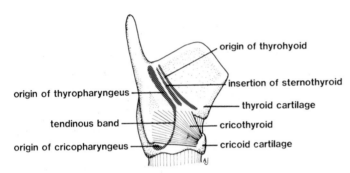

Fig. 4.100. Lateral view of the cricothyroid muscle.

Thyroarytenoid

This is a thin sheet of muscle which arises from the lower part of the inner surface of the angle of the thyroid cartilage and is inserted into the anterolateral surface of the arytenoid cartilage. The lower fibres run lateral to the vocal ligament (i.e. the free edge of the cricothyroid membrane) while the upper fibres pass lateral to the sinus and saccule (see below). It is an opponent of the cricothyroid, its contraction approximating the angle of the thyroid and the arytenoid cartilage and so shortening the vocal fold.

Vocalis

The lower and more medial fibres of thyroarytenoid, which lie immediately lateral to the vocal ligament, form a distinct band of muscle which is sometimes named separately as vocalis.

Posterior cricoarytenoid

Sometimes described as being the most important muscle in the body because it is the only dilator of the rima glottidis, the posterior crico-arytenoid arises from the concavity on the posterolateral surface of the cricoid lamina. Its fibres pass upwards and laterally and converge to be inserted into the muscular process of the arytenoid cartilage. The muscle dilates the rima glottidis in two ways. Contraction of its upper, more horizontally orientated, fibres rotates the arytenoid about its vertical axis so causing the vocal process to move laterally.

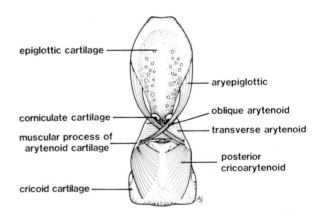

Fig. 4.102. Posterior view of the laryngeal muscles.

corners of the cricoid lamina. It is an opponent of the lower part of the posterior cricoarytenoid muscle.

Oblique arytenoid and aryepiglottic

The oblique arytenoid muscles are situated superficially to the transverse arytenoid. Each consists of a band of fibres running from the muscular process of one arytenoid cartilage to the apex of the opposite cartilage, the two bands crossing each other like the limbs of the letter X. A proportion of the fibres in each band continues forwards into the corresponding aryepiglottic fold and is inserted into the side of the epiglottic cartilage. These fibres constitute the aryepiglottic muscle. The oblique arytenoids and aryepiglottic muscles act as the sphincter of the laryngeal inlet by approximating the arytenoid cartilages and posterior surface of the epiglottis and drawing together the aryepiglottic folds.

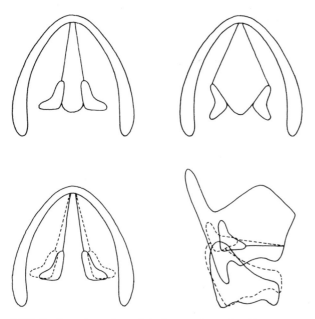

Fig. 4.103. To show the actions of the laryngeal muscles. Upper left, vocal folds in resting position; upper right, arytenoid cartilages rotated by contraction of the horizontal (upper) fibres of the posterior cricoarytenoid; lower left, arytenoid cartilages moved laterally by contraction of the vertical (lower) fibres of the posterior cricoarytenoid; lower right, relative movements of the cricoid and thyroid cartilages (with accompanying changes in the length of the vocal folds) brought about by the alternate contraction of the cricothyroid and thyroarytenoid muscles.

Thyroepiglotticus

This small group of muscle fibres arises from the upper part of the inner aspect of the angle of the thyroid cartilage and passes upwards, lateral to the quadrangular membrane, to be inserted into the aryepiglottic fold and lateral edge of the epiglottis. It is sometimes described as an upward continuation of the thryoarytenoid. With its fellow its action is to pull the epiglottis downward, thus approximating it to the arytenoid cartilages, but at the same time to widen the laryngeal inlet by pulling the aryepiglottic folds apart.

The cavity and mucous membrane of the larynx

The whole of the interior of the larynx is lined with mucous membrane. At the laryngeal inlet it is continuous with the mucous membrane of the pharynx and below it is continuous with that lining the trachea. Much of the mucous membrane above the vocal folds as well as that covering the folds themselves has an epithelium of the stratified squamous variety. Elsewhere the epithelium is ciliated columnar.

Within the larynx the mucous membrane is draped over the structures of the laryngeal wall to produce a number of elevations and indentations. The inlet to the larynx is bounded anteriorly by the posterior surface of the epiglottis, posteriorly by a fold of mucous membrane stretching between the arytenoid cartilages and laterally by the aryepiglottic folds reaching from the apices of the arytenoids

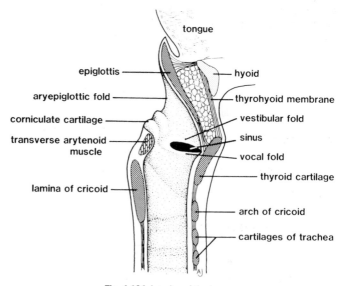

Fig. 4.104. Interior of the larynx.

to the sides of the epiglottis. Projecting into the laryngeal cavity some distance below the inlet are the vestibular and vocal folds, produced by the underlying vestibular and vocal ligaments respectively. The vocal folds are sharper, project further and are whiter in appearance (because of the adherent nature of the mucous membrane) than the vestibular folds. The anterior, or intermembranous, part of the rima glottidis lies between the vocal folds and its posterior, or intercartilaginous, part between the vocal processes and bases of the two arytenoid cartilages. The intermembranous part makes up over half of the total length of the rima glottidis.

The vestibular and vocal folds provide the boundaries between the three divisions of the cavity of the larynx. The part between the laryngeal inlet and the vestibular folds is called the **vestibule**. Its anterior wall is formed by the posterior surface of the epiglottis and is much longer than the posterior wall which consists of just the mucous membrane stretching between the two arytenoid cartilages. The lateral wall is provided by the mucous membrane covering the quadrangular membrane.

The middle part of the laryngeal cavity extends from the vestibular to the vocal folds. Opening into this part of the cavity on each side through a narrow slit between the two folds is a recess called the **sinus of the larynx**. It is lined by mucous membrane and is closely related laterally to the thyroarytenoid muscle. Extending from the anterior end of the sinus is a pouch, the **saccule of the larynx**, which ascends for a variable distance between the vestibular fold and the lamina of the thyroid cartilage.

The lower part of the laryngeal cavity extends from the vocal folds to the lower border of the cricoid cartilage. Its walls are formed, beneath the mucous membrane, by the cricothyroid membrane superiorly and the inner surface of the cricoid inferiorly.

Blood and nerve supply

The blood supply of the larynx is through the laryngeal branches of the superior and inferior thyroid arteries. The venous drainage is to the superior thyroid vein and thence to the internal jugular vein and through the inferior thyroid vein into the brachiocephalic vein. Lymph drains to the deep cervical nodes.

The innervation of the larynx is through the superior and recurrent laryngeal branches of the vagus. The superior laryngeal nerve divides into internal and external branches as it passes medial to the internal carotid artery. The internal laryngeal nerve descends to the thyrohoid membrane which it pierces above the superior laryngeal vessels and then supplies sensory fibres to the mucous membrane of the epiglottis, aryepiglottic folds, and interior of larynx down to the level of the vocal folds. The external laryngeal branch is motor to the cricothyroid muscle. The recurrent laryngeal nerve passes upwards deep to the inferior constrictor and supplies all the intrinsic muscles except cricothyroid and the mucous membrane below the vocal folds.

As well as being the boundary between the two areas of nerve supply, the vocal folds are a watershed in the arterial supply and venous and lymphatic drainage of the larynx. Above the folds these are through the superior laryngeal vessels and accompanying lymph channels; below the folds they are through the inferior laryngeal vessels and lymph channels.

Functions

The larynx guards the lower airway by its sphincteric action and by its roles in the mechanism of swallowing and the cough reflex. It is also the organ of phonation which is of special importance in man because it is a component of speech. Descriptions of both of these aspects of laryngeal function are better dealt with as part of the total mechanisms of swallowing and speech and are therefore delayed until Chapter 4.9.

Should food or other foreign bodies enter the larynx their contact with the laryngeal mucosa stimulates the cough reflex. Coughing is also stimulated by the presence of foreign bodies or inflammatory changes in the trachea, especially in the region of the bifurcation. The act of coughing consists of a short inspiration followed by immediate closure of the rima glottidis and a forcible expiratory effort. Pressure thus builds up below the vocal folds. The rima glottidis is then suddenly opened causing a powerful flow of air to be produced within the trachea and larynx which serves to expel the foreign body.

Clinical aspects

The most significant clinical aspect of the larynx, as far as the dental student is concerned, stems from the fact that the rima glottidis is the narrowest part of the upper respiratory tract so that inhaled foreign bodies tend to impact there. The entry of a foreign body into the upper part of the larynx of a conscious patient will precipitate a violent coughing reflex which is usually sufficient to eject it. In the unconscious subject (e.g. the anaesthetized patient), however, the coughing reflex is in abeyance and a foreign body entering the larynx may well obstruct the airway at the rima. Such an obstruction can be bypassed by making an incision through the neck and the anterior wall of the trachea and inserting a cannula, the operation of tracheostomy. The technique used in carrying out this operation is a clinical matter and will not be described here but from an anatomical viewpoint it is important to remember that the trachea is situated in the midline and, even if its rings cannot be felt, damage to major structures is unlikely if the incision is kept strictly to this plane.

Lymph drainage of pharynx and larynx and deeper structures of face

Lymph from the deeper structures of the head and neck, like that from more superficial parts, empties eventually into the deep cervical group of nodes. Some of this drainage is direct but in other cases the lymph passes first through one of the groups of lymph nodes surrounding the pharynx and trachea. These include the following.

Retropharyngeal nodes

These are found between the prevertebral fascia and the posterior wall of the pharynx. They receive lymph from the posterior part of the nasal cavity, paranasal air sinuses, nasopharynx, soft palate, and auditory tube. Their efferents open into the upper deep cervical nodes.

Paratracheal nodes

This group lies alongside the trachea and oesophagus and receives lymph from the oral and laryngeal parts of the pharynx and from the cervical part of the oesophagus.

Pretracheal nodes

Much of the lymph from the larynx, trachea, and thyroid gland passes to the pretracheal nodes which are located in front of the trachea deep to the investing layer of the deep fascia. The remainder of the lymph from these structures passes directly into the deep cervical nodes.

Both the para- and pretracheal nodes drain into the deep cervical group.

9

Mastication, swallowing, and speech

MASTICATION

Amongst the many characteristics distinguishing mammals from other vertebrates are the possession of a single-bone lower jaw, a temporomandibular jaw joint, a heterodont dentition, in which the post canine teeth bear multiple cusps, and a well developed and highly differentiated jaw musculature. The possession of these structural features has allowed the masticatory apparatus to undergo evolutionary specialization to produce the diverse and efficient feeding mechanisms encountered in placental mammals. The three principal feeding specializations in modern land mammals are (i) adaptation to a herbivorous diet by the development of extensive side-to-side movements of the mandible, (ii) adaptation for the capturing and devouring of prey by the development of a powerful scissor-like jaw action, and (iii) the rodent gnawing type of jaw action in which the predominant movement of the mandible is to-and-fro in the anteroposterior plane.

In one large group of mammals, however, the masticatory apparatus has remained relatively unspecialized both in its structure and function. As a result the jaws retain a wide range of usage but lack the ability to deal with any particular diet with the efficiency seen in the specialized feeders. This group comprises the most primitive living placentals, the insectivores, and also bats and primates. Man is a typical primate in most respects, the only outstanding feature of our jaws being their weak development. We have the same dental formula as our nearest living relatives, the Old World monkeys and apes, but our teeth, especially the canines, are much smaller in size relative to body mass. The upper lateral incisors, lower first premolars, and third molars appear to be still undergoing evolutionary reduction, being highly variable in size and congenitally absent in a considerable proportion of individuals. The jaw-closing muscles are also much reduced in relative size although conforming to the same general plan seen in other Old World primates. Despite these apparent structural disadvantages, the human masticatory apparatus can cope with a remarkable range of foodstuffs.

Understanding the mechanism of mastication requires a knowledge of the anatomy of the temporomandibular joint and jaw musculature. This is covered in Chapters 4.1, 4.3, and 4.6. If necessary you should revise these sections. The only additional anatomical fact that needs emphasizing is that, because the maxillary molars and premolars incline buccally while the corresponding teeth in the lower jaw incline lingually, the upper dental arcade is wider than the lower, a condition known as **anisognathy**. In consequence we can chew on only one side at a time.

Mandibular movements

Mastication involves simultaneous movements at the two temporomandibular joints. The basic movements at these joints are hinge (rotation) and translation. These are combined in various ways to produce the functional movements of depressing, elevating, protrud-

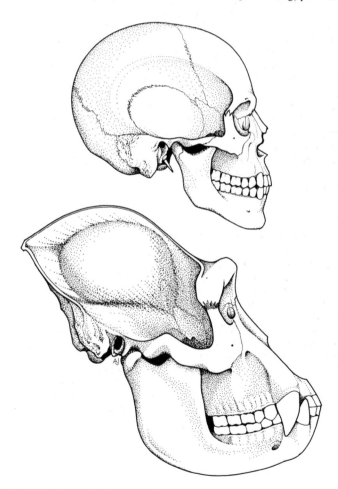

Fig. 4.105. The skulls of man and the gorilla (male) to illustrate the small size of the human jaws.

ing, retruding, and laterally deviating the mandible. The functional movements are, in turn, combined to produce the masticatory movements of incision and chewing.

Basic movements

In the **hinge movement** the head of the mandible rotates about a transverse axis. This transverse axis of rotation does not coincide exactly with the long axis of the head since the latter diverges posteromedially from the transverse plane. The movement of rotation occurs in the inferior compartment of the joint cavity.

Translation involves the mandibular head and disc sliding together forwards and downwards out of the mandibular fossa on to the articular tubercle. It takes place, therefore, in the upper compartment of the joint cavity.

If you attempt to depress the mandible by hinge movement alone, that is with the mandible forcibly held in the retruded position, you will find that you can open your mouth only a short distance. The posterior border of the mandibular ramus soon starts to compress the structures (principally the parotid gland) behind it and once their compressibility is exhausted no further movement is possible. Continued opening past this point requires that the mandibular head be allowed to translate forwards on to the articular tubercle. Verify

this for yourself by palpating the lateral poles of the mandibular heads whilst depressing the mandible to its full extent.

Functional movements

Depressing the mandible from the position of **maximum intercuspation** (in which there is maximum contact between the upper and lower teeth) to the **habitual** or **resting jaw position** (in which the teeth are separated by a few millimetres) involves a movement at the jaw joints which is so slight that it is difficult to define. It is widely held that this slight movement is virtually pure hinge but it is possible that a degree of translation is also involved. From the habitual position onwards, depression consists of a smooth and progressive combination of hinge and translation, the mandibular heads rotating against the under surface of the discs as the latter slide forwards onto the articular tubercles. During this phase the axis of rotation of the mandible moves downwards from its initial position through the mandibular heads to lie approximately between the right and left mandibular foramina. For most of the range of depression therefore, the region of the mandibular foramen is the part of the mandible which moves least. It may be significant that it is here that the major nerves and blood vessels enter the lower jaw.

The sequence of events in **elevating** the mandible is the reverse of that in depression.

Protrusion and **retrusion** are produced by symmetrical translation at the two temporomandibular joints.

In **lateral swing** the head of the mandible on the side to which movement is taking place (the ipsilateral head) is retained in the mandibular fossa while the contralateral head is translated forwards onto the articular tubercle. The mandible rotates about a vertical axis which passes just behind the ipsilateral head, not directly through it. In consequence the ipsilateral head makes a small lateral movement, called the 'Bennett' movement.

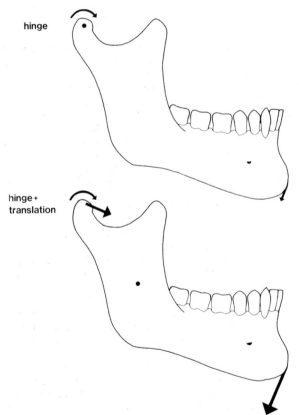

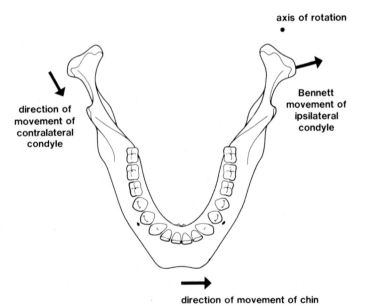

Fig. 4.106. Above, the movement from occlusion to the resting position may be pure hinge; below, depression of the mandible below the resting position is a combination of hinge and translation. Note change in location of axis of rotation (shown as small solid circle) from head of mandible to centre of ramus.

Fig. 4.107. To illustrate the 'Bennett' movement.

Masticatory movements

Modern investigations of human masticatory movements employ techniques, such as cinephotography and cineradiography, which allow the movements of the upper and lower dentitions, relative to each other, to be analysed stage by stage. These studies have made it clear that each individual possesses a characteristic chewing pattern which is established early in life. Within individuals the chewing pattern varies with the type of food being consumed. Malocclusion or dental procedures which change the shape of the occlusal surfaces can modify the chewing pattern either temporarily or permanently. In the following account of the masticatory movements, the average or typical pattern is described.

During mastication a portion of food is first bitten off by the anterior teeth (incision) and then transferred to the posterior teeth where it is finely divided by a number of chewing cycles. At this stage it is also thoroughly insalivated. In modern life, the use of knife and fork frequently obviates the need for incision.

Incision

This is a relatively simple movement in which the mandible is first moved forwards and depressed. It is then elevated so that the incisors slice through the food and meet either edge-to-edge or with the edges of the lower incisors sliding upwards against the palatal surfaces of the upper incisors. The severed portion of food is then transferred to the posterior teeth, of one or other side, by the action of the tongue.

Chewing

Once the food is in place a series of chewing cycles is initiated. Each chewing cycle consists of an **opening stroke** in which the mandible is lowered and usually moved laterally to some extent towards the working side (the side on which chewing is to take place). This may be preceded by a brief lateral movement towards the balancing side (the side opposite to that on which chewing is to take place). With the bolus held in position between the teeth on the working side by the action of the tongue and cheeks the mandible is then elevated (the **closing stroke**) with a marked deviation towards the working side. In the final stages of elevation the mandible starts to move back towards the midline so that as the upper and lower teeth come into contact, or close proximity, through the food, the occlusal surfaces of the lower teeth glide medially on, or immediately adjacent to, the corresponding surfaces of the upper teeth. During this phase, often referred to as the **power stroke**, powerful isometric contraction of the jaw-elevating muscles keeps the teeth in contact or closely approximated so that the food is ground between the opposing occlusal surfaces. The proportion of chewing cycles in which the teeth make contact is still uncertain but recent evidence suggests that it is high, probably greater than 50 per cent, and increases towards the end of a sequence of cycles.

The power stroke appears to be a particularly variable part of the human chewing cycle. It usually consists of two phases. In phase I, or buccal phase, the lower teeth move medially and somewhat superiorly from their first contact with the upper dentition to the position of maximum intercuspation. In the shorter phase II, or lingual phase, the lower teeth continue moving medially for a short distance but are now displaced inferiorly as their buccal cusps slide against the slopes of the lingual cusps of the upper teeth.

Because of the presence of anisognathy each chewing cycle is unilateral. In some subjects a whole sequence of chewing cycles takes place on one side but in others the chewing cycles, together with the food, are switched in rapid, and often irregular succession, between the two sides. In a few cases chewing takes place exclusively on the left or right.

The duration of the chewing cycle varies from about half a second to just under one second, with the power stroke occupying approximately one-quarter of the total time.

Action of the jaw muscles

The action of individual jaw muscles can be inferred from the disposition of their attachments and the general direction of their fibres. However the jaw muscles do not act singly but combine in various ways to produce the complex movements of which the jaws are capable. The analysis of the contributions made by the individual muscles to each of these movements has been advanced considerably by the technique of electromyography. This involves placing electrodes in or over the muscles being investigated and recording their electrical activity while appropriate movements are made. A non-contracting muscle is electrically quiescent whereas one that is contracting produces a burst of electrical activity which can be detected and recorded. The interpretation of electromyographical data is often difficult because the electrodes tend to pick up activity from more than one muscle; this is undoubtedly the principal reason for the frequent discrepancies between the findings of different authors.

There have been numerous electromyographical studies of the jaw muscles. The principal findings during functional movements of the mandible can be summarized as follows.

1. During depression of the mandible there is bilateral activity in the lateral pterygoid muscles accompanied, in the later stages of the movement, by activity in the digastric and other suprahyoid muscles.

2. Elevation involves the co-ordinated contraction of the temporalis, masseter, and medial pterygoids of the two sides. A certain amount of elevation is achieved by the passive tension in the elevator muscles and in the ligaments and consequently there may be little electrical activity in the muscles during the initial phase of closing.

3. Protrusion involves the bilateral contraction of the lateral and medial pterygoids.

4. Retrusion is brought about by the bilateral contraction of the middle and posterior fibres of the temporalis muscles.

5. Lateral movements are produced by contraction of the contra-lateral lateral and medial pterygoids and of the posterior fibres of the ipsilateral temporalis muscle.

During a chewing cycle the muscles combine in a rather more complex manner. In the opening stroke the two lateral pterygoid muscles are active but that on the balancing side predominates, especially towards the end of opening, so that the mandible is swung laterally towards the working side. The digastric and mylohyoid muscles are also active during the opening stroke. In closing the medial pterygoid muscles are the first elevators to contract, activity beginning first in the muscle of the balancing side but eventually reaching a higher level in the working side muscle. The masseter muscles show similar differential activity between the two sides although the onset of activity on the balancing side is later than in the corresponding medial pterygoid. The degree of activity in the temporalis muscles is about the same on the two sides but begins earlier on the working side. These patterns of activity can be readily correlated with the observed jaw movements during the closing stroke. The early contraction of the balancing side medial pterygoid and masseter is concerned with directing the mandible towards the working side. This is aided by contraction of the balancing side lateral pterygoid. The early contraction of the working side temporalis, especially the posterior fibres, aids this lateral swing by holding the ipsilateral head of the mandible in a relatively retruded position. During the later stage (i.e. the power stroke) of closing, the powerful contraction of the working side masseter and medial pterygoid serves to forcefully approximate the teeth and, together with the contraction of the balancing side temporalis, causes the mandible to return towards the median plane. At this stage, activity in the balancing side lateral pterygoid is replaced by activity in the corresponding muscle of the working side.

As would be expected, the electromyographical activity in the jaw closing muscles is greater when hard food is being chewed than when the food is soft and tends to decrease with successive chewing cycles as the food is progressively broken down and softened.

Factors influencing jaw movements

The range and direction of the movements at most joints are controlled to a large extent by the character of the articular structures, especially the size and shape of the articular surfaces and the disposition and tightness of the capsule and ligaments. This is less obviously the case in the temporomandibular joint where the articular surfaces lack congruence and the capsule and ligaments are rather weak, slack structures. This has led to the widespread belief that the structure of the jaw joints is not the prime factor controlling the position and movements of the mandible.

Although the matter cannot be considered finally settled it seems likely that the structure of the jaw joints determines the ultimate limits of mandibular movement but that within these limits other factors are more important. With the teeth separated the principal factor is probably the interplay of the jaw musculature. This would mean that jaw movements over a wide range are the outcome of learned patterns of muscle activity which would explain why the character of the chewing cycle is established at such an early age and why there is so little subsequent alteration despite age changes in the jaws, dentition, and neighbouring soft tissues. It would also explain why there is so much variation between individuals in the nature of the masticatory movements.

When the teeth are within intercuspal range, however, it appears inevitable that the shape of their occluding surfaces, or more specifically the direction of the gliding contacts between the opposed cusps, must become the major factor determining the jaw movements. As would be expected the small but powerful movements taking place during the power stroke can be influenced by changes in the shape of the dentition resulting from eruption or loss of teeth or from dental procedures. That this pattern is not easily disturbed, however, is indicated by the frequent clinical observation that an isolated filling left 'high' on the occlusal surface of a tooth will soon lead to soreness in the supporting tissues as a result of the continual trauma inflicted upon them as the lower jaw attempts to move in its accustomed path directed by the contacts between the remainder of the dentition.

The functional significance of the articular tubercle is still debated. Probably the most widely held view has been that it is related to the presence of overbite (the overlapping, in the vertical plane, of the lower incisors by the uppers) and overjet (the protrusion of the upper incisors relative to the lowers) in the human dentition. When the mandible is protruded the tubercles cause the mandibular heads to move inferiorly as well as forwards so that the lower jaw is depressed by a small amount. This has the effect of separating the occlusal surfaces of the posterior teeth when the incisors meet edge-to-edge and so allows incision to take place without interference from occluding molars or premolars.

Doubt is thrown upon this view by the fact that exactly the same effect could be achieved in the absence of the tubercle merely by combining a little opening with protrusion of the mandible, as well as by the observation that an articular tubercle is found in the jaw joints of ancient forms of humanity and of great apes in all of which the incisors meet edge-to-edge in the position of maximum intercuspation. An alternative possibility is that the presence of a tubercle is related to the lateral excursions that the mandible makes during chewing. Since the posterior teeth are tilted so that the occlusal plane on each side slopes downwards and medially, the lingual cusps project more than the buccal cusps in the upper molars and conversely in the lower molars. As the mandible is swung laterally and the teeth on the working side are brought into contact it is essential, therefore, that the balancing side of the jaw is depressed somewhat so that the projecting lingual cusps on the upper molars of that side do not collide with the buccal cusps on the lower molars. The presence of the articular tubercle, by depressing the mandibular head on the balancing side as it translates forwards, ensures that this occurs.

Statics of the mandible

One of the major controversies in the analysis of jaw function has been whether or not the mandible acts as a lever when the elevating muscles contract against resistance at the dentition, as when the teeth are closely approximated during the power stroke or when biting on a hard object. The early view was predominantly that it did and that the jaw joint provided the pivot or fulcrum. As seen in lateral view (Fig. 4.108) the resultant of the forces produced by the combined action of the elevator muscles is located between the fulcrum and the load (i.e. the bite point) so the lever would be of the class III variety. In such a system the relative magnitudes of the distances from the jaw joint to the resultant of the jaw-elevating muscles and to the bite point indicate that between one-third and two-thirds of the force generated by muscle contraction will be effective at the teeth, with the amount increasing from the premolars to the molars, and that the remainder, or reaction force, will be borne by the joint.

In the early decades of the century this view fell into disfavour largely because detailed examination of the temporomandibular joint revealed a structure which was thought to be inappropriate for stress-bearing. In particular it was observed that the bone in the roof of the mandibular fossa is very thin, that the mandibular neck is an apparently fragile structure and that the articular disc contains blood vessels and lymphatics and is covered by a synovial layer – all features thought to be incompatible with the bearing of compressive stresses. It was also pointed out that the articular surfaces are too poorly fitting to provide a stable fulcrum. It was suggested instead that the jaw-elevating muscles contract in such a way that the resultant passes directly through the bite point at the molar teeth. Thus the distances from the jaw joint to the resultant and to the main chewing teeth are identical in magnitude so that all the force is transmitted through the bite point and none through the joint.

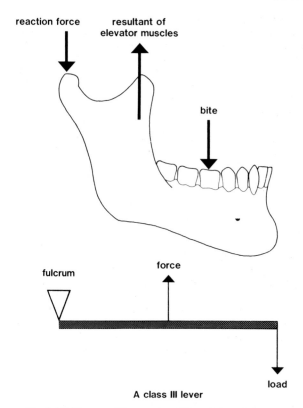

Fig. 4.108. The mandible as a class III lever in lateral view.

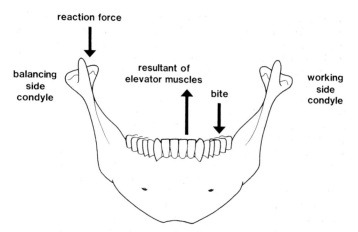

Fig. 4.109. The mandible as a class III lever in frontal view.

4.109) the mandible is acting as a class III lever with the fulcrum at the balancing side jaw joint, the force applied a little to the working side of the midline and the load borne at the bite point on the working side.

Since the mandible is swung laterally towards the working side during the power stroke, the balancing side condyle lies in a forward position on the articular tubercle in which condition the joint is best adapted to bear compression. The argument that the human temporomandibular joint is too loosely structured and its articular surfaces too poorly fitting to act as a fulcrum of a lever system is countered by the observation that even the loosest articulation can be fixed at any point by an appropriate combination of muscle action and effectively converted to a fulcrum. The reaction force at the balancing side jaw joint does not, therefore, represent wasted muscular effort; it is necessary to convert the joint into a stable fulcrum.

An alternative modern view, but one leading to rather similar conclusions, is that the mandible functions as a stationary beam during the power stroke. This is based on the fact that during this phase of the chewing cycle vertical movement is minimal. The postulated beam has three supports when viewed in frontal projection: at the working side joint, at the bite point and at the balancing side joint. If it is assumed that the resultant of the forces produced by bilateral contraction of the elevating muscles is located close to the midline, the magnitude of the distances between these three supports and their relationship to the resultant indicate that the reaction force will be about four times greater at the balancing side jaw joint than at the joint on the working side.

Recent work in experimental animals and especially in the macaque monkey has indicated that a reaction force is present at the balancing side joint during the power stroke, a finding which supports both lever and stationary beam hypotheses of jaw function. The essential similarity between the masticatory apparatus of the macaque monkey and man suggests that a comparable situation exists in the human jaws but confirmation of this awaits further investigation in man.

It will be noted that the description of the mandible as a lever or stationary beam applies only during the power stroke of the chewing cycle at which time the amount of movement taking place is very small. The fact that when the lower teeth have moved beyond the habitual position elevation and depression of the mandible take

More recently still opinion has tended to swing back towards the lever hypothesis, albeit in modified form. This has resulted from two groups of observations. First, it has been shown that the temporomandibular joint is better adapted to stress bearing than had been supposed for, in the working position of the mandible, the head articulates with the posterior face of the robust articular tubercle from which it is separated by an avascular part of the disc lacking a synovial layer (see p. 150), and the mandibular neck, despite its delicate appearance, has a strong mechanical structure. Secondly the suggestion that the resultant of the forces produced by contraction of the jaw-elevating muscles passes through the molar teeth, which is a fundamental premise of the argument that the jaw joint is non-stress-bearing, is anatomically incorrect; in fact it passes behind the last molar teeth.

The principal weakness of the original version of the lever hypothesis was that the lower jaw was considered in lateral view only and was treated as a unilateral structure with the fulcrum, force, and load all situated on one side. In fact the mandible is connected to the cranium by the two jaw joints and the elevating muscles of both sides contract during the power stroke. The resultant of the forces produced by this bilateral contraction is situated close to the median plane (since the working side elevators contract more powerfully than the balancing side muscles, the resultant probably lies somewhat to the working side of the median plane). Consequently with the bite point situated at the teeth on the working side, the reaction force will be borne by the head of the mandible on the balancing side which becomes, therefore, the fulcrum. As can be seen in frontal view (Fig.

place about a transverse axis passing through the mandibular foramina, with the mandibular heads translating as well as rotating on the squamous articular surfaces, must mean that the jaw cannot be functioning as a lever during this wider range of movement. As already emphasized it is almost certainly the pattern of muscle activity which then controls jaw movements. When the teeth come into intercuspal range, however, further elevation (or depression) takes place predominantly about a transverse axis through the mandibular heads. There is thus no inconsistency in the mandible acting as a lever or, given the very small range of movement, as a stationary beam during the power stroke and rotating about an axis through the mandibular foramina during the wider range of opening and closing.

Nervous control of mastication

Mastication is usually carried out without constant conscious effort, proceeding for most of the time in a semiautomatic manner. Since it involves complex and rapidly executed movements of the jaws, during which the teeth are moved in close contact and with powerful force against their opponents, a precise neural control is clearly required. In order that such control be exerted the brain must constantly receive information about the state of the jaw muscles and jaw joints, the position of the mandible in space and the degree of force being exerted on the supporting tissues of the teeth.

Information about muscle length is relayed from the numerous neuromuscular spindles found in the jaw musculature. The afferent fibres from the spindles in the elevating muscles pass in the mandibular division of the trigeminal nerve and enter the brainstem in the motor root of the nerve, bypassing the trigeminal ganglion. They terminate in the mesencephalic nucleus of the trigeminal. The neurons that end here are unique amongst sensory fibres in that their cell bodies are contained within the central nucleus not in the peripheral (i.e. trigeminal) ganglion.

Nerve receptors are present in large numbers in the capsule and ligaments of the temporomandibular joint. The most abundant are free nerve endings which are believed to be pain receptors. Unencapsulated spray type endings are also numerous in the capsule. There is evidence that these have a low threshold and are slowly adapting. They may well provide, therefore, a principal source of impulses concerned in the perception of mandibular position. A third type of ending present in the capsule is of the encapsulated variety. This has a higher threshold, is rapidly adapting and is thought to respond briefly to movements of the joint. The afferents of these various types of receptors pass to the brainstem via the auriculotemporal nerve and the mandibular division of the trigeminal. The pain fibres probably have their cell bodies located in the trigeminal ganglion and end in the nucleus of the spinal tract. The connections of the other types of fibre are uncertain but it seems likely that the mesencephalic nucleus is involved.

The periodontal tissues contain numerous receptors which respond to mechanical forces acting on the teeth. They are of several morphological types including encapsulated, unencapsulated, and free endings. They appear to be quite specialized in their function, some having a high threshold and being rapidly adapting while others have a low threshold and are slowly adapting, and to possess a measure of directional sensitivity (i.e. respond maximally to forces acting in one particular direction). The afferents of these receptors pass to the brainstem in the mandibular and maxillary nerves. Their central connections are uncertain. Some probably end in the mesencephalic nucleus but others appear to have their cell bodies in the trigeminal ganglion.

The manner in which the information received through these routes is utilized in controlling jaw position and movement has been investigated experimentally in anaesthetized and decerebrate animals and by the use of electromyography, to accurately determine muscle responses, in the human subject. The mechanisms are still far from completely understood but some of the simpler reflexes involved have been worked out.

Sustained downward pressure on the mandible of a decerebrate animal provokes a powerful **jaw-closing reflex** contraction of the elevator jaw muscles. Since this reflex is not abolished by sectioning the sensory root of the trigeminal nerve it seems likely that its afferent limb is from the elevator neuromuscular spindles (the fibres from which pass in the motor root). The motor limb is, of course, the innervation of the elevator muscles through the mandibular nerve. During the jaw-closing reflex the activity of the depressor muscles is suppressed. The jaw-closing reflex probably plays a part in determining the resting position of the mandible, the slight stretching of the elevator muscles produced by the effect of gravity on the mandible causing a few neuromuscular spindles to fire so maintaining a degree of postural tone in the elevating muscles. A sudden downward movement of the lower jaw, by contrast, evokes a brief burst of activity in the elevator muscles. This is the **jaw-jerk reflex** and is similar to the well known knee-jerk elicited by tapping the patellar ligament. As with the jaw-closing reflex, the afferent limb of the jaw-jerk is from the elevator neuromuscular spindles and the efferent limb is via the mandibular nerve. The reflex arcs for the knee-jerk and similar reflexes involving limb muscles are known to be monosynaptic (i.e. comprise an afferent and an efferent neuron with a single synapse between them and no connector neuron) and the same may be true for the jaw-jerk. Pressure applied to the teeth, gingivae, or hard palate of a decerebrate animal provokes a **jaw-opening reflex,** followed by a rebound closure. The opening is brought about by contraction of the depressor and inhibition of the elevator muscles and the closure by contraction of the elevators. It appears that the afferent limb of this reflex is made up of the fibres from the periodontal receptors.

The jaw-jerk reflex is present in the human subject where it is routinely tested in the physical examination of patients in order to investigate the integrity of the mandibular division of the trigeminal nerve. It is elicited by placing a finger on the patient's chin and then tapping the finger sharply with the fingers of the other hand or with a patellar hammer. If you try this on yourself you will find that the tap is followed by a small upward jerk of the chin. Electromyographic studies have shown that the slight downward movement of the mandible caused by the tap is followed, after a very brief interval, by a short burst of activity in the elevator muscles.

Another response which is readily elicited in man is the **unloading reflex.** This consists of a swift cessation of contraction of the elevator muscles following very rapid closure. It occurs, for example, when biting hard on a brittle substance which suddenly gives way and takes place so quickly that the unexpected movement of the jaw is arrested before the teeth make contact. It clearly has a protective action in safeguarding the teeth from sudden violent contact and is the result, presumably, of the interruption of firing of the elevator neuromuscular spindles consequent upon their shortening during the rapid upward movement of the mandible.

Once a chewing sequence is initiated it tends to proceed rapidly and regularly. In this respect chewing resembles other cyclical and semiautomatic activities such as walking. How the oscillatory pattern of jaw movement is produced is still uncertain. One view is that it is largely the result of reflex activity, being maintained by the alternate stimulation of the periodontal receptors and the receptors in the gums and hard palate as the jaws come together, which evokes the jaw-opening reflex, and of the elevator neuromuscular spindles as the lower jaw is depressed, which elicits the jaw-closing reflex. The alternative view is that the oscillatory pattern is dependent upon a central mechanism operating within the brain. It has been variously suggested that the centres involved are the primary motor area of the cerebral cortex, the basal ganglia, the hypothalamus and areas within the brainstem. It could well be that both reflex and central mechanisms are involved in initiating and maintaining a sequence of chewing cycles. A widely accepted modern view is that a correlation centre exists in the brainstem which can be driven by action potentials arriving from higher centres, such as the motor cortex, or from nerve endings in the mouth and adjacent tissues. It is possible that this centre coordinates the whole feeding mechanism, including the transport of food within the mouth and swallowing as well as the chewing cycles.

FURTHER READING

Ahlgren, J. (1966). Mechanisms of mastication. *Acta odont. scand.* **24**, Suppl. 44, 1–109.
—— (1976). Masticatory movements in man. In *Mastication* (ed. D. J. Anderson and B. Matthews). Wright, Bristol.
Hiiemae, K. M. (1978). Mammalian mastication, a review of the activity of the jaw muscles and the movements they produce in chewing. In *Development, function and evolution of teeth* (ed. P. M. Butler and K. A. Joysey). Academic Press, New York.
Hylander, W. L. (1975). The human mandible: lever or link? *Am. J. phys. Anthrop.* **43**, 227–42.
Matthews, B. (1976). Reflexes excitable from the jaw muscles in man. In *Mastication* (ed. D. J. Anderson and B. Matthews). Wright, Bristol.
Mills, J. R. E. (1978). The relationship between tooth pattern and jaw movements in the Hominoidea. In *Development, function and evolution of the teeth* (ed. P. M. Butler and K. A. Joysey). Academic Press, New York.
Thexton, A.J. (1992). Mastication and swallowing: an overview. *Br. dent. J.* **173**, 197–206.

SWALLOWING

In the new-born child feeding is primarily a process of transport in which milk is transferred to the back of the mouth and swallowed in one continuous action. It is not until solid food is introduced into the diet that a chewing phase becomes necessary. After weaning liquids and very soft foods are still transported through the mouth and swallowed without any interruption for chewing. The extent to which harder foods are chewed varies considerably from one individual to another, some chewing the food until it is finely divided while others swallow after only a few chewing cycles.

Once the food has been chewed and insalivated sufficiently to meet the individual's criteria for swallowing it is formed into a single mass, called a **bolus**, and transferred to the dorsum of the tongue. The subsequent act of swallowing consists of two stages, the first being voluntary and the second reflex.

First stage

The formation of the bolus and its transference to the dorsum of the tongue is brought about by the action of the intrinsic lingual musculature. The bolus is next squeezed rapidly backwards into the oral part of the pharynx by the tongue being forced upwards against the hard palate. The first contact is between the tip of the tongue and the part of the hard palate immediately behind the incisor teeth. The area of contact moves swiftly in a posterior direction under the influence of the intrinsic musculature of the tongue. At the same time the hyoid bone, and with it the tongue, is raised by the contraction of the suprahyoid muscles. At the end of the first stage the posterior part of the tongue is elevated by contraction of the styloglossi and palatoglossi. The tongue stays in this position during the first part of the second stage and so seals the oropharyngeal isthmus and prevents the re-entry of food into the mouth.

During the first stage of swallowing the lips are usually brought together and the teeth into occlusion but there is a great deal of individual variation and some subjects swallow with the lips or teeth, or both, apart.

Second stage

The arrival of the bolus in the pharynx stimulates the onset of the second stage of swallowing. The series of reflexes controlling this stage is elicited by the contact of the bolus with certain sensitive 'trigger' areas of the mucous membrane. These are situated on the palatoglossal arches and on the side and posterior walls of the oropharynx.

During the second stage the soft palate is tensed and elevated, by contraction of the tensor and levator palatini muscles, and so brought into contact with the posterior pharyngeal wall. The seal is completed by contraction of the palatopharyngeal sphincter. Food is thus prevented from entering the nasopharynx. Simultaneously the larynx is pulled upwards, behind the hyoid, by the action of stylopharyngeus, palatopharyngeus, and salpingopharyngeus muscles. The aryepiglottic folds are tightly approximated by the action of the aryepiglottic and oblique arytenoid muscles, thus sealing off the entrance to the larynx.

The fibres of the pharyngeal constrictor muscles now contract in sequence from above downwards propelling the bolus of food downwards over the closed inlet of the larynx. This action is aided by gravity (when in the erect or sitting posture) and by the elevation of the laryngeal part of the pharynx which accompanies the upward displacement of the larynx. Once the food has entered the oesophagus it is moved onwards by peristalsis. This oesophageal phase is sometimes called the third stage of swallowing.

The movements of the epiglottis during the second stage of swallowing have been much disputed. The most recent radiological investigations suggest that the epiglottis turns downwards over the closed laryngeal inlet but not until most of the bolus has passed. It has been suggested that the function of the epiglottis when in the upright position is to act as a barrier which diverts food into the channels either side of the laryngeal inlet and then, after turning downwards, to provide cover for the inlet as it re-opens.

The afferent limb of the reflexes involved in the second stage is made up of the sensory fibres from the oropharynx. These travel to the brainstem mainly in the glossopharyngeal nerve. The efferent limbs comprise the motor nerves supplying the many muscles involved in the reflexes.

The total duration of the first and second stages of swallowing is about one second.

Clinical aspects

Considering the complex sequence of events involved, swallowing is rarely at fault. When it does go wrong it is usually because we are trying to talk or laugh at the same time. On these occasions the seal produced by the soft palate may be incomplete so that food or drink enters the nasopharynx, or the laryngeal inlet may not be completely closed so that aliment enters the upper part of the larynx. In the latter case, the cough reflex is stimulated and the offending food or drink soon expelled.

Difficulty in swallowing, or dysphagia, may result from a mechanical obstruction of the pharynx or oesophagus or from a disorder of the nervous system involving the cranial nerves and central nuclei involved in the swallowing reflex. Obstruction may be caused by tumours of the pharynx or oesophagus or of structures, such as the thyroid gland or lymph nodes, bordering these passages, an impacted foreign body, or a pharyngeal pouch. The last is an outpouching of the lining of the pharynx through Killian's dehiscence, the weak area between the thyropharyngeus and cricopharyngeus parts of the inferior constrictor. A proportion of the food being swallowed passes into the pouch which gradually enlarges and presses on the oesophagus. Diseases of the nervous system which may be accompanied by dysphagia include multiple sclerosis and poliomyelitis.

Swallowing may also be rendered difficult by anomalies of development of the palate or tongue. This is particularly true in infants with severe clefts of the palate and special feeding procedures may have to be adopted until a surgical repair of the defect can be made.

SPEECH

Speech is to all intents and purposes a human characteristic and is of the utmost importance in the social life of the individual and of the community. We learn to speak during the first few years of our lives and for most of us speech soon becomes the natural means of communication. Although we may have difficulty in choosing the most appropriate words and in arranging them in grammatical sequence, especially when trying to express complicated thoughts, the process of uttering words usually causes no problem. Nevertheless the mechanism of speech is highly complex involving the muscles of the thorax, larynx, and mouth and being under the control of higher centres of the brain. Speech is usually accompanied, and its meaning emphasized, by changes in facial expression and movements of the head and upper limbs.

The production of sound begins in the larynx, a process called **phonation.** Normally phonation takes place during expiration. Phonation during inspiration is possible but is inefficient and cannot be maintained for long. When not speaking and at rest, breathing tends to be regular and each breathing cycle is divided about equally between inspiration and expiration. The rate of breathing is subject to great variation, both between individuals and within individuals from time to time, but averages about 15 cycles per minute. During speech this rhythm is drastically changed. Inspiration is timed to take place during a natural pause in talking, such as the end of a sentence or clause, and takes place very rapidly. Expiration, on the

other hand, is greatly prolonged. The amount of air inspired and expired during speech, even when talking loudly, is not significantly greater than during quiet breathing.

Phonation consists of converting the unidirectional, even flow of expired air passing through the larynx into an oscillating flow with a frequency within the range of human hearing (about 16–20 000 Hz in adults). This is achieved by adducting the vocal folds and so obstructing the flow of air from the lungs. Pressure then builds up below the folds and eventually reaches a point where it forces the folds apart, allowing air to escape through the rima glottidis. As soon as the pressure is released the vocal folds return to the adducted position and the cycle is repeated. In consequence, the flow of air is converted to a series of puffs occurring with a frequency determined by the level of subglottal pressure and the mass, length, and tension of the vocal ligaments, these being the principal factors determining the rate at which the folds will open and close.

The frequency with which the air oscillates determines the pitch of the voice. This varies during speech to add intonation and expression to the voice and also varies on average between individuals, some people having deeper voices than others. Although the ranges overlap the pitch of the voice in women and children is generally higher than that in men. This sex difference first becomes apparent during adolescence when the male voice deepens, or breaks, due to the greater growth of the larnyx and hence greater elongation of the vocal folds.

The quality or timbre of the voice is influenced by the interplay of the factors already mentioned as determining the pitch of the voice. Thus, for example, increasing the tension of the vocal folds, accompanied by compensating changes in the other factors, leads to harshness of the voice, as when speaking in anger, without necessarily increasing the pitch. Voice quality is also influenced by subtle alterations in the way the vocal folds open and close. These include variations in the extent of vertical contact between the folds, local variations in tension along the length of the folds, and changes in the relative amounts of time the rima glottidis is in the open and closed states.

The loudness of the voice is controlled primarily by the pressure of the expired air.

The sound produced in the larynx thus has pitch, quality, and loudness. In its passage to the exterior through the upper part of the larynx, the oropharynx and the mouth its quality is modified by the acoustic characteristics of these chambers which are known collectively as the **vocal tract.** The last part of the vocal tract is particularly important in this respect because it is surrounded by the highly mobile tongue and lips which are capable of continuously changing its shape and so modulating the sound passing through. This process is called **articulation** and is the basis of word formation. A sequence of speech consists of periods of relatively high sound intensity alternating with periods of low intensity. In the former the vocal tract is unrestricted but its shape is modified by the action of the tongue to produce the vowel sounds; in the latter the tract is constricted or completely occluded by the action of the tongue or lips to produce a consonant sound. Typically each vowel sound that we make is preceded and succeeded by a consonant sound, the whole making up a syllable. Some words consist of one syllable, others are made up of a combination of several syllables.

By making the sounds yourself it is quite easy to work out how the various vowels and consonants are produced. The following summary may be helpful.

Vowels

The vowel sounds (A,E,I,O,U) are formed by a continuous air flow passing through the oral cavity, the shape of which is modified by the dorsum of the tongue being elevated to some extent. Movements of the lips also modify the shape of the oral cavity.

Consonants

The consonant sounds are classified according to the point of maximum constriction of the vocal tract:

1. labials (e.g. B,P,M) – the point of maximum constriction is between the lips;

2. labiodentals (e.g. F,V) – the constriction occurs between the lower lip and the upper incisors;

3. linguopalatals – the point of constriction may be between the tip of the tongue and the anterior part of the hard palate (e.g. D,T,R), between the dorsum of the tongue and the posterior part of the hard palate (e.g. J,L), or between the dorsum of the tongue and the soft palate (e.g. K). The sibilants (S, Sh, and Z) are produced by the passage of expired air through a narrow space between the tip of the tongue and the anterior part of the hard palate.

In the sounds M and N a proportion of the air is expressed through the nose to give the sound a nasal quality.

Modification of the shape of the mouth, as occurs, for example, in the loss of teeth or fitting of a denture, may profoundly affect articulation. Fortunately most patients are adaptable and rapidly become accustomed to the change in the shape of their mouths so that there is little or no permanent alteration in the quality of the voice. Nevertheless correct design of the denture, especially in the palatal region and in the positioning of the teeth, makes the period of adjustment much easier and shorter. Anomalies of development, such as cleft palate or lip and an unduly short lingual frenulum, termed tongue-tie, may interfere with voice production to the point where speech is unintelligible.

10

Radiological anatomy of the head

The radiographs most frequently taken in general dental practice are of the teeth and their immediate supporting tissues. Such radiographs are obtained by using a dental X-ray machine and small films, wrapped in a light-proof and water-resistant covering, which are positioned in the mouth close to the teeth being investigated. More general views of the jaws, or of the whole skull, involve the use of larger films which are positioned extraorally. Most extraoral views require a more powerful X-ray machine than is usually available in the dental surgery and the employment of intensifying screens (which fluoresce on exposure to X-rays and therefore intensify the image) placed either side of the film in a cassette. In recent years there has been a rapid expansion in the use of panoramic radiography in which views of the entire dentition and its supporting structures are obtained on a single film. For certain purposes these have replaced the more traditional intraoral and extraoral views.

Since there is considerable fine detail to be appreciated in dental radiography, some of the general principles governing the radiographic appearance of anatomical structures must be briefly mentioned. The most important points to bear in mind are that a radiograph is no more than a record of the radiodensity of the structures through which the X-ray beam has passed (radiodensity decreases in the following sequence—enamel, dentine + cemetum, cortical bone, trabecular bone, soft tissue, and finally air) and that it is a two-dimensional representation of three-dimensional objects. Clearly, therefore, the orientation of the anatomical structures relative to the beam is a major factor determining their appearance on the film (the orientation of the film relative to the beam also affects radiographic appearance but distortion from this source is minimized by placing the film as nearly as possible perpendicular to the central axis of the beam). For example, directing the beam through the long axis of a structure, rather than through a shorter axis, will produce a whiter shadow on the film (because more X-rays are absorbed) as well as one of different shape. Orientation also affects the degree to which the outlines of structures are superimposed on the radiograph so that it is frequently necessary to carefully position the part being X-rayed so that the area to be viewed is not obscured by a superimposed radio-opaque structure.

A third important factor governing the radiographic appearance of anatomical structures is magnification. The X-ray beam begins at a small area in the X-ray tube and spreads outwards in a cone (or fan in panoramic radiography). Therefore the further the film from the structure the greater will be the magnification. For this reason the film is always positioned as close as possible to the structure being investigated. It is inevitable, however, that some magnification will occur and that this will be greater for structures more remote from the film than for those closer to it.

Intraoral radiographs

Bitewing and similar types of radiographs (Plate 3A and and Fig. 4.110)

The principal purpose of these types of radiograph is to disclose caries on the approximal surfaces of the posterior teeth (which are inaccessible to mirror and probe). The wrapped films measure approximately 4.5 × 3 cm and have a 'wing' or flange along the middle of the sensitive side or are held in a suitable holder. In either case the film is immobilized by the patient's bite and held so that it is internal and immediately adjacent to the crowns of the upper and lower teeth (Fig. 4.111). The X-ray beam is directed at right angles to the centre of the film.

The view obtained is of the crowns and coronal parts of the root of the upper and lower molars and premolars plus adjacent bone. The enamel, dentine, and pulps of the teeth are readily differentiated on account of their differing degrees of radio-opacity. Metal fillings show up as very radio-opaque areas and carious cavities as radiolucent areas. The lamina dura (the layer of dense bone) lining each tooth socket appears as a clearly defined white line and between this and the root of the tooth is the dark line produced by the periodontal ligament.

Periapical radiographs (Plate 3B, C and Fig. 4.110)

As the name suggests these are used to examine the roots of the teeth and the surrounding tissues. The crowns of the teeth are usually also visible. Film of the same size as that used in bitewing radiography but lacking the flange is used. The film is placed on the internal aspect of the teeth with one of its long edges level with the biting surfaces and with the sensitive side facing outwards. It is then brought as nearly parallel to the long axis of the teeth as the oral structures will allow. This can be more completely achieved for the lower teeth than for the upper, where the presence of the hard palate results in the film being at a considerable angle to the teeth. In order to reduce distortion to a minimum the X-ray beam is directed perpendicular to the plane that bisects the angle between the long axes of the teeth and the film (Fig. 4.111).

In order to radiograph a full permanent dentition at least 14 films are required—one for the central incisors and then, on each side, one for the lateral incisor and canine, one for the premolars and one for the molars in both the upper and lower jaws.

As in the bitewing films the enamel, dentine, and pulp of the teeth can be clearly seen in the periapical view. Cementum has the same radiodensity as dentine and cannot normally be distinguished from it. The periodontal ligament and lamina dura of the tooth socket are readily apparent. In the absence of disease the lamina dura is intact

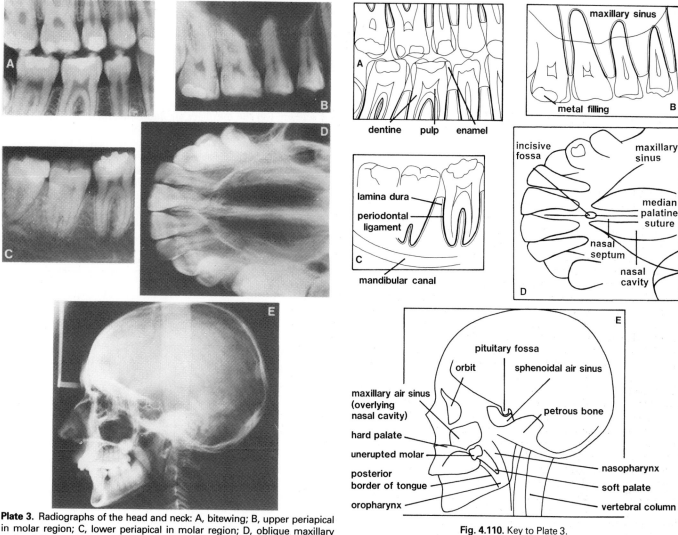

Plate 3. Radiographs of the head and neck: A, bitewing; B, upper periapical in molar region; C, lower periapical in molar region; D, oblique maxillary occlusal; E, true lateral.

Fig. 4.110. Key to Plate 3.

Fig. 4.111. Positioning of tube and film for (left) a periapical radiograph and (right) a radiograph for examining approximal surfaces with the film held in a special holder.

around the whole of the root. Deep to the lamina dura is seen the trabeculated pattern of the cancellous bone of the alveolar process.

In the periapical view of the upper molar region the maxillary paranasal air sinus appears as a rounded area of radiolucency surrounded by its wall of cortical bone. The size of the sinus is extremely variable (p. 120), with corresponding variations in its radiographic appearance. The apices of the roots of the teeth may be superimposed on the sinus. The presence of an intact lamina dura around the apices indicates that they are not projecting into the cavity of the sinus. Overlying the shadow of the sinus and the roots of the molar teeth is a radio-opacity produced by the root of the zygomatic process of the maxilla. Behind the last molar tooth is the maxillary tuberosity and further posteriorly still the pterygoid hamulus may sometimes be seen.

In the radiograph of the upper incisor region the incisive foramen on the bony palate appears as a dark area between the roots of the central incisors. Posterior to this is a linear radio-opacity produced by the nasal septum. On either side of the nasal septum are dark shadows representing the two halves of the nasal cavity.

The principal non-dental features of radiographs of the lower jaw are (i) the mandibular canal, a dark band, bordered by radio-opaque cortical bone running forwards below the posterior teeth to end at (ii) the mental foramen which appears as a dark area between the roots of the premolars, and (iii) the genial tubercles seen as small white areas either side of the midline.

Confusion may sometimes be caused by the superimposition of a foramen over the root of a tooth giving a radiolucent appearance similar to that seen in a chronic dental abscess. The two conditions can be distinguished by the fact that in the former case the lamina dura of the socket is intact whereas in a chronic abscess it will be interrupted adjacent to the radiolucency.

Occlusal radiographs (Plate 3D and Fig. 4.110)

To take an **oblique maxillary occlusal radiograph** the film (measuring approximately 7.5×5.5 cm) is held horizontally, sensitive side upwards, between the teeth and the X-ray beam directed obliquely downwards through the bridge of the nose at an angle of about 65° to the film. This gives a scan view of the anterior part of the hard palate and anterior teeth. The principal anatomical features, other than the teeth, which may be seen are (i) the nasal septum in the midline; (ii) superimposed upon the septum a dark line produced by the median palatine suture; (iii) the two halves of the nasal cavity either side of the septum; (iv) the maxillary air sinuses lateral to the nasal cavity; (v) the incisive fossa at the anterior end of the nasal septum; and (vi) the greater palatine foramina immediately medial to the second molars.

Occlusal views of the mandible are taken by extending the patient's head, with the film held between the teeth (sensitive side downwards) and the X-ray beam directed at right angles to it through the floor of the mouth. They are used to determine the position of unerupted lower teeth and to show stones in the submandibular ducts.

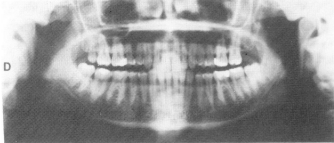

Plate 4. Radiographs of the head and neck: A, posterior/anterior; B, occipito-mental; C, lateral oblique; D, panoramic view.

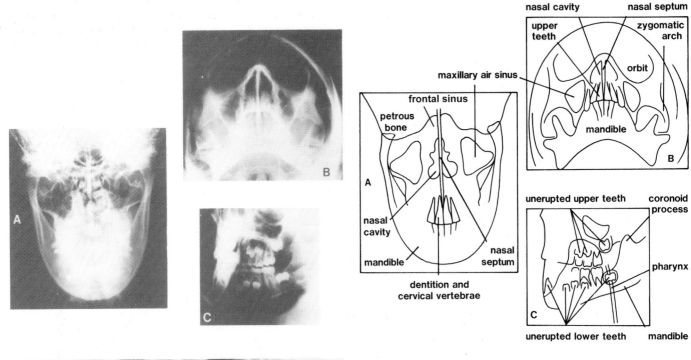

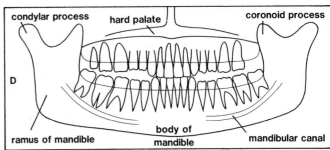

Fig. 4.112. Key to Plate 4.

Panoramic radiography (Plate 4D and Fig. 4.112)

Dental panoramic machines work on the principle of tomography. This involves simultaneously moving the film and the X-ray source in opposite directions relative to each other around the patient's head. The result is a radiograph in which a curved layer of tissues, including the teeth, mandible, and maxillary alveolar process, has a sharp image while structures in all other planes are blurred and effectively invisible.

The advantages of panoramic radiography include the much wider area of the jaws that can be viewed and the generally greater speed and comfort with which the procedure can be carried out. Its principal disadvantage is that the teeth and supporting structures are not shown with the sharpness and detail seen in conventional intraoral radiographs. The panoramic radiograph is a particularly useful diagnostic aid when dealing with large lesions and fractures of the jaws. Here fine detail is often not required and panoramic radiography has the great advantage that it can be performed quickly and easily and without the need to open the mouth.

Extraoral radiographs

Numerous extraoral views may be used in dentistry, many specially designed to give a clear picture of a particular region such as the temporomandibular joint or the base of the skull. These specialized views are more appropriately dealt with as part of clinical instruction in dental radiography and are not described in the following account where the emphasis is on standard and commonly used views displaying important anatomical features.

True lateral radiograph (Plate 3E and Fig. 4.110)

A true lateral radiograph is taken with the patient's head erect, the cassette positioned to one side of the head parallel to the median plane and touching the angle of the jaw, and the X-ray beam directed at right angles to the film through the molar teeth. It is a view of limited use in dentistry because of the superimposition of the two sides of the jaws and dentition.

It is important to realize that in extraoral radiographs prominent outlines are produced by the soft tissues as well as by bony structures. In Plate 3E the outline of the dorsum of the posterior one-third of the tongue can be clearly seen and behind this the dark area representing the pharynx. A short distance behind the posterior part of the tongue the shadow of the soft palate is apparent continuous with the more clearly defined outline of the bony palate. The nasal part of the pharynx can be seen continuing upwards above the soft palate to communicate with the nasal cavity while below the soft palate the oral part of the pharynx is continuous with the oral cavity. The outlines of the soft tissues and associated spaces are especially noticeable where they cross bony structures – note in Plate 3E, for example, the sharp outline of the pharynx as it crosses the ramus of the mandible. If the patient is in the process of swallowing when the radiograph is taken the anterior and posterior walls of the pharynx may be closely approximated, not wide apart as in Plate 3E, giving the impression of a fracture line across the ramus of the mandible.

Posterior–anterior radiograph (Plate 4A and Fig. 4.112)

For this view the cassette is placed in front of the patient touching the nose and forehead (a line drawn from the external acoustic meatus to the lateral canthus of the eye should be perpendicular to the film). The X-ray beam is aimed through the nape of the neck at an angle of about 20° to the perpendicular to the film. This gives a relatively clear picture of the mandibular rami but the central parts of the jaws are obscured by superimposition of the cervical vertebrae.

Occipitomental radiograph (Plate 4B and Fig. 4.112)

The occipitomental view is taken with the cassette touching the chin but with the head tilted backwards so that the line from the external acoustic meatus to the lateral canthus is at 45° to the film. The X-ray beam is centred perpendicular to the film through the occipital region of the head (Fig. 4.113). This orientation has the effect of projecting the shadows of the maxillary sinuses above the dense radio-opacities of the petrous parts of the temporal bones and thus gives an unobscured view of these chambers, which is frequently not available in the posterior/anterior view.

Lateral oblique radiograph (Plate 4C and Fig. 4.112)

This extraoral view of the mandible gives a clear picture of the posterior part of the body and most of the ramus, an area in which pathological conditions commonly occur (especially unerupted third

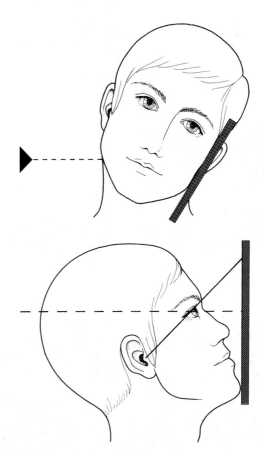

Fig. 4.113. Positioning of tube and film for occipitomental (lower) and lateral oblique radiographs.

molars), and has the further advantage that it can be taken with a dental X-ray machine.

This view is taken with the patient's head inclined towards the side to be X-rayed and the cassette placed against the cheek of that side. The X-ray beam is aimed at the centre of the film through the soft tissues below the angle of the mandible of the opposite side (Fig. 4.113).

The ramus and body of the mandible from the first molar to the angle can be seen unobscured by the opposite half of the mandible (the inferior border of which may be seen as a white line running obliquely upwards and backwards across the crowns of the lower first molar and upper third molar). The posterior part of the ramus has the outlines of the cervical vertebrae superimposed upon it. Running forwards beneath the roots of the molar teeth is the mandibular canal. In the posterior part of its course this is delineated by sharp white lines produced by the cortical bone lining the canal. Anteriorly the cortical bone is often less apparent. The body of the hyoid bone may be seen just below the angle of the jaw. Anterior to the cervical vertebrae, crossing the ramus of the mandible in a vertical direction, is the dark shadow of the pharynx and in front of this is the dorsum of the posterior third of the tongue. As in the true lateral view these shadows can sometimes give a misleading impression of bone pathology. At the upper border of the ramus is the coronoid process and behind this the mandibular incisure. The neck and head of the mandible are often obscured by the cervical vertebrae but may be shown by careful positioning of the patient's head and X-ray tube. Running across the mandibular incisure is the outline of the zygomatic arch.

Section 5

Central nervous system

1

Introduction

THE IMPORTANCE OF NEUROANATOMY

A knowledge of the anatomy of the nervous system is needed by the dental practitioner for several reasons. Probably the most obvious of these is that a full understanding of the cranial nerves innervating the dental region is not possible without reference to their central connections. This in itself demands a wide knowledge of the central nervous system. In addition the practitioner will frequently encounter patients suffering from one or other of the many diseases affecting the central and peripheral parts of the nervous system. Satisfactory dental management of these patients requires some understanding of their illness which in turn requires a knowledge of the general structure of the nervous system. Yet again some of the important drugs used in dentistry (notably the general anaesthetics) act upon the nervous system and their safe administration depends upon understanding their effects. Finally the nervous system plays a major role in controlling body function and no student of human biology could consider their understanding complete without a good knowledge of its structure and function.

The following chapters are written with these points in view, the emphasis being on the ten 'true' cranial nerves (i.e. third to twelfth inclusive) and their central connections, the major sensory and motor pathways, the areas of the cerebral hemispheres concerned with the perception of sensory input and the control of motor function, and the autonomic part of the nervous system. In Chapters 5.2 to 5.4 the regional structure of the central nervous system is described to provide the basis upon which these vocationally important topics, which are reviewed in Chapters 5.5 and 5.6, can be understood.

In order to facilitate description, it is customary to divide the nervous system into parts, the nature of the subdivision depending upon the purpose of the description. It is helpful to appreciate that the various systems of subdivision do not necessarily coincide morphologically with one another. Sometimes, for example, a distinction is made between the central (brain plus spinal cord) and peripheral parts, at other times it is convenient to distinguish the autonomic (concerned with the control of visceral function) from the somatic parts while at yet other times the motor and sensory components are separated. Within the central nervous system the various regions are named separately and within each region the various areas of grey and white matter each receive their own name. Useful though such subdividing and naming are, both in description and understanding, it must be stressed that the nervous system is in reality a highly integrated structure and that the course of a single neuron may run through several of the various subdivisions and named structures of the system. It is important, therefore, that you should develop the habit of thinking in terms of **whole neurons**. When considering any part of the nervous system you should make sure that you know the origin, course, termination, and the location of the cell bodies of the constituent neurons.

It will probably be helpful to briefly indicate at the outset the major subdivisions of the central part of the nervous system. The principal division is into **brain** and **spinal cord**, the two being continuous with each other at a level just below the foramen magnum. The brain itself consists of the **brainstem** (or bulb), **cerebellum** and **cerebrum**. The brainstem is the upward continuation of the spinal cord and is clearly divisible, on the basis of both external appearance and internal structure, into **medulla oblongata, pons,** and **midbrain** (in ascending order). The cerebellum is attached to the dorsal aspect of the brainstem by the three paired **cerebellar peduncles**. The cerebrum consists of the **diencephalon** and the paired **cerebral hemispheres**. The diencephalon is the central core of the cerebrum. It contains such important components as the **thalmus** and **hypothalamus**. The cerebral hemispheres have undergone enormous expansion in man. They are composed of an external layer of grey matter termed the **cerebral cortex** and an internal mass of white matter. Within this internal white matter are further masses of grey matter called the **basal nuclei**.

The regional anatomy of the cerebellum has little relevance to clinical dentistry and no formal description of this structure is included here. Mention is made, however, of some of the connections of this functionally important part of the brain.

One final but very important point to be made in this introductory section is that the investigation of the structure and function of the nervous system is one of the most active and yet most difficult areas of research in the whole of anatomy. In recent years the methods available for carrying out this work have become very much more powerful and refined. In particular it is now often possible to use non- (or minimally) intrusive methods to study the living, human nervous system directly rather than have to extrapolate from animal studies. For these reasons our views of the structure and functions of the brain and spinal cord are being constantly revised. It is essential to bear this in mind when reading the following chapters and to realize that descriptions of many aspects of the central nervous system are inevitably somewhat out of date even as they are written.

The cellular components of the nervous system

The nervous system contains two main groups of cells. The **neurons** are specialized for the reception of nerve impulses (which may lead either to excitation or inhibition of the cell) and for impulse conduction. Each neuron consists of a **cell body** (or **soma**), containing the nucleus, and a number of processes or fibres. One process, often of considerable length, conducts impulses away from the cell body. It is termed the **axon.** Impulses reach the cell body through one or more

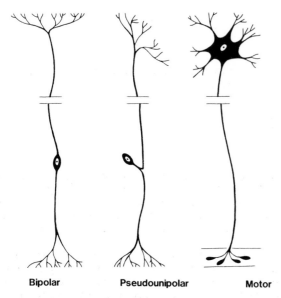

Bipolar   **Pseudounipolar**   **Motor**

Fig. 5.1. Some types of neuron.

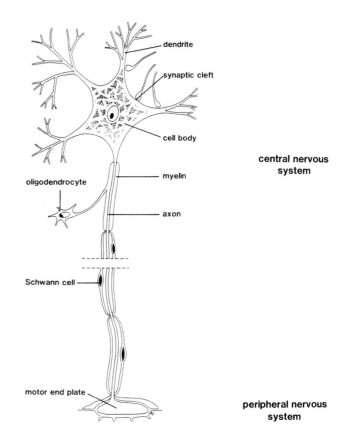

processes called **dendrites**. In peripheral sensory neurons there is a
single large dendrite which, close to the cell body (typically located in
a sensory ganglion), becomes fused with the axon during development (Fig. 5.1). Such neurons are termed **pseudounipolar** (or **unipo-
lar**). Similar types of sensory neurons are found in the central
nervous system in the mesencephalic nucleus of the trigeminal nerve
(p. 258).

Neurons connect with each other at **synapses** which are specialized
areas of contact where the plasma membranes of the two neurons are
separated from each other by a narrow **synaptic cleft**. Areas
containing a large number of cell bodies have a greyish appearance
and hence are known as grey matter. White matter consists mainly of
the long processes of neurons, the white appearance being due to the
presence of the myelin sheaths enclosing the processes.

Although all possess the general features just described, neurons
vary greatly in their detailed size and structure. The diameters of the
cell bodies range from as little as 5 μm to more than 100 μm while the
processes may at one extreme be fine fibres less than a millimetre
in length and at the other extreme be of considerable diameter (up to
20 μm including the myelin sheath) and approach a metre in length.
The larger fibres are usually enclosed in a myelin sheath. The number
and pattern of branching of the dendrites are particularly variable.

These variations in the morphology of the neurons can often be
related to their function. Large neurons with long fibres, for
example, are the principal component of the long tracts within the
central nervous system. Small neurons, on the other hand, are
usually involved in forming complex circuits where they are termed
connector neurons. Such circuits play a major part in the more
complex neural functions.

The second major group of cells within the central nervous system
is composed of the non-excitable, supporting **neuroglial cells**. These
include the **astrocytes** and **oligodendrocytes** (together known as
macroglia), the **microglia** and the **ependymal cells**. The microglia are
derived from mesoderm. The remainder of the neuroglia develop
from neurectoderm.

Astrocytes are present in large numbers throughout the brain and
spinal cord. They have numerous cytoplasmic processes (hence their
name) many of which terminate on small blood vessels, usually the
capillaries, while others end close to the surface of neurons. As well
as having a supporting role the astrocytes are involved in the
transport of chemicals within the brain. The oligodendrocytes
provide the myelin sheaths for nerve fibres within the central nervous
system (in the peripheral part of the nervous system this function is
taken over by the Schwann cells – see below). The plasma membrane
of the oligodendrocyte is wrapped around the fibre to provide several
covering layers, the actual number of which determines the thickness
of the myelin sheath. One oligodendrocyte provides the myelin
sheaths for up to 50 fibres. The microglia are small cells scattered
throughout the grey and white matter. They have a scanty cytoplasm
and a number of short processes. They are actively phagocytic and
are usually regarded as part of the macrophage system. The
ependymal cells form a thin epithelium lining the ventricles of the
brain and the central canal of the brainstem and spinal cord. In many
areas they are ciliated.

The principal non-excitable cells in the peripheral nervous system
are the **Schwann cells** which provide sheaths for the peripheral nerve
fibres. The smaller fibres are unmyelinated, running singly or in
groups in longitudinal grooves in a succession of Schwann cells. The
larger fibres are surrounded by a myelin sheath formed by Schwann
cells, the sheath for each internodal region being formed by a single
cell.

2

Spinal cord

EXTERNAL FEATURES

The spinal cord is cylindrical in shape and in adults occupies the vertebral canal from the upper border of the atlas down to the level of the disc between the first and second lumbar vertebrae. At its caudal extremity the cord narrows to a sharp tip, the **conus medullaris,** from which a fine filament, the **filum terminale,** continues downwards in the vertebral canal to attach to the first coccygeal vertebra. In the early fetus the vertebral canal and spinal cord are virtually of equal length but during later fetal life and, to a lesser extent, during childhood the vertebral column elongates more rapidly than the cord.

The spinal cord is surrounded by three meningeal layers arranged in a similar manner to the coverings of the brain (see page 131). The **spinal dura** (equivalent to the meningeal layer of the cranial dura) provides a loose sheath around the spinal cord and is separated from the periosteum lining the vertebral canal (equivalent to the endosteal layer of the cranial dura) by the **extradural (or epidural) space** containing adipose tissue and a venous plexus. The spinal dura provides sheaths for the roots of the spinal nerves as they pass through the intervertebral foramina. The sheaths continue for a short distance on the proximal parts of the nerves themselves before fusing with the covering epineurium.

The **spinal arachnoid mater** lies against the inner surface of the dura, the two being separated by the narrow **subdural space** which normally contains no more than a thin film of fluid. The **pia mater** closely invests the spinal cord and the surfaces of the roots of the spinal nerves. Between the pia and the arachnoid is the **subarachnoid space** containing cerebrospinal fluid. The spinal cord is suspended within the subarachnoid space by the **denticulate ligaments**. These are linear structures which run, one on each side of the cord in the interval between the dorsal and ventral roots of the spinal nerves, from the upper cervical to the lumbar region. Medially each ligament is continuous with the pia on the lateral surface of the cord while laterally it presents a number of tooth-like projections which are attached to the dura between the exits of successive spinal nerves.

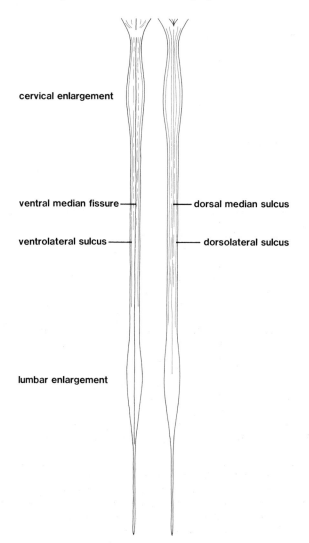

cervical enlargement

ventral median fissure —

— dorsal median sulcus

ventrolateral sulcus —

— dorsolateral sulcus

lumbar enlargement

Fig. 5.3. Ventral (left) and dorsal (right) views of the spinal cord.

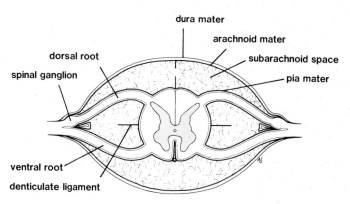

dura mater

arachnoid mater

subarachnoid space

dorsal root

spinal ganglion

pia mater

ventral root

denticulate ligament

Fig. 5.4. Transverse section to show the arrangement of the spinal meninges.

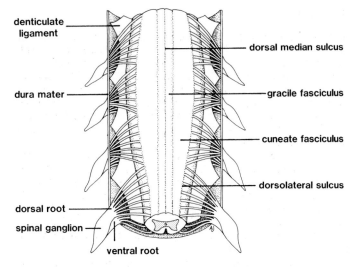

Fig. 5.5. The denticulate ligament. The dura mater dorsal to the cord has been removed.

The spinal cord is somewhat flattened dorsoventrally while its transverse width varies considerably from region to region, undergoing a general reduction in a cranial to caudal direction but with two enlargements associated with the emergence of the thick spinal nerves supplying the limbs. The **cervical enlargement** is the bigger of the two and corresponds to the lower cervical and upper thoracic nerves which form the brachial plexus through which the upper limb is innervated. The **lumbar enlargement** corresponds to the lumbar and sacral nerves forming the lumbar and sacral plexuses which supply the lower limb. Because of the discrepancy between the growth of the spinal cord and veretebral column, the lumbar enlargement in the adult lies opposite the ninth to twelfth thoracic vertebrae.

The external surface of the cord is marked by a **ventral median fissure** and a **dorsal median sulcus**. The latter is continuous internally with the dorsal median septum which extends ventrally through the white matter of the posterior part of the cord so dividing it into right and left halves. There are also shallow **dorsolateral** and **ventrolateral sulci** on each side. ·

Attached to the cord are 31 bilaterally paired **spinal nerves** (eight **cervical**, twelve **thoracic**, five **lumbar**, five **sacral**, and one **coccygeal**). Each nerve is formed by the fusion of a dorsal and a ventral root. Each root arises as a series of rootlets which leaves the corresponding segment of the cord along the dorsolateral sulcus in the case of a dorsal root and along the ventrolateral sulcus in the case of a ventral root. The pairs of dorsal and ventral roots pass laterally, pierce the dura mater, from which they receive a covering, and then leave the vertebral canal through the intervertebral foramina, the roots making up each pair uniting as they do so to form a spinal nerve. Just before uniting with the ventral root each dorsal root bears a swelling, the **spinal** or **dorsal root ganglion**. The dorsal roots contain sensory fibres (the cell bodies of which are in the spinal ganglia) and the ventral roots motor fibres. The spinal nerves are, therefore, mixed sensory and motor.

The convention used in naming the spinal nerves should be carefully noted. Each of the spinal nerves C1 to C7 leaves the vertebral canal through the intervertebral foramen **above** the corresponding vertebra. The eighth cervical nerve emerges through

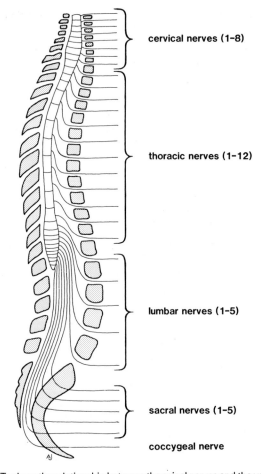

Fig. 5.6. To show the relationship between the spinal nerves and the vertebrae.

the foramen between the seventh cervical and first thoracic vertebrae. Each of the remaining spinal nerves leaves through the intervertebral foramen **below** the corresponding vertebra.

Because the spinal cord is shorter than the vertebral column the roots of the more caudal spinal nerves run downwards for a considerable distance to reach their exit from the vertebral canal. The roots of the fifth lumbar nerve, for example, leave the spinal cord opposite the twelfth thoracic vertebra and then pass downwards to their exit from the canal through the intervertebral foramen below the fifth lumbar vertebra. The roots of the second lumbar and subsequent spinal nerves run caudal to the lower end of the spinal cord to reach their corresponding intervertebral foramina and, in so doing, form a leash around the filum terminale called the **cauda equina**.

The cauda equina is surrounded by subarachnoid space. When a sample of cerebrospinal fluid is required for examination it is usually taken from this region by means of a lumbar puncture in which a needle is inserted between the arches of the third and fourth lumbar vertebrae and advanced until its tip enters the subarachnoid space. Inserting the needle at this level avoids any possibility of damaging the spinal cord.

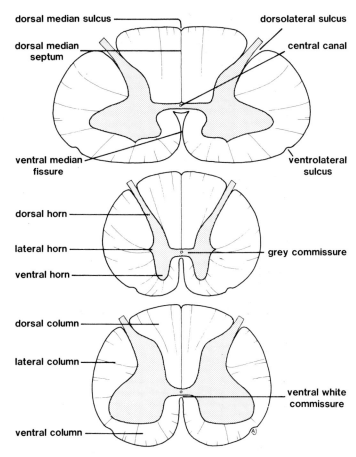

Fig. 5.7. Transverse sections of the spinal cord in the cervical (above), thoracic (middle) and lumbar (below) regions.

INTERNAL STRUCTURE

When seen in transverse section there is a clear distinction between the grey and white matter of the spinal cord. The grey matter, containing neuronal cell bodies, forms a single, continuous mass which is H-shaped in transverse section. The transverse connecting part of the grey matter (equivalent to the cross-bar of the H) is called the **grey commissure**. Projecting dorsally and ventrally on each side are the **dorsal** and **ventral horns** (or **columns**) of the grey matter. In the thoracic and upper lumbar regions a small **lateral horn** projects on each side from the junction of the dorsal and ventral horns. The grey commissure is traversed by the fine **central canal**, the derivative of the lumen of the original neural tube.

The white matter consists principally of nerve fibres (plus neuroglia) and is arranged in three columns on each side. Between the dorsal grey horn and the posterior median septum is the **dorsal column** (or **funiculus**) of white matter. Lateral to the dorsal and ventral horns is the **lateral column (funiculus)** which is continuous anteriorly with the **ventral column (funiculus)**. There is no clear demarcation between lateral and ventral columns. Anterior to the grey commissure is the narrow **ventral white commissure**.

Grey matter

The spinal grey matter is made up of populations of cell bodies of different neuron types. These populations are arranged in long columns which run, in most cases, the whole length of the spinal cord. In cross-section they appear as layers which are termed **laminae** (of **Rexed**). Ten laminae are recognized, designated by Roman numerals beginning at the tip of the dorsal horn (Fig. 5.8). This terminology has now largely replaced that based on named nuclei, but in the description which follows some of the older terms are given where they are still widely used.

True lamination is confined to the dorsal horn of the grey matter which contains six laminae. A further four laminae are described in the remaining grey matter, but here the layered arrangement is not so obvious. The simplified account of the laminae which follows is intended as a basis for understanding the major sensory and motor pathways described in Chapter 5.5. For a detailed description of the cytoarchitecture of the spinal grey matter you should consult a textbook of neuroanatomy.

It is perhaps worth emphasizing again at this point that views on the structure and functions of the grey and white matter of the spinal cord are being continually refined and, in some cases, substantially revised as research in these areas continues. This must be borne constantly in mind in reading the remainder of this chapter.

Dorsal horn

Many of the **first-order sensory neurons** (see p. 245 for an explanation of the terms first-, second-, and third-order sensory neurons) entering the spinal cord in the dorsal roots of the spinal nerves end in the dorsal horn which is concerned, therefore, with the reception of sensory impulses.

Lamina I is a thin layer of neurons capping the dorsal horn. Some of the dorsal root fibres mediating pain and temperature end in this layer. Lamina I contains some **second-order sensory (tract) neurons** which contribute to the contralateral **spinothalamic tract**.

Lamina II (substantia gelatinosa) receives numerous branches from dorsal root fibres, again mostly concerned with mediating pain and temperature. The axons of the cells in this layer are much branched and synapse with neurons in the other dorsal horn laminae in the same and adjacent segments of the cord. Lamina II also receives descending fibres from the reticular formation of the medulla. It is believed to play an important part in modifying the perception of pain.

Lamina III also receives fibres from the dorsal roots.

Lamina IV contains tract cells which connect with laminae II and III and send axons which enter the contralateral spinothalamic tract. It receives many dorsal root fibres.

Laminae V–VI form a single lamina in man. This contains numerous tract cells which contribute to the opposite spinothalamic tract. Their dendrites make synaptic connection with the first-order sensory neurons for pain, temperature, simple touch and pressure which end in the dorsal horn. Large numbers of corticospinal fibres end in lamina V–VI. Laminae IV and V–VI are known collectively as the **nucleus proprius**.

Intermediate zone and ventral horn

The ventral part of the grey matter is concerned with motor functions. It contains the large cell bodies of the **alpha lower motor neurons** whose axons pass out in the ventral roots of the spinal

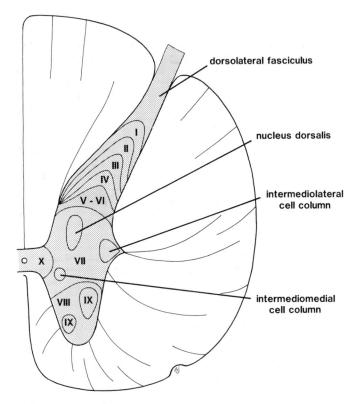

Fig. 5.8. Transverse section of the spinal cord in the thoracic region to show the laminae of the grey matter.

the vestibulospinal and reticulospinal tracts. Its cells project to laminae VII and IX of the same and opposite sides.

Lamina IX is composed of several columns in the ventral horn. It is the site of the cell bodies of the alpha and gamma motor neurons.

Lamina X surrounds the central canal and contains numerous fibres which are crossing from one side of the spinal cord to the other.

In the lateral region of the ventral horn in the upper cervical segments and extending into the lower part of the medulla is a special collection of motor cells termed the **spinal accessory nucleus.** The axons of these cells emerge, as a series of rootlets, from the lateral surface of the upper cervical cord. The rootlets unite to form the **spinal accessory nerve** which ascends in the subarachnoid space along the side of the cord to enter the cranial cavity through the foramen magnum. It re-emerges from the cranial cavity, in company with the cranial accessory, through the jugular foramen and supplies the sternocleidomastoid and trapezius muscles.

Lateral horn

A small lateral horn is found in the spinal segments from the first thoracic to the second or third lumbar inclusive. It is occupied by the intermediolateral cell column. The **preganglionic sympathetic fibres** begin in this column from cell bodies rather smaller than those of the alpha motor neurons in the ventral horn. Similar cells in the base of the ventral horn of the second to fourth sacral segments form the **sacral autonomic nucleus** from which the preganglionic fibres of the sacral part of the parasympathetic system arise.

White matter

It is known from experimental and clinical observations that the fibres in the white matter are aggregated into tracts, each with a distinct and separate function. Such tracts may be ascending to supraspinal destinations, descending from supraspinal sources or may be connecting different segments of the spinal cord.

Here, as in the account of the internal structure of the brainstem, attention will be focused on those tracts of particular importance to the dental student. With the help of the review of the motor and sensory systems given in Chapter 5.5 you should try to build up a three-dimensional picture of the routes followed by the neurons making up these tracts.

Ascending tracts

Within the dorsal roots of the spinal nerves the **first-order sensory fibres** concerned with the different sensations are intermingled. They are axons of pseudounipolar neurons with cell bodies situated in the spinal ganglia. As they enter the spinal cord the more heavily myelinated fibres, transmitting impulses for simple and discriminative touch, pressure, vibration, and proprioception, come together to form the **medial division** of the root, which continues into the dorsal white column, while the less heavily myelinated fibres, conducting pain and temperature sensation, form the **lateral division** and enter the **dorsolateral fasciculus** situated between the dorsal grey horn and the external surface of the cord.

Within the dorsolateral fasciculus the pain and temperature fibres divide into short ascending and descending branches, each giving off numerous collaterals. These branches terminate in the dorsal grey horn in the segment of entry or in the neighbouring segments by contacting **second-order sensory (tract) cells,** either directly or indirectly

nerves to supply striated muscles. They are acted upon by numerous descending fibres including those of the corticospinal tract (the cell bodies of which are located predominantly in the opposite cerebral hemisphere) and by neurons involved in spinal reflexes. Also present in the ventral horns are the smaller cell bodies of the **gamma lower motor neurons** which supply the intrafusal fibres of the neuromuscular spindles. As would be expected, the venal horns are much enlarged in the segments corresponding to the limb plexuses.

Lamina VII is the biggest of the layers in the spinal grey matter, occupying much of the ventral horn and the area between the ventral and dorsal horns. It contains numerous connector neurons, the axons of which run to the grey matter of other spinal segments. Many of the corticospinal fibres end in this lamina. Within lamina VII are three cell columns – the **intermediolateral column** (see lateral horn), the **intermediomedial column** (whose precise function is still debated) and the **nucleus dorsalis** (Clarke's column). The last is found in the most dorsal part of lamina VII, from the lower cervical to the upper lumbar segments of the cord being biggest in the lower thoracic segments. The afferents to the nucleus include sensory fibres from the lower limb ascending in the dorsal white column. Efferents from the nucleus enter the lateral white column where they form the **dorsal spinocerebellar tract.** It is an important nucleus in the relay of proprioceptive information from the lower limb to the cerebral cortex and cerebellum.

Lamina VIII is located in the ventral part of the ventral horn and receives the endings of many descending fibres, including those of

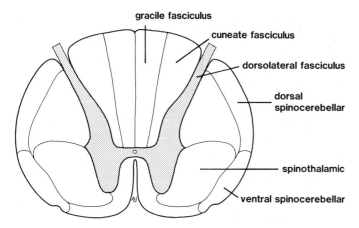

gracile fasciculus

cuneate fasciculus

dorsolateral fasciculus

dorsal spinocerebellar

spinothalamic

ventral spinocerebellar

Fig. 5.9. Transverse section of the spinal cord in the upper thoracic region to show the principal ascending tracts in the white matter.

through connecting neurons. Most of the tract cells are located in the nucleus proprius. First-order sensory neurons for simple touch and pressure (which enter the cord in the medial divisions of the spinal nerve roots—see below) contact similarly located tract cells. The axons of the tract cells immediately cross the midline in the grey and white commissures, then pass through the contralateral grey matter to reach the ventrolateral area of white matter where they turn rostrally and enter the **spinothalamic tract.** This tract is present at all levels of the cord but increases progressively in size as it ascends as more fibres are added in each segment. The spinothalamic tract traverses the brainstem, where it is known as the **spinal lemniscus,** to reach the thalamus. Here its constituent fibres end. Thalamocortical or **third-order neurons** complete the pathway to the cerebral cortex.

The fibres of the medial division of the dorsal root enter the ipsilateral dorsal white column medial to the dorsolateral fasciculus. Here they divide into ascending and descending branches. The descending fibres, which may be several segments in length, give off many collateral branches and synapse with numerous connector neurons and with tract cells in the dorsal grey horn. Many of the ascending fibres after passing up the cord for a number of segments terminate in a similar manner. A considerable proportion of the ascending fibres, however, continues upwards in the dorsal white column to reach the medulla. These fibres constitute the bulk of the **cuneate fasciculus** and **gracile fasciculus,** the two main tracts of the dorsal column. These tracts lie side by side with the cuneate fasciculus the more lateral of the two. Since fibres are added to the lateral aspect of the dorsal column in each segment the more medially located gracile fasciculus contains fibres from the lower levels of the body (below midthoracic level) while the cuneate fasciculus contains fibres from the upper levels. The fasciculi end above at the **cuneate nucleus** and **gracile nucleus** which are situated in the dorsal part of the lower medulla. In these nuclei the ascending fibres connect with **second-order sensory neurons** whose axons cross the midline of the medulla and continue upwards, as the **medial lemniscus,** to the thalamus. From here **third-order sensory fibres** pass to the cerebral cortex. Through this pathway information about discriminative touch and vibration reaches consciousness. Proprioceptive sense from the upper part of the body follows a similar pathway. Pro-

prioception from the lower limb, however, is now known to follow a different route – this is described on page 247.

Many of the ascending and descending fibres of the dorsal column that end in the spinal cord are involved in spinal reflexes concerned with the control of body position and movement and response to touch. Some, however, connect with tract neurons, principally of laminae V–VI. These are concerned with the sensations of simple touch and pressure, and their axons cross the midline and ascend in the contralateral spinothalamic tract.

Other fibres in the dorsal column, including collateral branches of the long fibres ascending to the gracile and cuneate nuclei, connect with the neurons of the nucleus dorsalis. The axons of the latter ascend, on the same side, as the **dorsal spinocerebellar tract,** to eventually reach the cerebellum. This tract begins at the lower level of the nucleus dorsalis (located in the upper lumbar region). The nucleus dorsalis and the dorsal spinocerebellar tract are also involved in the proprioceptive pathway from the lower limb to the cerebral cortex (p. 247). The **ventral spinocerebellar tract** consists of crossed fibres originating in the region of the lumbar enlargement. Through the spinocerebellar tracts the cerebellum receives sensory data for proprioception, touch, and pressure.

Descending tracts

Two major tracts contain fibres descending from the cerebral cortex to the grey matter of the spinal cord. These are the **lateral** and **ventral corticospinal tracts.** The former occupies an area in the lateral column just in front of the dorsal horn of grey matter; the latter is situated in the ventral column alongside the anterior median fissure. Both tracts diminish in size as they descend, the larger lateral tract becoming indiscernible at about the level of the third sacral segment and the ventral tract at about the midthoracic level.

Before reaching the spinal cord the corticospinal fibres of each side descend from the cortex of the cerebral hemisphere through the internal capsule within the hemisphere and then through the corresponding side of the midbrain, pons, and medulla. Their presence in the medulla produces an elongated swelling, termed the **pyramid,** on its anteromedial aspect. In this region the majority of the corticospinal fibres crosses over to the opposite side in the pyramidal decussation. These crossed fibres enter the lateral column of the white matter where they constitute the **lateral corticospinal tract.** The uncrossed fibres continue in a more ventral position and make up the **ventral corticospinal tract.** Thus, on say the right side of the cord, the lateral corticospinal tract consists of fibres which began in the left cerebral hemisphere while the ventral tract consists of fibres from the right hemisphere. Many of the fibres in the ventral tract cross the midline before terminating so these too eventually reach the side opposite to that on which they began.

Most of the corticospinal fibres end in laminae V–VI and VII, and make connection with the lower motor neurons which begin in lamina IX through the intermediary of connector neurons. A few pass into lamina IX and synapse directly with the lower motor neurons. The corticospinal fibres are often known as **upper motor neurons.**

The fibres making up the corticospinal tracts vary greatly in diameter (from 1 μm to about 20 μm) and most of them are myelinated. Just under half begin in the motor cortex of the frontal lobes of the cerebral hemispheres, the remainder in other cortical areas. Through their connections with the lower motor neurons they are concerned with the control of voluntary movement.

Because the corticospinal fibres pass through the pyramid of the

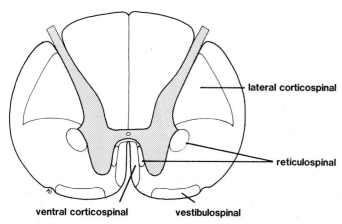

lateral corticospinal

reticulospinal

ventral corticospinal   vestibulospinal

Fig. 5.10. Transverse section of the spinal cord in the upper thoracic region to show the principal descending tracts in the white matter. The tectospinal tract ends in the cervical part of the cord but its equivalent position is shown.

medulla the tracts which they enter in the spinal cord are often referred to as **pyramidal.** For reasons which are discussed in the review of the motor system in Chapter 5.5 this term is unsatisfactory from an anatomical, functional, and clinical standpoint.

Several descending tracts begin in the brainstem. These include the **vestibulospinal tract**, from the lateral vestibular nucleus of the same side, and the **reticulospinal tracts**. The position of some of these tracts is shown in Fig. 5.10.

The vestibulospinal tract descends the whole length of the cord, its fibres ending in mainly lamina VIII of successive segments of the ventral grey horn. It is involved in the maintenance of equilibrium through the control of muscle tonus in response to stimuli from the organs of balance. The reticulospinal tract in the lateral funiculus begins in the reticular nuclei of both sides of the medulla; that in the ventral funiculus begins in the ipsilateral reticular nuclei in the pons. Many of their fibres end in laminae VII, VIII, and IX of the spinal grey matter.

Dispersed between the other tracts, especially in the lateral white columns are numerous crossed and uncrossed autonomic fibres. Most originate in the reticular formation of the brainstem and pass to the lateral horn of the grey matter and to the sacral autonomic nucleus and constitute a pathway by which the visceral centres of the brainstem and hypothalamus influence sympathetic and parasympathetic function.

Intersegmental tracts

The intersegmental tracts are situated next to the grey matter in all three white columns. They consist of crossed and uncrossed fibres whose function is to connect segments at different levels of the cord.

3

Brainstem

From a vocational viewpoint the brainstem is especially important for the dental student because this part of the brain contains the nuclei of the ten 'true' cranial nerves. Understanding the arrangement of this rather complex region will be facilitated if it is remembered that the brainstem is continuous with the spinal cord and that it contains the upward continuations, or the equivalents, of many of the structures present in the cord. All the major tracts in the white columns of the spinal cord, for example, traverse at least part of the brainstem to reach their destinations.

The principal differences between the brainstem and the spinal cord are that (i) whereas the grey matter in the cord forms a single continuous mass, in the brainstem it is broken up into discrete nuclei, (ii) the central canal, which is of narrow diameter throughout the cord, is greatly expanded in the middle region of the brainstem to form the fourth ventricle, (iii) the cranial nerves emerge from the brainstem in a manner which appears to be less regular than that in which the spinal nerves leave the cord (although there is, in fact, an underlying similarity in the way the two sets of nerves are arranged), and (iv) attached to the posterior aspect of the brainstem by three pairs of peduncles in the cerebellum.

The brainstem is divided into three parts. In ascending order these are the **medulla oblongata, pons,** and **midbrain.** Ventrally the brainstem is related to the basilar part of the occipital bone and the body of the sphenoid while its principal dorsal relationship is with the cerebellum. The medulla and pons are situated in the posterior cranial fossa and the midbrain occupies the hiatus in the tentorium cerebelli.

The fourth ventricle is located in the upper part of the medulla and in the pons. Above and below the ventricle the central canal is narrow, as it is in the spinal cord. The part of the medulla associated with the fourth ventricle is often referred to as 'open' and that containing the narrow central canal as 'closed'.

The old name for the brainstem was the bulb. It is still encountered in terms such as 'corticobulbar' which is applied to the tract passing from the cerebral cortex to the motor nuclei of the cranial nerves.

EXTERNAL FEATURES

Medulla

The junction of the spinal cord and medulla is taken, for descriptive purposes, as being at the level of the upper rootlet of the first cervical spinal nerve (corresponding to the upper border of the atlas). This is a purely arbitrary dividing line since the transition in internal structure is not abrupt. The upper limit of the medulla is at its junction with the pons and is clearly marked on the ventral surface of the brainstem. The medulla has a total length of about 3 cm and becomes progressively wider in a rostral direction.

On the ventral surface of the medulla the **ventral median fissure** and **ventrolateral sulci** can be seen continuing upwards from the spinal cord. On each side of the ventral median fissure, between it and the ventrolateral sulcus, is an elongated swelling, the **pyramid.** It is produced by the corticospinal fibres passing caudally through the medulla close to its ventral surface. Lateral to the ventrolateral sulcus in the upper part of the medulla is a second elongated swelling, the **olive.** This marks the position of the **inferior olivary nucleus.** The rootlets of the **hypoglossal nerve** leave the medulla between the pyramid and olive and the rootlets of the **glossopharyngeal, vagus,** and **cranial accessory nerves** emerge, in that order from rostral to caudal, dorsolateral to the olive.

The dorsal surface of the medulla is hidden by the overlying cerebellum. With this removed, by severing the cerebellar peduncles, the **gracile** and **cuneate fasciculi** can be seen running upwards from the cord on to the dorsal surface of the closed medulla. The gracile fasciculi of the two sides are separated by the **dorsal median sulcus.** The fasciculi terminate at low swellings, the **clava** marking the position of the underlying **gracile nucleus** and the **cuneate tubercle** marking the position of the underlying **cuneate nucleus.**

On the lateral aspect of the medulla between the olive and the cuneate fasciculus, is a smoothly rounded area called the **tuberculum cinereum** (not to be confused with the tuber cinereum – see page 237). It marks the position of the spinal tract of the trigeminal nerve and its nucleus.

The dorsal surface of the open medulla is formed by the caudal part of the roof of the fourth ventricle. This is extremely thin, consisting of a layer of ependyma with a closely adherent layer of pia mater, and is almost invariably torn in removing the cerebellum so that a view is obtained of the floor of the ventricle (as in Fig. 5.12).

Pons

When the brainstem is viewed from its ventral aspect, the pons has the appearance of a bridge (hence its name) connecting the right and left cerebellar hemispheres (an appearance which is misleading so far as the internal structure of the pons is concerned). It is little more than 2 cm in extent between its caudal and rostral borders, both of which are clearly marked. Running along its ventral surface, in the median plane, is the shallow **basilar sulcus.** Laterally the pons continues, as the middle cerebellar peduncle, into the corresponding cerebellar hemisphere. Medial to the middle cerebellar peduncle are the inferior and superior peduncles (see Fig. 5.12). The dorsal surface of the pons forms the rostral part of the floor of the fourth ventricle and is described further below.

Leaving the brainstem at the junction of pons and medulla are the **abducent, facial,** and **vestibulocochlear nerves,** in that order from medial to lateral. The facial nerve is attached to the brainstem by a

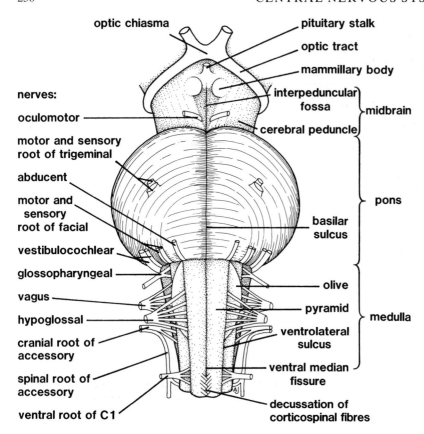

optic chiasma

pituitary stalk

optic tract

mammillary body

interpeduncular
fossa

} midbrain

nerves:

oculomotor

cerebral peduncle

motor and sensory
root of trigeminal

abducent

motor and
sensory
root of facial

} pons

basilar
sulcus

vestibulocochlear

glossopharyngeal

olive

vagus

pyramid

} medulla

hypoglossal

ventrolateral
sulcus

cranial root of
accessory

spinal root of
accessory

ventral median
fissure

ventral root of C1

decussation of
corticospinal fibres

Fig. 5.11. Ventral view of the brainstem.

large motor and a small sensory root. The latter, sometimes called **nervus intermedius,** lies between the motor root and the vestibulo-cochlear nerve. The **trigeminal nerve** leaves the ventral surface of the pons in the region where it is continuous with the middle cerebellar peduncle. The trigeminal nerve also has motor and sensory roots but in this case the sensory root is the larger and lies caudolateral to the motor root.

Midbrain

The midbrain is a relatively short part of the brainstem, being less than 2 cm in length, and connects the pons to the cerebrum. It is approximately cylindrical in shape. The central canal is narrow and is called the **cerebral aqueduct** or, less confusingly, the **aqueduct of the midbrain.** On its ventral surface are two prominent swellings, the **cerebral peduncles.** They contain the major descending tracts. Between the peduncles is a deep midline depression, the **interpeduncular fossa.** On the dorsal surface of the midbrain are two pairs of swellings, the **superior** and **inferior colliculi.** These contain nuclei concerned with visual reflexes and the auditory pathway, respectively. Running downwards from the lateral surface of the midbrain to the cerebellum is the **superior cerebellar peduncle.** It passes medial to the middle cerebellar peduncle to reach the corresponding cerebellar hemisphere.

The **oculomotor nerve** leaves the ventral surface of the midbrain in the depths of the interpeduncular fossa. The **trochlear nerve** is

unique amongst the cranial nerves in that it emerges on the dorsal surface of the brainstem. Its point of exit is immediately caudal to the inferior colliculus.

Fourth ventricle

The fourth ventricle is the expanded central canal of the brainstem in the region of the upper medulla and pons. The expansion of the cavity has taken place in a predominantly dorsal direction so that the bulk of the nervous tissue lies ventral to the ventricle and all that is left dorsal to the ventricle (i.e. forming its roof) is a thin layer of ependyma.

The ventricle is broadest in its middle region and narrows sharply superiorly and inferiorly where it is continuous respectively with the aqueduct of the midbrain and the central canal of the closed medulla. The floor of the fourth ventricle, formed by the open medulla and the pons, is therefore diamond-shaped when viewed from the dorsal aspect and is known as the **rhomboid fossa.** It is divided into right and left halves by a shallow median sulcus. Each half of the floor is itself divided into medial and lateral areas by the **sulcus limitans.** The part of the floor lateral to the sulcus limitans is called the **vestibular area** and marks the position of the vestibular nuclei. The medial area, between the median sulcus and the sulcus limitans, is slightly elevated to form the **medial eminence** which marks the position of several motor nuclei. The lower part of the medial eminence contains the hypoglossal nucleus medially and the dorsal nucleus of

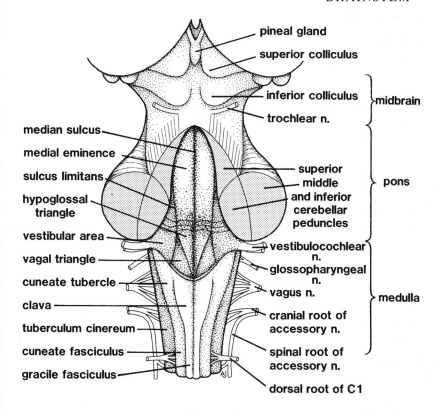

Fig. 5.12. Dorsal view of the brainstem with the cerebellum removed by cutting the cerebellar peduncles.

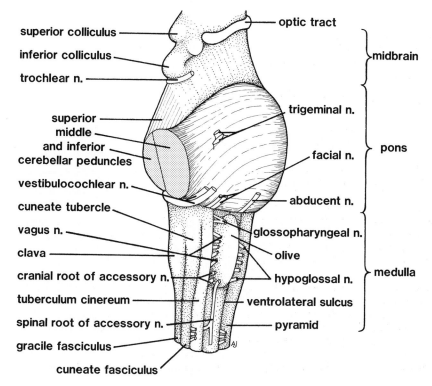

Fig. 5.13. Lateral view of the right side of brainstem with cerebellum removed.

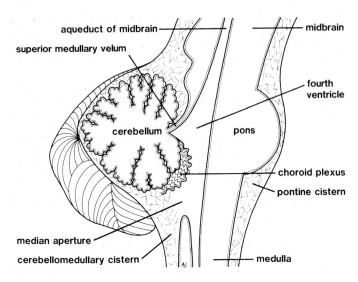

Fig. 5.14. Median section through the brainstem and cerebellum to show the fourth ventricle.

the vagus laterally. The position of these nuclei is indicated by two triangular areas – the **hypoglossal** and **vagal triangles** – which can be seen on each side of the caudal part of the floor of the fourth ventricle between the median sulcus and the sulcus limitans. Beneath the more rostral part of the medial eminence is the nucleus of the abducent nerve with fibres of the facial nerve looping over it, an arrangement producing an elongated swelling called the **facial colliculus.**

The lateral walls of the fourth ventricle are formed on each side, from caudal to rostral, by the clava, the cuneate tubercle, the inferior cerebellar peduncle, and the superior cerebellar peduncle.

The rostral part of the roof of the fourth ventricle is provided by the superior cerebellar peducles, which although entering mainly into the lateral boundaries of the ventricle also overlap its dorsal aspect, with the **superior medullary velum** filling the angular gap between them. The latter is a thin sheet consisting of juxtaposed layers of ependyma and pia mater. The caudal part of the roof is provided by a similarly constituted **inferior medullary velum.** The rostral and caudal parts of the roof incline dorsally to meet at a ridge running transversely beneath the cerebellum. This arrangement can be understood by comparing Figs 5.12 and 5.14.

Between the cerebellum and the caudal part of the ventricular roof the pia mater is reflected upon itself to form the **tela choroidea** of the **fourth ventricle.** Vascular fringes, covered by an ependymal layer, project from the tela into the cavity of the ventricle. These fringes are known collectively as the **choroid plexus of the fourth ventricle** and, with similar plexuses in the third and lateral ventricles, are concerned in the production of cerebrospinal fluid (see p. 139).

The caudal part of the ventricular roof is pierced by three apertures – a large **median aperture** (or **foramen of Magendie**) and two smaller **lateral apertures** (or **foramina of Luschka**). The median aperture communicates with the subarachnoid space in the region of the cerebellomedullary cistern and provides the principal route by which cerebrospinal fluid passes out of the ventricular system. The lateral apertures also communicate with the subarachnoid space but are occupied to a large extent by extensions of the choroid plexus.

INTERNAL FEATURES

The principal components of the brainstem can be grouped under four headings. First there are the nuclei of the ten 'true' cranial nerves. These are mostly situated close to the central canal or fourth ventricle in a manner which corresponds broadly with the arrangements of the grey matter in the spinal cord. Secondly there are other named nuclei such as the **red nucleus, substantia nigra,** and **inferior olivary nucleus.** These serve various functions, some of which are discussed on p. 250. Thirdly there are the ascending and descending pathways. Many of these are continuations of the tracts already described in the spinal cord and together make up the bulk of the white matter in the brainstem. Finally, there is the **reticular formation** composed of those parts of the brainstem not occupied by the named nuclei or tracts.

In the following account emphasis is placed upon the nuclei and central connections of the cranial nerves and, as in the description of the spinal cord, upon the corticospinal tract amongst the descending pathways and upon the spinothalamic and dorsal column tracts amongst the ascending pathways. The nuclei of the cranial nerves are described individually as they are encountered at each level of the brainstem. In Chapter 5.6 these nuclei and their connections are described collectively. With the help of this chapter and also Chapter 5.5, in which the motor and sensory systems are reviewed, you should try to build up a complete picture of the neurons associated with the nuclei and tracts of the brainstem.

Medulla

Closed part

As would be expected the internal structure of the lower part of the medulla resembles that of the cervical region of the spinal cord. The white columns are still recognizable and contain the same tracts as they do in the cord. The outline of the grey horns is also discernible but becomes modified even in the lowest levels of the medulla. The ventral grey horns continue upwards for a short distance into the medulla where they contain cell bodies of the lower motor neurons of the first cervical nerve and the spinal root of the accessory nerve.

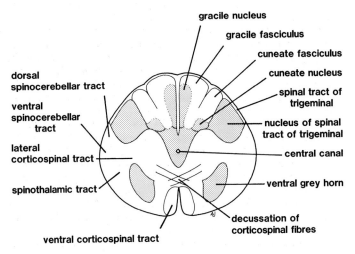

Fig. 5.15. Transverse section through the lower part of the closed medulla.

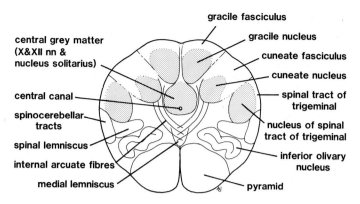

Fig. 5.16. Transverse section through the closed medulla above the decussation of the corticospinal fibres.

They are, however, separated from the grey matter around the central canal by decussating corticospinal fibres passing from the pyramid of one side to the lateral white column of the opposite side. The dorsal grey horns are represented in the medulla by the nucleus of the spinal tract of the trigeminal nerve and the gracile and cuneate nuclei.

Above the decussation of the corticospinal fibres the similarity to the spinal cord is lost. In a section through the closed medulla at the caudal end of the olive the following general arrangement is found. The **central canal** is surrounded by a layer of grey matter containing, on each side, the **hypoglossal nucleus** ventromedially and the **dorsal nucleus of the vagus** more laterally. Dorsolateral to the dorsal nucleus of the vagus is the **tractus solitarius** and its **nucleus** (Fig. 5.16). The tract consists of sensory fibres from the facial, glossopharyngeal, and vagus nerves. Their cell bodies are located in the sensory ganglia of the nerves and they terminate in the nucleus of the tract. The fibres from the facial nerve and some of those from the glossopharyngeal and vagus are for taste. They end in the rostral part of the nucleus (often referred to separately as the **gustatory nucleus**). The remainder of the fibres from the glossopharyngeal and vagus are general visceral sensory and end in the caudal part of the nucleus.

Dorsolateral to the central grey matter are the gracile and cuneate nuclei and their associated fasciculi. The axons of the first-order sensory neurons for discriminative touch and vibration as well as for proprioception from the upper limb which ascend in the gracile and cuneate fasciculi of the dorsal white columns of the cord, end by synapsing in the corresponding nuclei with second-order neurons. The axons of these second-order neurons leave from the ventral aspect of the nuclei and run medially, as the **internal arcuate fibres,** in front of the central grey matter where they decussate with corresponding fibres from the opposite side. They then turn upwards and ascend to the thalamus as a prominent tract, the **medial lemniscus,** situated close to the median plane. Fibres conveying proprioceptive information from the lower limb synapse in **nucleus Z** which is located immediately rostral to the gracile nucleus. The cells of nucleus Z give rise to internal arcuate fibres which cross the midline and join the medial lemniscus.

The fibres of the spinothalamic tract (for simple touch, pressure, pain, and temperature) continue in the brainstem as the **spinal lemniscus** which runs upwards in the lateral part of the medulla.

These fibres are the axons of second-order neurons whose cell bodies lie in the laminae (principally V–VI) of the dorsal grey horn of the spinal cord. Like the second-order neurons in the medial lemniscus, they are crossed (having decussated shortly after their origin in the cord) and end in the thalamus.

Ventrolateral to the central grey matter is the **inferior olivary nucleus.** This nucleus stretches from the upper part of the closed medulla into the open part, lying beneath the olive seen on the external surface of the brainstem. In section it has the appearance of a somewhat crumpled bag with its opening facing posteromedially. Fibres from the nucleus (and from the associated **accessory olivary nuclei**) cross the midline to reach the cerebellar hemisphere of the opposite side through the **inferior cerebellar peduncle.** The olivary complex receives afferents from the cerebral cortex and from the red nucleus and other areas of the midbrain. It is involved in the cerebellar control of movement.

Medial to the inferior olivary nucleus is the pyramid. This is situated immediately adjacent to the median plane, separated from its fellow of the opposite side by the ventral median fissure. It extends virtually the whole length of the medulla. The pyramid contains the corticospinal fibres descending from the motor cortex of the cerebral hemisphere of the same side. At the lower end of the pyramid most of these fibres decussate and continue downwards into the cord as the lateral corticospinal tract. The uncrossed fibres form the ventral corticospinal tract and most eventually cross the midline within the cord. The corticospinal fibres end mainly in laminae V–VI and VII of the spinal grey matter and constitute the upper motor neurons of the pathway for voluntary movement.

Lateral to the central grey matter, and ventral to the cuneate nucleus, is the prominent **nucleus of the trigeminal spinal tract.** This runs the whole length of the medulla and into the upper part of the cervical spinal cord where it is continuous with the dorsal grey horn. It is often called by the shorter name of trigeminal spinal nucleus. Between the nucleus and the external surface of the medulla is the **spinal tract** itself. The tract consists of the central processes of finely myelinated and unmyelinated first-order sensory neurons which enter the brainstem through the sensory root of the trigeminal nerve (their cell bodies being located in the trigeminal ganglion). Like the nucleus, the tract descends through the whole length of the medulla and into the upper part of the cervical cord giving off, as it does so, terminals to the nucleus. The spinal nucleus also receives the small somatic sensory components of the facial, glossopharyngeal, and vagus nerves. The second-order neurons which begin in the spinal nucleus cross the midline and ascend to the thalamus in the **ventral trigemino-thalamic tract.**

Ventrolateral to the spinal nucleus of the trigeminal nerve are the **ventral** and **dorsal spinocerebellar tracts.** They are the upward continuations of the tracts of the same name already described in the spinal cord.

Dorsal to the inferior olivary nucleus is the **vestibulospinal tract** from the vestibular nuclei of the same side.

Open part

The expansion of the central canal to form the fourth ventricle leads to some rearrangement of the internal structures in the upper part of the medulla. Because this expansion has taken place in a dorsal direction virtually all the substance of the brainstem lies ventral to the ventricle and structures which are situated dorsally in the closed medulla tend to lie laterally in the open medulla. The continuity

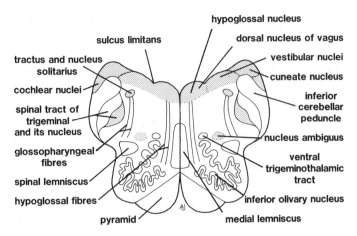

Fig. 5.17. Transverse section through the open medulla.

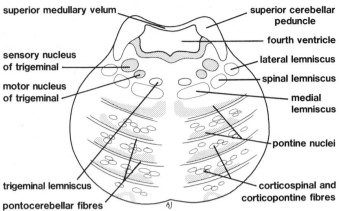

Fig. 5.18. Transverse section through the middle of the pons.

between the nuclei and tracts in the two parts of the medulla can thus be appreciated and requires no detailed description. It should be noted from Fig. 5.17 that the central grey matter is now located entirely in the floor of the fourth ventricle and that the cuneate nucleus is situated rather more laterally than it is at lower levels (the gracile nucleus having ended below this level).

Several structures additional to those described in the closed medulla are present in the open part. At the more rostral levels the **inferior cerebellar peduncles** can be seen. These are situated, one on each side, in the posterolateral part of the medulla and help form the side walls of the fourth ventricle in this region. Medial to the peduncle (i.e. immediately adjacent to the cavity of the ventricle) is a layer of grey matter containing the **nuclei of the vestibular component of the vestibulocochlear nerve.** This forms the **vestibular area** of the floor of the fourth ventricle and is bounded medially by the **sulcus limitans.** The dorsal and ventral cochlear nuclei, which receive fibres from the cochlear parts of the vestibulocochlear nerve, are situated in the grey matter in the dorsolateral part of the medulla superficial to the inferior cerebellar peduncle. The grey matter in the ventricular floor medial to the sulcus limitans forms the **medial eminence** and contains the **dorsal nucleus of the vagus** (including the salivatory nuclei) and the **hypoglossal nucleus.** Their positions are marked by the **vagal** and **hypoglossal triangles** respectively.

Some distance ventral to the grey matter in the floor of the ventricle is the **nucleus ambiguus.** This contains the cell bodies of lower motor neurons innervating the muscles derived from the third and subsequent branchial arches (through the glossopharyngeal, cranial accessory, and vagus nerves) and of preganglionic parasympathetic neurons supplying the heart (through the vagus). It extends caudally into the upper part of the closed medulla.

Close to the nucleus ambiguus and immediately dorsal to the medial part of the inferior olivary nucleus is the small but important **ventral trigeminothalamic tract.** As already described this contains fibres from the opposite spinal nucleus of the trigeminal conveying predominantly pain and temperature sensations.

Pons

The fourth ventricle continues throughout virtually the whole extent of the pons so that, as in the open medulla, the bulk of the substance

of this part of the brainstem lies ventral to the chamber. The pons is divisible into a dorsal or **tegmental** part, lying adjacent to the floor of the ventricle, and a ventral or **basal** part.

Tegmentum

The region of the pons adjacent to the fourth ventricle is recognizably similar to the corresponding area of the medulla. The floor of the ventricle is occupied by central grey matter and the sulcus limitans, separating the **vestibular area** from the medial eminence, is discernible. The medial eminence at this level contains the **abducent nucleus.** The **motor nucleus of the facial nerve** lies ventrolateral to the abducent nucleus and its fibres course dorsomedially and then form a loop dorsal to the latter nucleus (see Fig. 5.38, p. 258) before running ventrolaterally to emerge, as the **motor root of the facial nerve,** from the lateral part of the junction of pons and medulla. This looping arrangement of the facial motor fibres produces a swelling on the rostral part of the medial eminence, the **facial colliculus.**

In the caudal part of the pons the spinal trigeminal tract and its nucleus occupy the lateral part of the tegmentum. The rostral end of this nucleus is expanded to form the **chief sensory nucleus of the trigeminal nerve.** This is located in the upper part of the pons and receives heavily myelinated fibres for discriminative touch from the sensory root of the nerve. Like the fibres terminating in the spinal nucleus, the cell bodies of these heavily myelinated fibres are in the trigeminal ganglion. Second-order neurons from the chief sensory nucleus join the contralateral **ventral trigeminothalamic tract** (also containing second-order neurons from the spinal nucleus) and both the ipsilateral and contralateral **dorsal trigeminothalamic tracts** (consisting exclusively of fibres from the chief sensory nuclei). These pathways ascend to the thalamus through the pons and midbrain, close to the medial lemniscus, and are often known together as the **trigeminal lemniscus.** Continuing rostrally from the chief sensory nucleus is a thin column of grey matter called, since most of it lies in the midbrain, the **mesencephalic nucleus of the trigeminal nerve** (see Fig. 5.37, p. 256). This nucleus receives fibres concerned with proprioception which are unusual in that their cell bodies are found in the nucleus, not in the trigeminal ganglion (the cell bodies of first-order sensory neurons typically have their cell bodies located in a peripheral ganglion not a central nucleus). Most of their peripheral fibres pass in the motor root of the trigeminal nerve to reach the mandibular division through which they are distributed to the temporomandibular joint, supporting tissues of the lower teeth and muscles of mastication. Because of their unusual features they were at one time assumed to be motor in function and the mesencephalic nucleus was accordingly regarded as a motor nucleus. Some of the peripheral fibres from the mesencephalic nucleus traverse the sensory root and maxillary division of the trigeminal nerve to reach the supporting tissues of the upper teeth (see also pp. 247 and 257).

The **motor nucleus of the trigeminal nerve** is located medial to the chief sensory nucleus in the rostral part of the pons. The fibres from this nucleus, together with those from the mesencephalic nucleus, form the motor root of the trigeminal nerve.

The **medial lemniscus** is situated in the ventral part of the tegmentum and has rotated through 90° so that it is widest, when viewed in transverse section, in the mediolateral rather than in the dorsoventral plane as it is in the lower part of the brainstem. Near its lateral edge are the **spinal lemniscus** and the **lateral lemniscus**. The latter is a tract of mostly crossed fibres connecting the cochlear nuclei with the inferior colliculus of the midbrain. Close to the medial edge of the medial lemniscus are the trigeminothalamic tracts.

Running from the dorsolateral aspect of the pons to the cerebellum are the three paired cerebellar peduncles. The **inferior peduncle** leaves from the caudal part of the pons and is an afferent structure containing the **dorsal spinocerebellar, olivocerebellar,** and **vestibulocerebellar tracts**. The **superior peduncle** leaves from the rostral part of the pons and the adjacent part of the midbrain and contains a preponderance of efferent fibres passing from the cerebellum to the red nucleus, thalamus, and cerebral cortex. Its principal afferent component is provided by the crossed fibres of the ventral spinocerebellar tract. The large **middle peduncle** lies lateral to the inferior and superior peduncles and carries afferent fibres from the pontine nuclei to the cerebellum.

Basal part

Conspicuous in the basal part of the pons are bundles of fibres, some running rostrocaudally and some transversely. The descending fibres enter the pons from the midbrain. Many of them belong to the corticospinal and corticobulbar pathways but there are also numerous **corticopontine fibres**. The latter terminate by making synaptic connection with the cells of the **pontine nuclei** which are scattered between the bundles of fibres. The axons of the cells in the pontine nuclei form the transverse **pontocerebellar fibre bundles** which cross the midline and enter the cerebellum through the contralateral middle cerebellar peduncle. The corticopontine fibres begin in many areas of the cerebral cortex and through their connections with the cerebellum play a part in ensuring that voluntary movements are carried out precisely and efficiently.

Midbrain

The midbrain can be conveniently divided into the **tectum**, which lies dorsal to the aqueduct of the midbrain, and the **cerebral peduncles** which lie ventral to the aqueduct. The cerebral peduncles are each divided into a dorsal and a ventral component by a transverse band of deeply pigmented grey matter termed the **substantia nigra**. Ventral to the substantia nigra, in each peduncle, is the **basis pedunculi**. The parts of the two peduncles between the nigral masses and the

aqueduct are known collectively as the **tegmentum**. This is continuous with the tegmentum of the pons.

Tectum

This part of the midbrain consists of the paired **inferior** and **superior colliculi** (also called **corpora quadrigemina**). The inferior colliculi are relay stations in the auditory pathway from the cochlear nuclei to the cerebral cortex. Axons from the cells of the inferior colliculus pass to the **medial geniculate nucleus of the thalamus,** whence further neurons project to the **auditory area** of the cortex of the temporal lobe of the cerebral hemisphere.

The superior colliculi are nuclei involved in reflex response to visual stimuli and are not part of the visual pathway connecting the eyes to the visual cortex. Many of the afferent fibres to these nuclei come from the cortex surrounding the visual areas of the occipital lobes of the cerebral hemispheres. The superior colliculi also receive a few fibres directly from the optic tracts. Efferent fibres pass bilaterally to connect with the cranial nerve motor nuclei in the brainstem, especially the oculomotor, trochlear, abducent, and motor nucleus of facial. A few fibres go to the opposite side of the cervical spinal cord.

Just rostral to the superior colliculus is the pretectal area which is involved in the pupillary light reflex (see p. 248).

Tegmentum

The central (periaqueductal) grey matter contains the nuclei of the trochlear and oculomotor nerves and the upper part of the mesencephalic nucleus of the trigeminal nerve. As described above, the mesencephalic nucleus is a rostral continuation from the chief sensory nucleus of the trigeminal nerve and is concerned with proprioception. In the midbrain it occupies the lateral region of the central grey matter.

The **nuclei of the trochlear and oculomotor nerves** are situated in the ventral part of the central grey matter, the trochlear nucleus at the level of the inferior colliculus and the oculomotor nucleus at the level of the superior colliculus. The axons from the trochlear nucleus follow an unusual course in that they run dorsally around the central grey matter, decussate with their fellows of the opposite side, and emerge from the dorsal surface of the midbrain below the contralateral inferior colliculus. Fibres from the oculomotor nucleus run ventrally through the tegmentum to leave the midbrain in the interpeduncular fossa.

The **red nucleus,** so called because of its reddish tinge in the fresh specimen, is situated in the rostral part of the tegmentum. Important amongst its afferent connections are fibres from the cerebellum

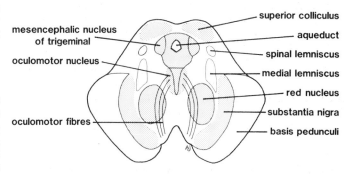

Fig. 5.19. Transverse section through the upper part of the midbrain.

(passing in the superior cerebellar peduncle) and the cerebral motor cortex. A large number of efferents pass from the red nucleus to the inferior olivary nucleus. A few fibres pass to the cervical spinal cord and to the facial motor nucleus of the opposite side.

The **medial, spinal, lateral,** and **trigeminal lemnisci** continue upwards from the tegmentum of the pons into the tegmentum of the midbrain. They form a curved band, situated dorsal to the lateral part of the substantia nigra, with the lateral lemniscus lying dorsal, as well as lateral, to the medial lemniscus and with the spinal lemniscus between them. The trigeminal lemniscus runs close to the medial part of the medial lemniscus.

The **substantia nigra**, forming the boundary between the tegmentum and the basis pedunculi, is a large motor nucleus with a dark colouration produced by melanin granules in certain of its cells. It has connections, both afferent and efferent, with the basal nuclei (p. 243).

Basis pedunculi

This part of the cerebral peduncle consists of fibres descending from the cerebral hemisphere to the brainstem and spinal cord. The middle section is occupied by **corticospinal fibres** from the cerebral motor cortex of the same side. The medial and lateral parts are occupied respectively by **frontopontine** and **temporopontine fibres** passing from the cortex of the frontal and temporal lobes of the cerebral hemisphere to the pontine nuclei. Some corticobulbar fibres run in the basis pedunculi on the medial side of the corticospinal tract but many, including those to the midbrain nuclei, proceed to their destinations through the tegmentum.

The reticular formation

In primitive vertebrates a large part of the brain is made up of a diffuse network of neurons termed the reticular formation. During the course of evolution the fore part of the brain has developed enormously to give rise to the cerebral hemispheres and diencephalon while in the brainstem structures associated with the enlarged forebrain, such as the ascending and descending tracts and many of the large nuclei, have come to occupy an increasing proportion of its volume. The reticular formation, however, has persisted in those areas of the brainstem not occupied by the tracts and nuclei and remains a literally vital component of the mammalian brain since it is concerned with the control of visceral function. It also plays a part in determining the level of consciousness and the perception of pain and is important in controlling voluntary muscle action. It has connections with all levels of the central nervous system.

In the human brain the reticular formation occupies a considerable portion of the dorsal part of the brainstem. By definition it excludes the cranial nerve nuclei, the other conspicuous nuclei, and the long tracts. Its cells have unusually long dendrites which extend widely through the brainstem and make numerous connections with other reticular cells and with cells in non-reticular structures. The neurons of the reticular formation can be aggregated, on the basis of such features as cell architecture, connections, and functions, into groups which are named as nuclei although these are not obvious to the unaided eye. Noteworthy amongst these are centrally located nuclei in the pons which contribute fibres to the reticulospinal tract in the ipsilateral ventral funiculus of the cord and the gigantocellular nucleus in the central part of the medulla which contributes to the reticulospinal tract of the lateral funiculus of both sides. Through their afferent connections, direct and indirect, with the remainder of the reticular formation, the thalamus, cerebellum, and cerebral motor cortex, the neurons of these nuclei play an important part in controlling motor function. Centrally located reticular nuclei are also concerned in the modulation of pain sensation through their connections with the spinal cord, thalamus, and periaqueductal grey matter.

Certain collections of neurons within the reticular formation are specifically associated with visceral function. These 'vital centres' have been identified by electrical stimulation in animals and are not identifiable as anatomical entities. Centres have been demonstrated for respiratory rhythm, inspiration, expiration, and pressor and depressor effects on the cardiovascular system.

Knowledge of the structure and function of the reticular formation is increasing rapidly and many of our present ideas are undoubtedly simplistic and will be greatly modified as information increases.

4

Cerebrum

DIENCEPHALON

As described in Chapter 2.5 the cephalic part of the neural tube at an early stage of development presents three enlargements, termed the **prosencephalon, mesencephalon,** and **rhombencephalon,** which give rise respectively to the cerebrum, midbrain and hindbrain (medulla and pons). With continued development the prosencephalon becomes subdivided into a rostral vesicle, the **telencephalon,** and a caudal vesicle, the **diencephalon.** The telencephalon develops bilateral bulges, the cerebral vesicles, which rapidly enlarge to form the cerebral hemispheres. The diencephalon undergoes a more modest expansion but thickenings in its lateral walls come to form a group of important structures comprising, on each side, the **epithalamus, thalamus** and **subthalamus,** and inferiorly the **hypothalamus.** Also derived from the diencephalon are the neurohypophysis, optic pathways (tracts, chiasma, and nerves) and the retinae.

The thickening of the lateral walls of the diencaphalon results in its central cavity becoming compressed to form the median, slit-like **third ventricle.** The dorsal wall of the diencephalon undergoes no such thickening and remains as a thin layer of ependyma which eventually forms the roof of the third ventricle. Because of its fragility it is usually lost in bisecting the cerebrum but its line of attachment to the lateral wall of the ventricle is marked by a strand of nerve fibres called the stria medullaris (Fig. 5.21). The ependyma is invaginated by pia to form a small choroid plexus. The anterior wall of the ventricle is provided by the **lamina terminalis.** This represents the extreme rostral end of the neural tube before the development of the cerebral vesicles. It provides a link between the right and left cerebral hemispheres and in it develop several commissures composed of fibres connecting the two sides. The **anterior commissure** remains as a small bundle of fibres in the lamina terminalis but the **corpus callosum** enlarges greatly in a dorsal direction, above the roof of the third ventricle, from its original position in the upper part of the lamina terminalis. The floor of the third ventricle contains the **optic chiasma.** Behind this, the floor is formed by a sheet of grey matter, the **tuber cinereum.** Attached to the tuber cinereum is the hollow **pituitary stalk.** The floor then slopes upwards towards the opening of the aqueduct of the midbrain and bears a pair of small swellings, the **mammillary bodies.**

The third ventricle communicates on each side with the lateral ventricle within the cerebral hemisphere through the **interventricular foramen.** The lateral ventricle represents the cavity of the original cerebral vesicle while the interventricular foramen represents the communication between this cavity and the interior of the diencephalic vesicle and so indicates the site from which the cerebral vesicle expanded.

The extent of the diencephalon in the adult brain can now be appreciated. It is bounded laterally by the **internal capsule,** a thick

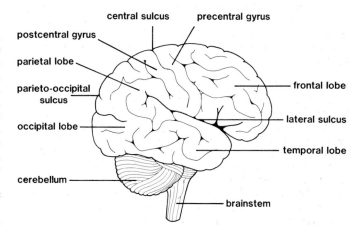

Fig. 5.20. Lateral view of the brain.

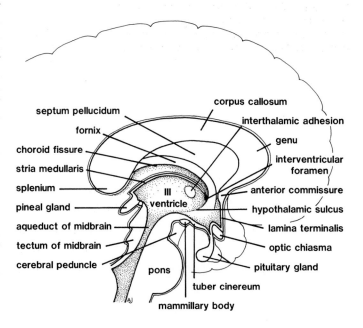

Fig. 5.21. Median section through the diencephalon.

band of ascending and descending fibres within the cerebral hemi-sphere; inferiorly it is continuous with the midbrain, the junction between the two being at a level just caudal to the mammillary bodies; superiorly and posteriorly its boundary is marked by the thin layer of ependyma forming the dorsal wall of the third ventricle while its anterior boundary is similarly marked by the lamina terminalis. The original junction of diencephalon and cerebral hemispheres is at the level of the interventricular foramina.

From the point of view of the dental student the parts of the diencephalon requiring special attention are the thalamus and hypothalamus – the former because it is an important relay station in the sensory pathways to the cerebral cortex and the latter because it is a principal higher centre for the control of visceral function. The epithalamus, a phylogenetically ancient part of the diencephalon, is situated dorsally and contains, amongst other components, the **pineal gland** which is attached to the roof of the third ventricle. The subthalamus is located ventral to the thalamus and contains the subthalamic nucleus which has connections with the basal nuclei.

Thalamus

The thalami are two ovoid masses of grey matter situated one each side of the third ventricle. They constitute the largest component of the diencephalon. Their medial surfaces provide the upper parts of the lateral walls of the third ventricle and are often connected across the midline by the **interthalamic adhesion**.

Each thalamus is divided into three main parts by an internal sheet of white matter consisting of fibres connecting different thalamic regions and called the **internal medullary lamina**. The lamina lies in a parasagittal plane and forks anteriorly in a Y-shaped manner (see Fig. 5.22). Lateral to the lamina is the **lateral nuclear mass**, medial to the lamina is the **dorsomedial nucleus** and enclosed within its fork is the **anterior nucleus.** The large lateral nuclear mass is divisible into dorsal and ventral groups of nuclei. The **intralaminar nuclei** are located within the internal medullary lamina while the **reticular nucleus** is a thin layer of cells between the lateral surface of the main mass of the thalamus and the internal capsule.

The thalamus sends fibres to all parts of the cortex. Reciprocal fibres run from the cortex to the thalamus. In addition the thalamic nuclei receive fibres from subcortical regions. Both the thalamocorti-cal and the corticothalamic fibres send collateral branches to the reticular nucleus which projects to the other thalamic nuclei.

The thalamic nuclei which require more detailed consideration are members of the ventral group of nuclei in the lateral mass. The **ventral posterior nucleus** is the relay nucleus for the fibres of the medial lemniscus and most of the fibres of the spinothalamic and trigeminothalamic tracts. It also receives fibres from the gustatory nucleus (rostral part of the nucleus of the tractus solitarius). The arrangement of the afferent fibres to the ventral posterior nucleus is such that the opposite half of the body has a **somatotopic** (or **topographical**) **representation** in the nucleus—the lower limbs being represented in the dorsolateral part and the head in the medial part of the nucleus. The third-order neurons leave the lateral aspect of the ventral posterior nucleus to run in the internal capsule to the sensory area of the cerebral cortex maintaining, as they do so, their somatotopic representation. The **medial geniculate nucleus** is part of the auditory pathway receiving afferents from the inferior colliculus and projecting to the auditory cortex in the temporal lobe of the cerebral hemisphere. The **lateral geniculate nucleus** is part of the visual path-

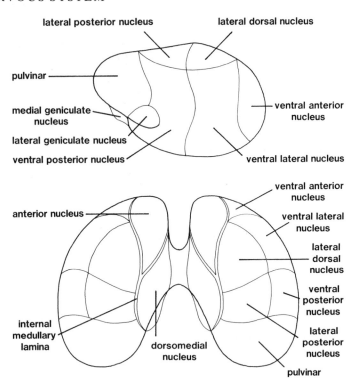

Fig. 5.22. Above, lateral view of the right thalamus; below, superior view of the thalami. Dorsal group of lateral nuclei = lateral dorsal, lateral posterior and pulvinar; ventral group of lateral nuclei = ventral anterior, ventral lateral, ventral posterior, lateral geniculate and medial geniculate nucleus.

way being the terminus for most of the fibres of the optic tract and projecting to the visual cortex of the occipital lobe. The position of these nuclei is indicated in Fig. 5.22.

The remaining nuclei of the ventral group of the lateral nuclear mass are involved in pathways from the cerebellum and corpus stria-tum to the motor areas of the cerebral cortex. They are believed to be important in the control of voluntary motor function.

The dorsal group of nuclei in the lateral nuclear mass and the dor-somedial nucleus have numerous connections with association areas of the cerebral cortex (i.e. areas not concerned specifically with sensory and motor functions). Their functions are poorly understood, but they may be involved in determining the level of activity of the cerebral cortex and in influencing moods and other emotional states. The lateral dorsal nucleus and the anterior nucleus are often included in the limbic system (see p. 244).

Hypothalamus

Although small the hypothalamic part of the diencephalon is of major functional and clinical significance because of its role in the control of visceral function. It surrounds the lower part of the third ventricle, its boundary with the thalamus being marked on the lateral wall of the ventricle by the shallow **hypothalamic sulcus**. The floor of the third ventricle in the hypothalamic region consists of the tuber cinereum and the mammillary bodies.

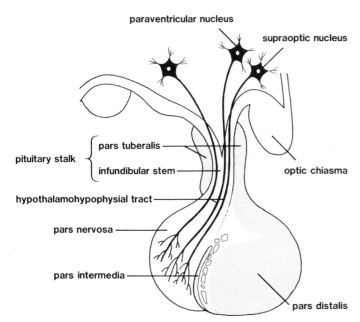

paraventricular nucleus

supraoptic nucleus

pituitary stalk

pars tuberalis

infundibular stem

optic chiasma

hypothalamohypophysial tract

pars nervosa

pars intermedia

pars distalis

Fig. 5.23. The pituitary gland and its connections with the hypothalamus.

Dependent from the inferior surface of the tuber cinereum is the **pituitary (hypophysial) stalk**. Around the attachment of the stalk the tuber cinereum is raised to form the **median eminence**. The stalk expands distally into an ovoid body, the main part of the **pituitary gland** (or **hypophysis cerebri**), which is lodged in the pituitary fossa of the sphenoid bone. The pituitary gland consists of two distinct parts – (i) the **neurohypophysis**, developmentally a downgrowth of the diencephalon, consisting of the median eminence, the **infundibular stem** (the central core of the pituitary stalk) and the **pars nervosa (pars posterior)** and (ii) **adenohypophysis**, a derivative of oral ectoderm, consisting of **pars distalis (pars anterior)**, **pars intermedia**, and **pars tuberalis** (the last surrounding the infundibular stem to complete the pituitary stalk).

The hypothalamus receives afferent fibres conveying information of visceral origin. These fibres follow poorly defined pathways within the central nervous system but many of them relay in the brainstem and thalamus. The hypothalamus also receives afferents from the olfactory cortex, the thalamic nuclei and, through the fornix, from the hippocampus (part of the limbic system). As well as being influenced by nervous factors, the hypothalamus responds to the properties of the circulating blood. This is particularly important in its control of body temperature and of the release of hormones by the adenohypophysis.

Fibres leave the hypothalamus in the **dorsal longitudinal** and **mammillotegmental fasciculi** and pass to the autonomic nuclei in the brainstem and spinal cord, many after relay in the reticular formation of the brainstem. The **mammillothalamic fasciculus** connects the mammillary body with the anterior nucleus of the thalamus.

The hypothalamus elaborates the hormones vasopressin (antidiuretic hormone) and oxytocin (a stimulator of the smooth muscle of the uterus) in its **supraoptic** and **paraventricular nuclei**. These hormones pass along the axons in the **hypothalamohypophysial tract** to the neurohypophysis where they are stored and eventually released into the bloodstream. Cells of the hypothalamus also produce releasing factors which are passed into capillaries in the median eminence. Blood from these capillaries passes through veins which open into a second set of capillaries, the **pituitary portal system**, in the adenohypophysis where the releasing factors stimulate (or in some cases inhibit) the secretion of hormones by the cells of the adenohypophysis. The production of releasing factors is influenced partly by nervous factors but more importantly by the blood levels of the hormones produced by the target organs. For example, if the blood level of thyroid hormone is low the production of thyrotrophin releasing factor by the hypothalamus is increased which, in turn, stimulates increased secretion of thyrotrophin (thyroid-stimulating hormone) by the adenohypophysis and so increases production of hormone by the thyroid gland. This is an example of a negative feedback mechanism.

CEREBRAL HEMISPHERES

The cerebral hemispheres develop from the cerebral vesicles of the telencephalon. They are much enlarged in all mammals but especially in man where they make up by far the greater proportion of the brain. Each hemisphere contains a cavity, the **lateral ventricle**, which represents the lumen of the original cerebral vesicle and communicates with the third ventricle through the **interventricular foramen**. The two hemispheres are separated from each other by a deep median cleft, called the **longitudinal cerebral fissure**, in which is lodged the falx cerebri of the dura mater.

The outer layer of the hemisphere, or **cerebral cortex**, is composed of grey matter and surrounds a central mass of white matter made up of **projection fibres** connecting the cortex with lower centres, **association fibres** connecting one part of the cortex with another and **commissural fibres** connecting the two hemispheres. Most of the commissural fibres cross from one side to the other in the **corpus callosum**. Buried within the central white matter are a number of subcortical masses of grey matter, the **basal nuclei** (or **ganglia**).

External surfaces

Each hemisphere has superolateral, medial, and inferior surfaces. They are much folded to form irregular eminences, the **gyri**, separated by furrows, the **sulci**. This folding greatly increases the total volume of the cerebral cortex. Its arrangement is sufficiently constant from one brain to another to have permitted the naming of the majority of gyri and sulci. Committing these names to memory adds little to the understanding of cerebral structure and function. In the following account only the names of those external features having a clear functional or topographical significance and of interest to the dental student will be given.

Superolateral surface

Two sulci need to be identified on this surface. The **lateral sulcus** is a deep and readily visible cleft that runs forwards and slightly downwards on the inferior part of the surface. It separates the **frontal lobe** above from the **temporal lobe** below. If the lips of the sulcus are prised apart, a buried area of cortex, termed the **insula**, can be seen. The insula is also clearly visible in coronal sections of the hemisphere (Fig. 5.30).

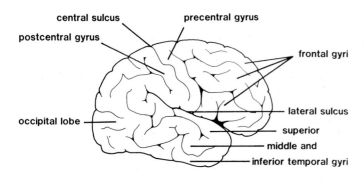

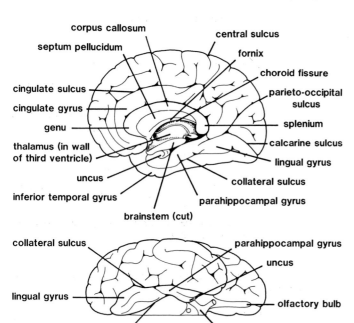

Fig. 5.24. Lateral (above), medial (middle) and inferior (below) surfaces of the right cerebral hemisphere with brainstem removed.

The **central sulcus** is not always so readily identifiable. It runs upwards and backwards from the posterior part of the lateral sulcus to cross the superior border of the superolateral surface, a little posterior to its midpoint, on to the medial surface (it is, in fact, the only major sulcus on the superolateral surface to cross on to the medial surface). It separates **frontal** and **parietal lobes**.

Immediately in front of the central sulcus is the **precentral gyrus**, the **primary motor area** of the cerebral cortex. Immediately behind the sulcus is the **postcentral gyrus**, the **primary sensory (somesthetic) area** of the cortex.

Medial surface

In order to view the medial surface, the two hemispheres have to be separated by cutting through the structures connecting them across the midline (principally the corpus callosum and the walls of the third ventricle – see Fig. 5.21). The full extent of the **corpus callosum** can now be seen. It is sharply curved on itself anteriorly at the **genu** while posteriorly it ends at the rounded **splenium**. Arching forwards a short distance below the corpus callosum is the **fornix**. This consists of a band of white matter running, on each side, from the hippocampus to the hypothalamus. Anteriorly the two bands converge to lie side by side and are conjoined, before diverging again to fuse with the mamillary bodies. Occupying the vertical interval between the corpus callosum and the fornix is a thin, median partition, the **septum pellucidum** (actually consisting of two laminae separated by a narrow central cavity). The anatomical relationships between the corpus callosum, fornix, and the roof of the third ventricle are best understood by reference to their development (see p. 63).

Either side of the septum pellucidum, within the cerebral hemispheres, are the bodies and frontal horns of the lateral ventricles. Below the fornix and immediately above the attachment of the roof of the third ventricle is a narrow area where the medial wall of the body and temporal horn of the lateral ventricle consists of a layer of ependyma invaginated by the covering pia mater to form the **choroid plexus of the lateral ventricle**. This area runs at first posteriorly and then curves around in a C-shaped manner to run forwards on to the medial surface of the temporal lobe. In cleaning the brain the choroid plexus is usually torn away leaving a C-shaped slit, the **choroid fissure**, leading into the ventricle.

The **cingulate sulcus** begins below the genu of the corpus callosum, runs forwards a short distance and then curves upwards and backwards to run posteriorly above the corpus callosum. Finally it turns upwards to reach the superior border of the hemisphere. Over most of its course it conforms with the curvature of the corpus callosum from which it is separated by the **cingulate gyrus**. Above the cingulate sulcus the upper end of the central sulcus can be seen cutting the superior border of the hemisphere.

The posterior part of the medial surface is marked by two important sulci. The **parieto-occipital sulcus** begins at the upper border of the hemisphere some distance anterior to the occipital pole. It runs downwards and forwards to meet the **calcarine sulcus** which curves upwards and forwards from the occipital pole. The parieto-occipital sulcus marks the boundary between the **occipital** and **parietal lobes** of the hemispheres. There is no clear cut boundary between these lobes on the superolateral surface of the hemisphere.

Inferior surface

This is made up anteriorly of the orbital surface of the frontal lobe and posteriorly of the inferior surface of the temporal and occipital lobes. Lying against the orbital surface of the frontal lobe are the olfactory bulb and tract.

Running anteroposteriorly on the inferior surface of the occipital and temporal lobes is the **collateral sulcus**. Posteriorly the collateral sulcus is separated from the **calcarine sulcus** by the **lingual gyrus**. Anteriorly the lingual gyrus is continuous with the **parahippocampal gyrus** which separates the collateral sulcus from the choroid fissure. The anterior end of the parahippocampal gyrus is hook-shaped and is known as the **uncus**. Along the lower border of the inferior limb of the choroid fissure can be seen a narrow strip of cortex termed the **dentate gyrus**. The uncus and adjacent area of the parahippocampal gyrus form the **piriform lobe** (p. 63). Anteriorly the collateral sulcus is continuous with the **rhinal sulcus** which marks the lateral boundary of the piriform lobe.

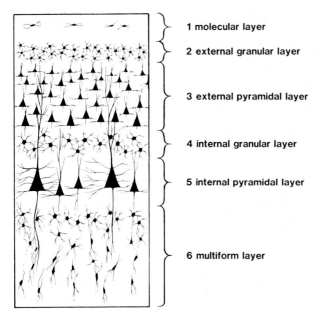

1 molecular layer

2 external granular layer

3 external pyramidal layer

4 internal granular layer

5 internal pyramidal layer

6 multiform layer

Fig. 5.25. The six layers of the neocortex.

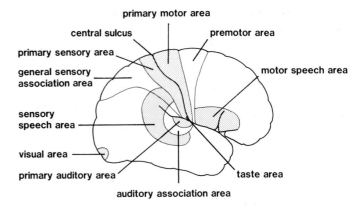

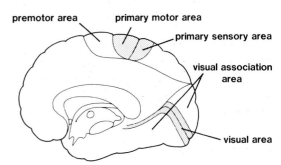

Fig. 5.26. The principal motor and sensory areas of the right cerebral cortex. Lateral view above; medial view below.

Cerebral cortex

Structure

The microstructure of the cerebral cortex is extremely complex and views on its functions change rapidly. The following brief account is greatly simplified and, like all simplifications, lacks total accuracy.

From both a phylogenetic and functional viewpoint the cortex of the mammalian brain can be divided into two basic parts – the ancient paleocortex and archicortex (= paleopallium and archipallium, respectively, page 62) and the newer neocortex (= neopallium). The neocortex predominates, constituting in man, for example, some 90 per cent of the total bulk of the cerebral cortex. It includes the primary areas for general sensation, motor function and the special senses (other than smell) and the cortex associated with these primary areas. In the human brain, especially, much of the neocortex is made up of such association areas. The paleocortex is found in the part of the cerebral hemisphere concerned with olfaction and the archicortex in the **limbic system.**

The paleocortex and archicortex are usually described as having three layers, the distinction between the layers depending upon the presence in greater or lesser numbers of certain cell types. On a similar basis the neocortex is described as being six-layered of which the second, third, and fourth layers (counting in from the surface) are relatively recent acquisitions (Fig. 5.25). It should be emphasized that the neocortex is, in fact, quite variable from one region of the cerebral hemisphere to another. The six layers are usually most distinct in the association areas. In the primary motor area (precentral gyrus) layers two to six appear as a single zone containing numerous pyramidal cells, many of the giant variety (pyramidal cells have a pyramidal body and an axon which enters the white matter as a projection, association, or commissural fibre). In the general sensory, visual, and auditory areas, by contrast, layers two to five appear as a single layer which contains many stellate cells (star-shaped cells with many short processes).

Functional localization

The **primary sensory (somesthetic) area** occupies the postcentral gyrus. The opposite side of the body is represented in inverted fashion, with the area for the head being most ventral and that for the lower limb and lower part of the trunk being most dorsal and extending over on to the medial surface of the hemisphere. This **somatotopic representation** reflects the fact that the fibres carrying sensation from the various parts of the body maintain an orderly arrangement within the ascending pathways in the cord and brainstem. As already noted (p. 238) somatotopic representation is maintained in the ventral posterior nucleus of the thalamus which is the main source of afferent fibres for the primary sensory area. Behind the primary sensory area on the superolateral surface of the hemisphere, is the **general sensory association area**. Here sensory data are integrated and interpreted. Destruction of the primary sensory area greatly reduces awareness and localization of sensory stimuli on the contralateral side of the body whereas damage to the association area, with the primary area intact, results in an inability to interpret the sensory input as, for example, the inability to recognize, with the eyes closed, an everyday object placed in the hand.

The **visual area** surrounds the calcarine sulcus. On section the visual cortex contains a prominent stripe (produced by tangentially running fibres) and is, therefore, described as striate. Destruction of the visual area on one side leads to loss of the opposite visual field (see p. 248). The **visual association cortex** surrounds the primary visual area. Damage here may lead to the inability to recognize objects in the opposite field of vision.

The **auditory area** lies on the superior surface of the temporal lobe (i.e. in the floor of the lateral sulcus) and only a small part of it is visible on the lateral surface of the hemisphere. Since there is bilateral projection from the organs of hearing, a unilateral lesion involving the auditory area leads to little impairment of hearing. The **auditory association area** is situated in the floor of the lateral sulcus behind the primary auditory area.

The **taste area** is located in the postcentral gyrus in the upper wall of the lateral sulcus and extends into the insula.

The **primary motor area** occupies the precentral gyrus with, as in the primary sensory area, the contralateral side of the body being represented somatotopically in an inverted manner. Destruction of the motor area is followed by voluntary muscle paralysis (see p. 251) on the opposite side of the body. Anterior to the motor area is the **premotor area.** It is believed to be concerned with the control of learned motor activities of complex nature.

The **motor speech area** is situated in the frontal lobe above the anterior end of the lateral sulcus. A lesion at this site results in distorted speech but comprehension remains good. The **sensory speech area** is in the parietal and temporal lobes around the posterior termination of the lateral sulcus and close to the auditory association cortex. Lesions in these sites lead to poor comprehension of language. The speech areas are usually located in the left hemisphere (i.e. in the hemisphere which is also dominant for handedness in right-handed people).

Outside these parts of the cortex with clearly defined functions are large cortical areas in the frontal, parietal, occipital, and temporal lobes whose functions are less precisely understood. Those in the frontal lobe are concerned with control of behaviour and relating it to judgement and previous experience. The areas in the other three lobes are involved in such complex processes as memory, the experience of emotions, and intellectual processes such as thinking and learning.

Lateral ventricle

The lateral ventricle is developed from the cavity of the original cerebral vesicle and communicates with the third ventricle through the interventricular foramen. It has a **frontal (anterior) horn** projecting into the frontal lobe, an **occipital (posterior) horn** projecting towards the occipital lobe, and a **temporal (inferior) horn** extending forwards and downwards into the temporal lobe. The main part of the ventricle from which these horns project is called the **body.**

The lateral ventricle does not lie centrally within the hemisphere but is much closer to its medial surface. This is the result of varying degrees of thickening of the walls of the cerebral vesicle during development. Above, below, and lateral to the ventricle the walls undergo great expansion to form the bulk of the grey and white matter of the hemisphere. Medial to the body and temporal horn of the ventricle there is virtually no thickening at all so that in this area the wall of the ventricle consists of a layer of ependyma only. It is invaginated by the covering pia to form the **choroid plexus of the lateral ventricle.** In cleaning the brain the thin medial wall of the ventricle is usually torn away but its position is marked by the choroid fissure. As would be expected this fissure follows the shape of the ventricle (or more precisely of its body and temporal horn),

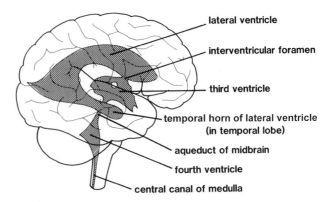

Fig. 5.27. The outline of the ventricular system superimposed on a lateral view of the brain.

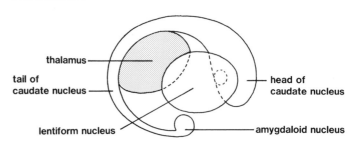

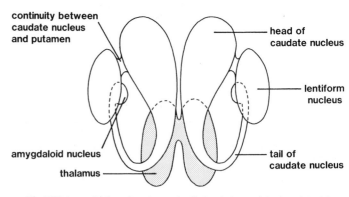

Fig. 5.28. Lateral (above) and superior (below) views of the basal nuclei.

appearing as a C-shaped slit curving around the structures of the diencephalon (Fig. 5.24). The medial wall of the remainder of the body and of the frontal horn of the ventricle is formed by the septum pellucidum with the fornix in its inferior margin.

Basal nuclei

The term basal nuclei (or ganglia) is used with different meanings by different authors. Here it is used to include the **caudate, lentiform,** and **amygdaloid nuclei** and the **claustrum.** The caudate and lentiform nuclei together are known as the **corpus striatum.** In the clinical context the term 'basal ganglia' is frequently used to refer to the corpus striatum, subthalamic nucleus, and substantia nigra.

Caudate nucleus

The caudate nucleus possesses a large bulbous head, a somewhat narrower body and a long, tapering tail. Seen in side view it is **C**-shaped, being situated adjacent to the lateral ventricle with whose curvature it conforms. The head and body of the caudate nucleus form a bulge in the floor of the frontal horn and body of the ventricle while the tail extends forwards in the roof of the temporal horn. Anteriorly the tail is continuous with the amygdaloid nucleus, part of the limbic system.

Lentiform nucleus

This nucleus was named after its fancied resemblance to a biconvex lens. In section it can be seen to consist of a lateral, darker part termed the **putamen** and a medial, paler part termed the **globus pallidus**. It lies deep within the white matter of the cerebral hemisphere with the internal capsule on its medial side.

Claustrum

The claustrum is a thin sheet of grey matter situated in the white matter between the lentiform nucleus and the insula.

Connections

The caudate nucleus and putamen (often referred to together as the **neostriatum**) receive fibres from a wide area of the cerebral cortex. Many of these fibres enter the nuclei from the internal capsule. The neostriatum also receives fibres from the thalamus and substantia nigra. The globus pallidus (or **paleostriatum**) receives its afferent supply principally from the neostriatum. Most of its efferent fibres pass to the ventral lateral nucleus of the thalamus. which projects in turn, to the motor and premotor area of the cortex.

The basal nuclei are involved in the control of motor activity (p. 250).

White matter

Much of the interior of the cerebral hemisphere is composed of white matter. As already mentioned, the fibres constituting this white matter may be of the projection, association, or commissural variety. The projection fibres may be either afferent (passing to the cortex) or efferent (passing from the cortex) and are concentrated into the internal capsule.

Corpus callosum

The main features of the corpus callosum are described on page 240. Fibres crossing in the body of the commissure radiate outwards into the hemispheres on each side, intersecting the association and projection fibres. From the splenium the fibres radiate posteriorly into the occipital lobes, the splenium and radiations constituting together the **forceps major**. Fibres from the genu radiate into the frontal lobes and constitute the **forceps minor**.

The **anterior commissure** is a small bundle of fibres crossing in the lamina terminalis.

These interhemispheric connections are concerned with bilateral learning processes such as being able to employ the left hand to carry out a task learned by use of the right hand.

Internal capsule

The internal capsule is a broad band of white matter passing medial to the lentiform nucleus. In a horizontal section (Fig. 5.29) it is seen

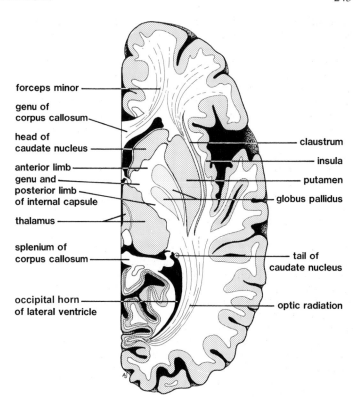

Fig. 5.29. Horizontal section through the right cerebral hemisphere.

to consist of **anterior** and **posterior limbs** continuous with each other at an angle termed the **genu**. The anterior limb is situated between the lentiform nucleus laterally and the head and body of the caudate nucleus medially. The posterior limb is again related to the lentiform nucleus laterally but medially it is bounded by the thalamus.

Above the internal capsule, the ascending and descending projection fibres, in their passage to or from the various areas of the cerebral cortex, radiate outwards in a fan-like arrangement called the **corona radiata**. As the internal capsule passes downwards it also tends somewhat medially to run between, on the one hand, the head and body of the caudate nucleus (which lie above and medial to the capsule) and, on the other, the tail of the nucleus (which lies below and lateral to the capsule). These relationships can be appreciated by consideration of Fig. 5.28. The capsule ends by running into the cerebral peduncle of the corresponding side of the midbrain.

The anterior limb of the capsule contains frontopontine fibres descending from the cortex of the frontal lobe to synapse with the cells of the pontine nuclei. The posterior limb contains the corticospinal and corticobulbar fibres. The corticobulbar fibres occupy a position closest to the genu and are followed, in anteroposterior sequence, by the corticospinal fibres concerned with innervating the upper limb, then those related to the trunk and finally those related to the lower limb. The internal capsule also contains numerous other descending tracts including fibres to the corpus striatum, red nucleus, substantia nigra, and inferior olivary nucleus.

Most of the ascending fibres in the internal capsule are passing from the thalamus to the cortex. In the anterior limb these project to the cortex of the frontal lobe. The ascending fibres in the posterior limb pass to the cortex of the occipital and parietal lobes and include the projection to the primary sensory area of the postcentral gyrus and the geniculocalcarine fibres (in the optic radiation) from the lateral geniculate nucleus to the visual cortex around the calcarine sulcus. Auditory fibres pass below the lentiform nucleus (where they form the sublentiform part of the internal capsule) to reach the auditory cortex of the temporal lobe.

The internal capsule is supplied with blood by the **striate arteries** which are branches of the middle cerebral artery. These branches are liable to thrombosis or rupture as a result of degenerative changes in their walls – events termed 'strokes' in lay terminology. If the subject survives, which is more likely with a thrombosis than with a haemorrhage, there are contralateral motor and sensory deficits consequent upon the destruction of the descending and ascending fibres in the internal capsule (see p. 251).

Limbic and olfactory systems

In lower vertebrates, the paleocortex and archicortex, both structures associated with olfaction, form a major part of the cerebrum, reflecting the importance of the sense of smell (p. 62). In higher mammals, the neocortex is greatly expanded, and the paleocortex and archicortex are much reduced in relative size. The paleocortex is still concerned with olfaction while the archicortex has become included in the limbic system, a group of structures related to emotional and instinctual urges of high survival value both for the individual and the species. The limbic system is also involved in the processes of memory, especially the memorizing of new information.

The human **olfactory system** consists of the olfactory cells of the nasal mucosa, the olfactory bulbs and tracts and the olfactory areas of the cerebral cortex. The olfactory cells are neurons specialized to be responsive to minute quantities of chemicals in the inspired air. Their axons pass, as the olfactory nerves, through the foramina in the cribriform plate of the ethmoid and end in the olfactory bulb by synapsing in a highly complex manner with the dendrites of mitral cells. The axons of the mitral cells travel to the olfactory areas of the cortex in the olfactory tract. The primary olfactory area is the paleocortex in the region of the uncus (the piriform lobe). There are numerous projections from the olfactory areas to other parts of the brain and especially to the hypothalamus and the limbic system. These connections explain the powerful effects that odours can have in stimulating or inhibiting visceral functions (such as appetite) and in arousing emotions.

The **limbic system** (or lobe) comprises a number of structures located around the junction of the diencephalon and cerebral hemispheres. These include the cingulate and parahippocampal gyri, the hippocampal formation, the amygdaloid nucleus, the mammillary bodies of the hypothalamus and the anterior nucleus of the thalamus. Its main tracts are the fornix, mammillothalamic fasciculus, and stria terminalis. Some authors include the olfactory structures in the limbic system.

The **hippocampal formation** comprises the hippocampus, dentate gyrus, and the adjacent area of the parahippocampal gyrus (Fig. 5.30). The hippocampus is located in the floor of the temporal horn of the lateral ventricle. The dentate gyrus is a narrow strip of grey matter situated between the hippocampus and the parahippocampal gyrus and is visible on the inferomedial aspect of the hemisphere immediately below the choroid fissure. The hippocampal formation receives numerous afferent fibres from the olfactory areas and the

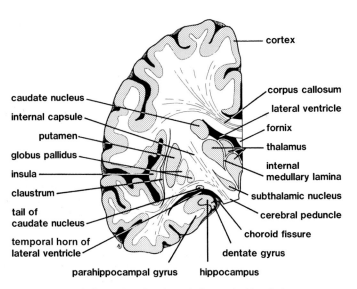

Fig. 5.30. Coronal section through the cerebral hemisphere.

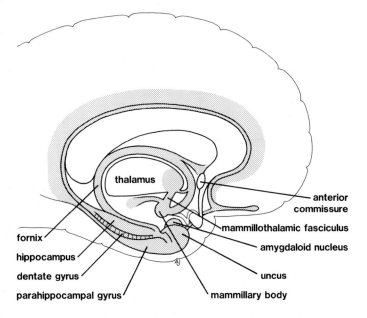

Fig. 5.31. Diagrammatric representation of the limbic and olfactory systems (both stippled) in medial view. Left cerebral hemisphere.

cingulate gyrus. Its principal efferent pathway is the fornix. This begins on each side at the posterior end of the hippocampus beneath the splenium of the corpus callosum. The tract curves around the posterior end of the thalamus and then runs forwards beneath the corpus callosum where it joins with its fellow of the opposite side to form the body of the fornix. Anteriorly it turns downwards, in front of the interventricular foramen, to end in the mammillary body of the hypothalamus. The latter is connected to the anterior nucleus of the thalamus by the mammillothalamic fasciculus.

5

Major sensory and motor systems

The purpose of this chapter is to bring together and review information about the sensory and motor pathways of importance to the dental student so that each can be understood in its entirety and without regard to the somewhat artificial divisions of the nervous system employed in describing its topography. It must be appreciated that, as with many aspects of the nervous system, our views of the structure and function of these pathways are being constantly revised as new clinical and experimental evidence comes to light. In some instances, the experimental findings in animals and the findings in human patients are at variance and here, especially, opinions are in a state of flux. The account that follows should be regarded, therefore, as a much simplified summary of current views written predominantly as a guide for the clinically orientated dental student. To understand it you will need to have a good grasp of the arrangement of structures within the spinal cord and brain and you are strongly urged, if necessary, to revise the account of these structures given in Chapters 5.2 to 5.4.

GENERAL SENSORY PATHWAYS

Sensory fibres enter the spinal cord in the dorsal roots of the spinal nerves. Their cell bodies are located in the spinal ganglia. In the cranial region the arrangement is essentially similar. General sensory fibres enter the brainstem in cranial nerves V, VII, IX, and X (traditionally taken to be equivalent to the dorsal roots of the spinal nerves) and have their cell bodies in the ganglia of these nerves. An exception to these general rules are the proprioceptive fibres from the cranial region. Although the pathways followed by these fibres are not fully elucidated it is believed that most, if not all, end in the mesencephalic nucleus of the trigeminal nerve where their cell bodies are located (see p. 257).

Impulses traversing sensory fibres may elicit reflex responses of various types. The central pathways involved in these responses may be local, being restricted to the spinal cord or brainstem, or involve the cerebellum and other higher centres. In other cases the impulses are conveying information destined to reach the cerebral cortex. It is the pathways followed by the latter impulses which are dealt with in this section. They may be divided into two main categories: (i) the pathway from the receptors responding to pain, temperature, simple (light) touch and pressure stimuli, and (ii) the pathway from receptors for proprioception (i.e. the endings in muscles, joints, and ligaments) and for fine (discriminative) touch and vibration. The evidence suggests that not all the fibres in these pathways are as modality-specific as previously assumed and that there is some overlap in function between the two systems, particularly in the case of the different types of touch.

In each of these pathways there are typically (but not always) three principal neurons between the end receptor and the cerebral cortex. These are called in order from receptor to cortex, the **first-order** (or **primary**), **second-order (secondary),** and **third-order (tertiary) neurons.** The cell bodies of the first-order neurons in the trunk and neck are located in the spinal ganglia. They have peripheral processes which pass out through the spinal nerves to the end receptors and central processes which pass into the cord through the dorsal roots to connect with the second-order neurons. In the cranial region the arrangement of the first-order neurons, except those travelling to the mesencephalic nucleus of the trigeminal nerve, is similar; their cell bodies are located in the ganglia of the 'dorsal root' cranial nerves, their peripheral processes pass to receptors in the head and neck and their central processes enter the brainstem. First-order neurons have a pseudounipolar structure (p. 222). The cell bodies of the second-order neurons are situated within the grey matter of the cord or brainstem. Their axons cross the midline and ascend to the thalamus where they connect with the third-order neurons. The axons of the latter traverse the posterior limb of the internal capsule and the corona radiata to reach the sensory area of the cerebral cortex. An important exception to the three-neuron arrangement is found in the pathway for proprioception from the lower limb (p. 247). Connector neurons often occur between the principal neurons of the sensory pathways.

The projection to the primary sensory cortex has a somatotopic representation such that each part of the body is represented in a specific area of the cortex. At this level all the modalities of sensation mediated by the ascending tracts come together in the appropriate cortical area. Thus impulses concerned with pain, temperature, simple and discriminative touch and proprioception from, say, the hand arrive at the same sensory area of the cortex.

Pathway for pain, temperature, simple touch and pressure (spinothalamic system)

The skin contains many types of sensory endings. Investigating their function has proved difficult but it seems likely that they have a high degree of selectivity, if not absolute specificity, for the various modalities of sensation. The pain receptors consist of unencapsulated nerve endings in the epidermis and in other epithelia and in deeper tissues such as ligaments and the capsules of joints. The afferents from these receptors are unmyelinated and finely myelinated fibres of small diameter. The finely myelinated fibres conduct the initial sensation of sharp pain while the unmyelinated fibres convey the wave of duller but intensely disagreeable pain which follows. The temperature receptors have not been certainly identified but may be similar to those for pain. The receptors for simple touch are of both the unencapsulated and encapsulated variety. The unencapsulated endings subserving this modality are Merkel endings (where the axonal ter-

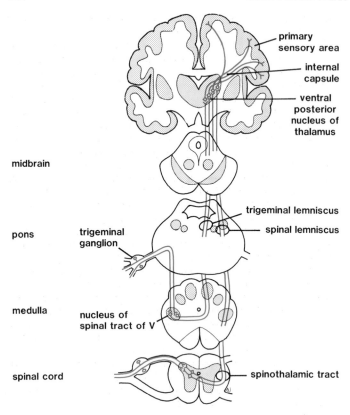

Fig. 5.32. The pathway for pain, temperature, simple touch and pressure.

minals contact specialized Merkel cells in the germinal layer of the epidermis) and peritrichial endings (where the axonal branches surround hair follicles). The encapsulated endings are Meissner corpuscles (each an ovoid body of epithelioid cells with three or four endings entering its deep pole and located in the dermis). Pacinian corpuscles (ellipsoidal, laminated bodies each surrounding a single nerve fibre, found widely distributed in subcutaneous tissues and in connective tissue adjacent to many synovial joints) and Ruffini endings (a greatly branched array of expanded axonal branches surrounded by capsular cells) respond to pressure. The afferents from the receptors for simple touch and pressure are medium-calibre, myelinated fibres.

The afferent fibres from the receptors for pain, temperature, simple touch and pressure in the limbs, trunk and neck are the peripheral processes of first-order sensory neurons of the **spinothalamic system.** Their cell bodies are located in the spinal ganglia. The central processes of the pain and temperature fibres pass in the lateral divisions of the dorsal roots of the spinal nerves to enter the dorsolateral fasciculus of the spinal cord where they divide into ascending and descending branches which travel for one or two segments before entering the dorsal grey horn. The central processes of the simple touch and pressure fibres enter the dorsal column of white matter through the medial divisions of the dorsal roots. They too divide into ascending and descending branches most of which terminate in the dorsal grey horn.

The first-order sensory neurons of the spinothalamic system make contact with numerous connector neurons for spinal reflex responses as well as, directly or indirectly, with the second-order tract neurons. The cell bodies of the latter are situated mainly in the nucleus proprius. The tract neurons receive numerous other contacts, notably with fibres descending from the reticular formation of the brainstem and with fibres from the parietal lobe cortex.

The axons of the tract cells immediately cross the midline in the grey and white commissures, then pass through the contralateral ventral horn of grey matter and ascend in the **spinothalamic tract** located in the ventrolateral part of the white matter of the opposite side of the cord. The spinothalamic tract continues upwards through the brainstem, where it is known as the **spinal lemniscus,** to end mainly in the lateral part of the **ventral posterior nucleus** of the thalamus. Here, the tract fibres connect with third-order neurons whose cell bodies are located in the thalamic nucleus. The processes of these tertiary neurons pass to the sensory area of the cortex through the posterior limb of the internal capsule.

Most of the pain, temperature, simple touch and pressure fibres from the cranial region travel in the trigeminal nerve and have cell bodies located in the trigeminal ganglion, although a few similar fibres run in the facial, glossopharyngeal, and vagus nerves with cell bodies in the corresponding ganglia. The central processes of all these first-order neurons enter the brainstem (in the case of the trigeminal and facial fibres travelling in the sensory roots of the nerves) to end in the sensory nuclei of the trigeminal nerve by connecting with second-order neurons. The arrangement of the endings is complex and is described on pp. 256–7.

The second-order fibres ascend in the **trigeminal lemniscus,** mostly of the opposite side, to end in the medial part of the ventral posterior nucleus of the thalamus whence third-order neurons project to the sensory cortex through the posterior limb of the internal capsule.

The perception of pain does not depend solely upon transmission along the spinothalamic route but is modulated by numerous neural mechanisms within the central nervous system including the activity of pathways descending from the cortex and reticular formation. For details of this complex but clinically important subject you should consult a textbook of neurophysiology.

Pathway for discriminative touch, proprioception, and vibration (medial lemniscus system)

The proprioceptive receptors include neuromuscular spindles, the neurotendinous organs and other endings in the capsules and ligaments of the joints. Meissner's corpuscles are the principal receptors involved in discriminative touch. Pacinian corpuscles are believed to be the principal receptors for the sense of vibration. The first-order neurons for this pathway are large-calibre, myelinated fibres. In the spinal region the central processes of these neurons enter the dorsal white columns, through the medial divisions of the dorsal roots, and bifurcate. The short descending and ascending branches, and their collaterals, synapse with connector neurons for spinal reflexes and with cells contributing fibres to the spinocerebellar tracts. The long ascending branches travel upwards to the medulla oblongata in the dorsal white column of the side on which they entered the cord. New fibres are added to the lateral side of the dorsal column in each segment of the cord. From the midthoracic level upwards the dorsal column is divided into a medial **gracile fasciculus** and a lateral **cuneate fasciculus** the former containing the fibres from the lower half of the body and the latter the fibres from the upper half.

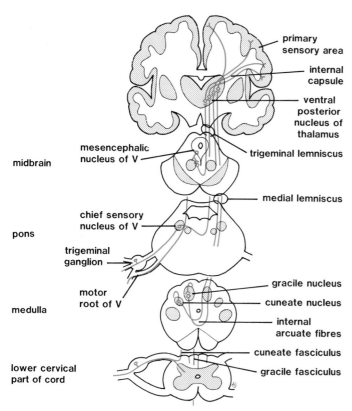

primary
sensory area

internal
capsule

ventral
posterior
nucleus of
thalamus

mesencephalic
nucleus of V

trigeminal lemniscus

midbrain

medial lemniscus

chief sensory
nucleus of V

pons

trigeminal
ganglion

motor
root of V

gracile nucleus

cuneate nucleus

medulla

internal
arcuate fibres

cuneate fasciculus

lower cervical
part of cord

gracile fasciculus

Fig. 5.33. The pathway for discriminative touch and vibration sensation and for proprioception from the upper limb; for proprioception from the lower limb see text.

The fasciculi end at the **gracile nucleus** and **cuneate nucleus** located in the dorsal part of the lower medulla. Here the ascending fibres synapse with the second-order neurons. The axons of these secondary neurons leave the nuclei by passing ventrally and medially, as the **internal arcuate fibres,** to cross the midline in the **decussation of the medial lemniscus.** They ascend, in the **medial lemniscus,** to the thalamus where they end in the lateral part of the **ventral posterior nucleus.** The third-order neurons project to the sensory area of the cortex through the posterior limb of the internal capsule.

The long ascending fibres in the dorsal columns to the gracile and cuneate nuclei are concerned with discriminative touch and vibration sense from the whole body. Proprioception from the upper limb follows the same pathway with the first-order neurons synapsing in the cuneate nucleus. Proprioception from the lower limb is now known to follow a rather different route which consists of four principal neurons in sequence not three. The ascending branches of the first-order neurons in the proprioceptive pathway from the lower limb connect with neurons in the **nucleus dorsalis** whose axons ascend in the ipsilateral **dorsal spinocerebellar tract** in the lateral white column. These fibres eventually pass through the inferior cerebellar peduncle into the cerebellum but before doing so, they give rise to collateral branches which end in **nucleus Z** (located just rostral to the gracile nucleus). The neurons in nucleus Z give rise to internal arcuate fibres which join the opposite medial lemniscus and ascend to the lateral

part of the ventral posterior nucleus of the thalamus from which thalamocortical fibres pass to the sensory cortex.

In the cranial region the pathways for discriminative touch and for proprioception are separated, at least so far as the trigeminal fibres are concerned. The first-order neurons for discriminative touch are typical sensory nerve cells in that their cell bodies are contained within a sensory ganglion (principally the trigeminal ganglion although there may be similar fibres in the facial, glossopharyngeal, and vagus nerves with their cell bodies in the corresponding ganglia). The central processes enter the brainstem, in the case of the trigeminal and facial nerves through their sensory roots, and end in the **chief sensory nucleus of the trigeminal.** From here the axons of the second-order neurons pass in the **trigeminal lemniscus** to the medial part of the **ventral posterior nucleus** of the thalamus. It appears that these fibres are both crossed and uncrossed. Third-order neurons project from the thalamus to the sensory cortex.

The proprioceptive pathways in the cranial region are not completely elucidated. In the case of the trigeminal nerve the first-order neurons for proprioception are unusual amongst sensory fibres in that their cell bodies are located not in the sensory ganglion of the nerve but in the **mesencephalic nucleus,** a central nucleus within the brainstem. Electrophysiological evidence suggests that fibres from the neuromuscular spindles in the muscles of mastication, the extraocular muscles, and possibly also the facial, lingual, and laryngeal muscles all terminate in this nucleus as do fibres from endings in the jaw joint and periodontal tissues (see also p. 257).

Central branches of the cells in the mesencephalic nucleus connect with cells in the reticular formation from which axons pass to the motor nucleus of the trigeminal nerve (for reflex action) and to the thalamus in the trigeminal lemniscus.

Clinical aspects

Because of the segregation of the two sensory pathways in the cord and brainstem it is possible for each to be involved in lesions which leave the other pathway unaffected. Degenerative changes in the region of the central canal of the spinal cord, for example, will interrupt the axons of the second-order neurons of the spinothalamic system as they decussate in the ventral commissures. This occurs in the disease syringomyelia which typically involves the cervical area of the cord and leads to bilateral loss of pain and temperature sensibility in the upper limbs – a severe disability in that the sufferer lacks the protective effects of these modalities of sensation. Loss of simple touch is less noticeable because discriminative touch, mediated through the dorsal columns, is still intact and because of the functional overlap between the different types of touch fibres. Lesions in the dorsal columns, on the other hand, will interrupt the ascending processes of the first-order neurons for discriminative touch, proprioception, and vibration. The most frequent cause of lesions in this site are demyelinating diseases such as multiple sclerosis. Degenerative changes in the dorsal columns are also a feature of tertiary syphilis. The pathways may also be interrupted in the brainstem as a result of demyelinating disease, diminished blood supply, or trauma

Section of the cord will, of course, affect the ascending pathways for all modalities of sensation from below the injury. Although section through only the right or left half of the cord is rare it is instructive to consider its effects. On the side of the section there will be interruption of the uncrossed axons of the first-order neurons ascending in the dorsal column and of the crossed second-order neurons ascending in the spinothalamic tract. There will, therefore, be loss of discriminative touch, position sense and vibration on the side of the hemisection and of pain and temperature sensibility on the opposite side. Any diminution of simple touch and pressure sense on the opposite side is difficult to detect because discriminative touch on that side is still appreciated through the intact dorsal column pathway. Hemisection also interrupts the descending pathways with consequent upper motor neuron paralysis of the muscles supplied from the affected side of the cord below the lesion. The combination of sensory and motor effects is known as the Brown–Sequard syndrome.

The third-order neurons for the two principal pathways travel to the cerebral cortex together, with maintenance of the somatotopic pattern of body representation. Localized lesions of the ascending pathways at a suprathalamic level will affect, therefore, all modalities of sensation from a particular part of the body. This occurs in a 'stroke', one of the commonest neurological disorders especially of older people. Its usual cause is a thrombus forming in one of the striate arteries supplying the internal capsule. As a result the internal capsule is deprived of its blood supply with consequent interruption of the fibres ascending and descending through it. Interruption of the ascending fibres leads to loss or modification (depending upon the extent of the neuronal damage) of all modalities of sensation on the opposite side of the body, the precise area affected being determined by the size and position of the lesion. The accompanying damage to the descending fibres results in muscle impairment, also on the opposite side of the body (see p. 251).

VISUAL, AUDITORY, AND VESTIBULAR PATHWAYS

Although of little direct relevance to the clinical practice of dentistry a brief outline of these pathways will be of general interest to dental students.

Visual pathway

The photoreceptors are the rods and cones of the retina of each eyeball. These connect, through the intermediary of bipolar cells, with ganglion cells which lie close to the surface of the retina (i.e. adjacent to the vitreous body in the interior of the eyeball). The axons of the ganglion cells leave the retina to constitute the **optic nerve.** At the **optic chiasma** the axons from the ganglion cells in the nasal half of each retina decussate. The fibres from the temporal half of the retina do not cross. Thus each **optic tract** (the continuation of the optic pathway from the chiasma) is made up of temporal fibres from the eyeball of its own side and nasal fibres from the opposite eyeball. Most of the fibres in the optic tract terminate in the **lateral geniculate nucleus** of the thalamus from which fibres pass in the **geniculocalcarine tract** (or **optic radiation**), through the posterior limb of the internal capsule, to the **visual cortex** in the upper and lower lips of the calcarine sulcus of the occipital lobe of the cerebral hemisphere. The retinal image of the visual fields is inverted and reversed right to left by the optics of the eye. In consequence each hemisphere receives information about the opposite field of vision (Fig. 5.34).

A few of the fibres in the optic tract bypass the lateral geniculate nucleus to end in the **pretectal area** and **superior colliculus** of the midbrain. These parts of the midbrain also receive fibres from the occipital lobe of the cerebral hemisphere. They are involved in reflex

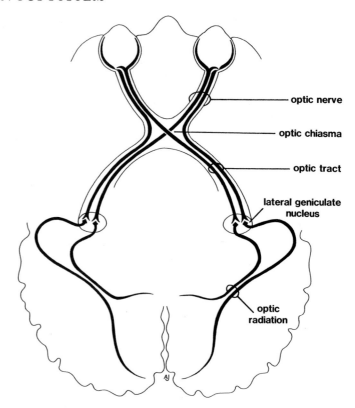

Fig. 5.34. The visual pathway. Note that the visual cortex of each hemisphere receives fibres from the corresponding side of each retina. Since the eyeball contains a biconvex lens, which, therefore, produces a reversed image, the visual cortex receives information from the opposite visual field.

responses to light including the pupillary light reflex (constriction of the pupil to bright light) and the accommodation reflex (ocular convergence, pupillary constriction, and change in the curvature of the lens when viewing close objects) as well as reflex movements of the eyes and body.

Clinical aspects

It should be clear from the above account that lesions at different parts of the optic pathway will produce different visual defects. A lesion in one eye or optic nerve may lead to blindness in that eye. Damage to the optic tract, geniculocalcarine tract, or visual cortex of one side will produce loss of the opposite visual field. Damage to the chiasma (from, for example, the pressure of an enlarged pituitary gland) will lead to interruption of the nasal fibres from each retina with consequent loss of both temporal visual fields, a condition called tunnel vision.

Auditory pathway

The sound receptors are located in the Organ of Corti within the cochlear part of the internal ear. These connect with the peripheral processes of first-order sensory neurons whose cell bodies are located in the **spiral** (or **cochlear**) **ganglion.** The central processes of these cells constitute the **cochlear nerve** which unites, in the lateral part of the internal acoustic meatus, with the nerve from the vestibular part of the internal ear to form the **vestibulocochlear nerve.** Each central process, on entering the brainstem, gives one branch to the **dorsal cochlear nucleus** and one to the **ventral cochlear nucleus.**

From these nuclei, the auditory pathway ascends to the **inferior colliculi** of the midbrain, many of its constituent fibres undergoing additional synaptic relay in the superior olivary nucleus (located at the level of the ponto-medullary junction) and nuclei of the lateral lemniscus. Although most of the fibres project to the contralateral inferior colliculus, those originating in the superior olivary nucleus project to both colliculi so that the pathway is partly uncrossed. The bundle of fibres ascending to the inferior colliculus is called the **lateral lemniscus.**

The fibres in the lateral lemniscus synapse in the inferior colliculus with neurons whose processes pass to the **medial geniculate nucleus** of the thalamus. Here, a further synapse occurs, in this case with neurons that project via the sublentiform part of the internal capsule to the **auditory cortex** of the temporal lobe of the cerebral hemisphere.

Fibres from the superior olivary nucleus and inferior colliculus connect, either directly or indirectly, with the nuclei of other cranial nerves for reflex responses to auditory stimuli.

Vestibular pathway

The vestibular part of the internal ear provides information to the central nervous system which, together with that arriving from the visual system and from the proprioceptive endings scattered throughout the body, plays a major part in maintaining equilibrium. The vestibular labyrinth consists of the utricle and saccule, concerned with the appreciation of the static position of the head, and the three semicircular canals which detect movements of the head. The cell bodies of the first-order neurons are situated in the **vestibular ganglion** which lies close to the lateral end of the internal acoustic meatus. These neurons connect with the receptor cells in the various parts of the vestibular labyrinth and have central processes which constitute the **vestibular nerve.**

Most of the central processes end in the **vestibular nuclei** of the brainstem. The remainder pass to the cerebellum through the inferior cerebellar peduncle. The connections of the vestibular nuclei are with the cerebellum, spinal cord, brainstem, and cerebral cortex.

The projection to the cerebellum, consisting of fibres directly from the vestibular nerve as well as from the nuclei, is concerned with the maintenance of equilibrium through the influence that this part of the brain has over muscle tone.

Fibres from the lateral vestibular nucleus descend in the ipsilateral **vestibulospinal tract** in the ventral white column of the spinal cord to connect with lower motor neurons in the ventral grey horn. They help to maintain balance by regulating muscle tone. Other fibres from the vestibular nuclei connect bilaterally with ventral horn cells in the cervical region of the cord and with the abducent, trochlear, and oculomotor nuclei. In this way movements of the head and eyes are co-ordinated to maintain visual fixation.

The **vestibular area** of the cerebral cortex is believed to lie adjacent to the general sensory area for the head. Fibres ascending to this area travel close to the medial lemniscus and are predominantly crossed.

MOTOR PATHWAYS

Corticospinal and corticobulbar pathways (pyramidal system)

These pathways play an important part in the voluntary control of movement. Their constituent fibres begin in the **primary motor area** and adjacent zones of the cerebral cortex, most being the axons of the pyramidal and fusiform cells of these areas. About 3 per cent of the fibres have a much larger diameter (more than 11 μm) than the remainder. These rapidly conducting fibres are believed to be the axons of the giant pyramidal cells of the motor area.

Fibres from the ventral part of the primary motor area join the corticobulbar tract while those from the more dorsal parts of the area join the corticospinal tract, as would be expected from the somatotopic representation of the body regions in the precentral gyrus. Together with contributions from the adjacent areas of the cortex, these fibres pass through the corona radiata, posterior limb of the internal capsule and basis pedunculi of the midbrain.

The corticospinal tract becomes broken up into several discrete bundles as it traverses the basal part of the pons and then comes together again in the medulla where it forms a prominent bulge, the **pyramid,** on the ventral surface. At the caudal end of the medulla many of the fibres decussate. The actual number crossing over in this way varies between individuals but averages more than two-thirds of the total. The crossed fibres continue downwards into the cord as the **lateral corticospinal tract** and the uncrossed fibres continue as the **ventral corticospinal tract** although it is believed that some may enter the lateral tract. Most of the fibres in the ventral tract eventually cross to the opposite side before terminating. Although the majority of corticospinal fibres decussate some control of ipsilateral muscle activity is exerted by the fibres of the ventral tract that do not cross as well as by uncrossed fibres that are believed to travel in the lateral tract.

The corticospinal fibres terminate in the grey matter of the spinal cord. They connect with the alpha and gamma motor neurons (whose cell bodies are located in lamina IX) mostly through the intermediary of connector neurons. A few, however, synapse directly with the motor neurons.

During their descent, the corticospinal fibres give collateral branches to the thalamus, neostriatum, red nucleus, pontine nuclei, and the reticular formation of the brainstem.

The corticobulbar tract descends through the brainstem along the medial side of the corticospinal tract. It dwindles rapidly in size as bundles of fibres leave it at intervals to supply the motor nuclei of the cranial nerves. Most of the corticobulbar fibres end in the reticular formation adjacent to the nuclei and connect with the motor neurons through connector neurons but a few enter the nuclei and terminate directly on the motor neurons. Most corticobulbar fibres cross to the opposite side but numerous ipsilateral connections also occur. The only exceptions to this are the lower part of the motor nucleus of the facial nerve and the hypoglossal nucleus where the connections are predominantly, if not exclusively, with the contralateral corticobulbar tract.

It will be noted that in the pathways for voluntary movement just described there are two principal neurons between motor cortex and muscle. The first begins in the cortex and ends in a motor nucleus in the brainstem or in the grey matter of the cord and, in most cases, crosses the midline before terminating; the second begins in a motor nucleus or in the ventral grey matter of the cord and traverses a peripheral nerve to reach the muscle. These are usually referred to

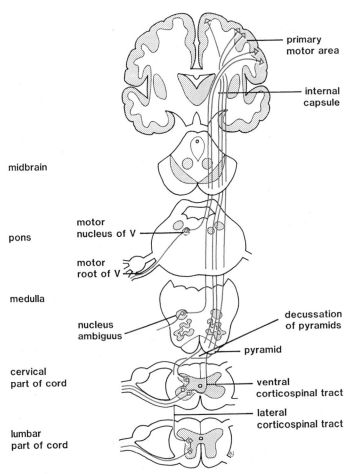

midbrain

pons

medulla

cervical
part of cord

lumbar
part of cord

primary
motor area

internal
capsule

motor
nucleus of V

motor
root of V

nucleus
ambiguus

decussation
of pyramids

pyramid

ventral
corticospinal tract

lateral
corticospinal tract

Fig. 5.35. The corticospinal and corticobulbar motor pathways. In the interests of clarity only the crossed fibres to the trigeminal nucleus and to the nucleus ambiguus are shown.

Other descending pathways

Pontine reticular nuclei give rise to fibres which travel ipsilaterally in the **reticulospinal tract in the ventral funiculus** of the cord while fibres from **medullary reticular nuclei** travel in the **reticulospinal tract in the lateral funiculus** of both sides. These two tracts end mainly in laminae VII, VIII (mostly pontine fibres), and IX (mostly medullary fibres). The reticulospinal fibres have many branches within the brainstem and spinal cord. Afferents to the reticular nuclei are known to come from the motor and sensory areas of the cerebral cortex, the spinal cord and the cerebellum.

The **vestibulospinal tract** originates in the **lateral vestibular nucleus** of the same side and terminates mainly in lamina VIII.

Functional and clinical aspects of voluntary control of muscle action

The voluntary control of muscle action is still far from fully understood but it will be clear from the foregoing that many parts of the nervous system are involved. The motor and associated areas of the cortex are obviously of great importance but their electrical stimulation produces much simpler movements than the normal voluntary movements resulting from conscious control. In the latter case, many more areas of the cortex are involved than with electrical stimulation and the thalamic nuclei, corpus striatum, and cerebellum also have important roles.

The cerebellum receives a copious input from the cerebral cortex, vestibular system, proprioceptive endings in muscles, tendons, and joints, reticular formation and from the inferior olivary nucleus (which, in turn, receives afferents from the red nucleus, motor cortex, and spinal cord). It projects to the ventral lateral nucleus of the thalamus, red nucleus, reticular formation, and vestibular nuclei. The thalamic nucleus also receives many efferents from the paleostriatum and itself projects to the motor areas of the cortex. The cerebellum plays an important part in the control of muscle activity including the maintenance of equilibrium (in response to vestibular stimuli) and of muscle tonus and synergy. Through its connections with the motor cortical areas, the cerebellum also helps ensure that voluntary movements are carried out smoothly, precisely and in the correct sequence.

Most of the afferents to the corpus striatum end in the neostriatum (i.e. caudate nucleus + putamen). These come from the neocortex of the cerebral hemisphere, thalamus and substantia nigra. Efferents from the neostriatum end in the paleostriatum (globus pallidus) and substantia nigra. The fibres leaving the corpus striatum arise mainly in the paleostriatum and project to the ventral lateral thalamic nucleus which projects, in turn, to the motor areas of the cerebral cortex. The paleostriatum also has reciprocal connections with the subthalamic nucleus.

Although the precise functions of the corpus striatum, and its connections are still poorly understood, it seems likely from clinical findings, that they are essential for the control of muscular activity. The numerous interconnections of these nuclei with each other and with other areas of the brain suggest that they are centres where much integrative activity occurs.

Disorders of movements take many forms. Perhaps the simplest is that produced by a lesion of the lower motor neurons. These neurons represent the final common pathway through which all the higher centres, and their descending tracts, exert their influence on the muscles. Their interruption, either by trauma to a peripheral

as **upper** and **lower motor neurons** respectively (the term upper motor neuron is now increasingly taken to include all the descending fibres involved in the voluntary control of muscle action, not just the corticospinal or corticobulbar fibres – see next section). Lesions involving these two parts of the pathway produce different effects upon muscle function (see next section).

Because the corticospinal tracts traverse the pyramids of the medulla they are frequently termed the pyramidal pathways. It is usual, although inaccurate, to include the corticobulbar tracts under this heading. As is described in the following section, the lower motor neurons are acted upon by many other fibres descending from higher centres besides those in the pyramidal tracts. It was at one time customary to call these other fibres the extrapyramidal system to distinguish them from the pyramidal fibres. This term, which was always vague and unsatisfactory, has now largely fallen into disuse.

nerve or as a result of infections (such as poliomyelitis which specifically affects ventral horn cells) effectively denervates the associated muscles leading to paralysis with muscle flaccidity and wasting and absent tendon reflexes.

The features of an 'upper motor neuron' lesion include absent (or weak) voluntary movements of the muscles, increased muscle tone (spasticity) and enhanced tendon reflexes. Wasting of the muscles is not marked. The type of 'upper motor neuron' lesion that the dentist is likely to encounter is caused by a cerebrovascular accident (thrombus or haemorrhage) in the region of the posterior limb of the internal capsule. Such an event – called a 'stroke' in lay terminology – is not uncommon in the elderly. After the initial effects wear off, the victim is left with some degree of voluntary paralysis (or weakness, termed paresis), hyperreflexia, and spasticity on the opposite side of the body to which the lesion occurred (there will also be an accompanying loss or modification of all modalities of sensation). Because the flexor muscles are stronger than the extensors in the upper limb while the reverse is true in the lower limb, the spasticity produces a characteristic gait in which the affected arm is carried with the elbow flexed and the forearm held across the chest and the corresponding leg is swung forwards with the knee and ankle joint extended. The bilateral projection to most of the motor nuclei in the brainstem usually prevents any marked effect upon the muscles innervated by the associated cranial nerves. The exceptions to this are the caudal part of the facial motor nucleus and the hypoglossal nucleus where the afferent corticobulbar fibres are crossed. Voluntary paralysis of the muscles of the lower part of the face, together with some weakness in the tongue, on the opposite side to the lesion is consequently a frequent clinical feature in strokes.

It was at one time thought that 'upper motor neuron' paralysis was caused specifically by interruption of corticospinal and corticobulbar fibres. However, experiments in animals have indicated that such a lesion produces reduced tone in the contralateral muscles with little or no effect upon the tendon reflexes. The principal deficit appears to be clumsiness in the use of the contralateral limbs. Lesions limited to the pyramidal pathway are rare in human beings but there are a few clinical observations suggesting that when they do occur they produce deficits similar to those in experimental animals. This has led to the view that the principal function of the pyramidal system is in the control of highly skilled movements. How the features of an 'upper motor neuron' type of paralysis are produced is still not fully understood but it seems likely from the experimental findings just described that interruption of pathways additional to the pyramidal must be involved.

Lesions, often of a degenerative nature, may affect the corpus striatum and related nuclei, and are associated with involuntary movements (called dyskinesias). These include choreiform movements (intermittent, purposeless twitching of individual muscles) and athetoid movements (slow sinuous writhings, especially of the limbs). The most common dyskinesia is Parkinson's disease (paralysis agitans) in which degeneration in the substantia nigra is accompanied by poverty of voluntary movement, tremor, and muscular rigidity.

AUTONOMIC NERVOUS SYSTEM

A large part of the nervous system is given over to the control of the internal viscera. Much of the activity of these organs is controlled reflexly at lower levels but there are also higher centres, notably the **hypothalamus** and the '**vital centres**' in the **reticular formation,** involved in governing the general tone of visceral activity. At these higher levels somatic and visceral functions are closely integrated as is obvious from the readiness with which emotional factors or the stimulation of somatic afferents can influence such visceral features as heart rate, blood pressure, and gastrointestinal activity.

So far as the dental student is concerned the most important part of the autonomic nervous system is the motor outflow from the brainstem and spinal cord (in fact the term autonomic nervous system is often used as though synonymous with just its motor side). In order to understand the total functioning of the system, however, it is necessary to add a brief outline of the pathways followed by the sensory fibres from the viscera.

Visceral efferents

Visceral efferents innervate the smooth muscle and secretory cells of the gastrointestinal and respiratory systems, the smooth and cardiac muscle of the cardiovascular system, the sweat glands and arrector pili muscles of the skin and the muscles of the ciliary body and iris of the eyeball. In many cases there is a dual supply from the **sympathetic** and **parasympathetic divisions** of the autonomic nervous system. The sympathetic efferents leave the central nervous system from the thoracic and upper lumbar segments of the spinal cord while the parasympathetic efferents leave from the brainstem and from the sacral segments of the cord. In both instances there is a sequence of two neurons between the central grey matter and the effector organ which synapse with each other in a peripheral autonomic ganglion (note that autonomic ganglia contain synapses but that sensory ganglia do not). The neuron proximal to the synapse is termed **preganglionic** and that distal to the synapse is called **postganglionic**. In the case of the gastrointestinal tract, a third neuron may be interposed between the postganglionic neuron and the effector cells. The third neuron is part of the enteric plexus within the wall of the tract.

The functional effects of the two divisions of the autonomic system are antagonistic but under normal circumstances there is a balance between them which maintains an appropriate level of visceral activity. In states of alarm or anger there is a massive stimulation of the sympathetic outflow which completely overrides the parasympathetic effects and results in the body being placed in a state of activity suitable for violent physical activity, the so called 'fight or flight' response. This effect is backed up and prolonged by increased secretion of adrenalin from the adrenal medulla.

The postganglionic parasympathetic fibres are cholinergic (i.e. release acetylcholine). Postganglionic sympathetic fibres are noradrenergic (i.e. release noradrenalin) apart from those to sweat glands which are cholinergic.

Sympathetic (thoracolumbar) outflow

Each sympathetic trunk consists of a chain of interconnected ganglia extending throughout the trunk and neck and situated just lateral to the vertebral column (Figs. 3.35 and 3.36). The number of ganglia varies but typically there are three in the cervical region, twelve in the thoracic region, four in the lumbar region, and four or five in the sacral region. The original one-to-one correspondence between the sympathetic ganglia and the spinal nerves has been lost by the phylogenetic tendency for adjacent sympathetic ganglia to fuse. Each ganglion is connected to the corresponding spinal nerve by a **grey ramus communicans** carrying postganglionic fibres. In regions where fusion of ganglia has occurred the ganglia are attached by grey rami to the nerves issuing from several spinal segments. Thus the first cervical ganglion, formed by fusion of the upper four sympathetic ganglia, is connected by a grey ramus to each of the upper four cervical nerves. The ganglia corresponding to the thoracic and upper two or three lumbar segments of the cord are each connected to their spinal nerve by a **white ramus communicans** as well as by a grey ramus. The white rami carry preganglionic neurons. In some segments the white and grey rami may fuse to form a mixed ramus.

In addition to the rami communicantes the sympathetic ganglia give off **visceral** and **vascular branches.** The visceral branches pass to large autonomic plexuses in the thoracic and abdominal cavities from which the viscera of the trunk receive their innervation. Vascular branches leave many of the ganglia of the sympathetic trunk and pass to nearby arteries where they form plexuses about the vessels and are so distributed to the periphery.

The cell bodies of the preganglionic sympathetic neurons are located in the **intermediolateral cell column** of the lateral grey horn of the thoracic and upper lumbar segments of the cord. Their myelinated axons pass to the sympathetic trunk through the ventral roots, spinal nerves, and white rami of these segments. Once within the trunk the fibres may end in the ganglion corresponding to the segment of exit, ascend or descend to terminate in a ganglion at a higher or lower level, or leave, without synapsing, through a visceral branch of one of these ganglia.

The fibres terminating in a ganglion of the sympathetic trunk do so by synapsing with the postganglionic neurons (probably in some instances through connector neurons). The axons of the postganglionic neurons are of small diameter and mostly unmyelinated. They may leave the ganglion through a grey ramus communicans or a visceral or vascular branch or they may ascend to a higher or lower level of the sympathetic trunk before leaving through one of these routes.

The fibres leaving through a grey ramus communicans join the corresponding spinal nerve and are distributed, through its branches, to the blood vessels, sweat glands, and arrector pili muscles of the area supplied by the nerve. Those that leave in a visceral branch are distributed to the viscera of the trunk. The fibres that pass in the vascular branches join the sympathetic plexuses on the arteries and supply the vessel and its branches and are also carried to the structures in the peripheral area of distribution of the vessels. This is a particularly important route for the postganglionic fibres supplying the head and neck.

The preganglionic fibres which traverse the sympathetic trunk without synapsing enter the visceral branches of the ganglia. Through these they reach the autonomic plexuses in the thoracic and abdominal cavities where they end in one of the associated ganglia by synapsing with postganglionic neurons.

The adrenal medulla is supplied directly by preganglionic sympathetic neurons. This is explained by the fact that the cells of the adrenal medulla are, in reality, modified postganglionic sympathetic neurons.

Cervical part

The cervical part of the sympathetic trunk (Fig 4.55) bears three ganglia, the **superior** representing the fused ganglia of the upper four segments, the **middle,** the fused ganglia of the fifth and sixth segments and the **inferior,** the fused ganglia of the seventh and eighth segments.

Continuing upwards from the superior ganglion is the **internal carotid nerve,** composed principally of postganglionic fibres from the ganglion. It runs upwards behind the internal carotid artery and terminates in the carotid canal of the temporal bone by dividing into medial and lateral branches which form a plexus around the internal carotid artery.

The **internal carotid plexus** gives communicating branches to cranial nerves III, IV, V, VI, and IX. It also communicates with the pterygopalatine and ciliary ganglia. The route to the pterygopalatine ganglion is through the deep petrosal branch of the plexus which enters the pterygoid canal and joins with the greater petrosal branch of the facial, forming the nerve of the pterygoid canal. The sympathetic fibres pass through the ganglion without synapse and are distributed in its branches. The branch to the ciliary ganglion contains vasomotor fibres which traverse the ganglion without synapse to be distributed to the blood vessels of the eyeball through the short ciliary nerves.

The superior cervical ganglion gives grey rami communicantes to the upper four cervical spinal nerves. Its visceral branches are the **laryngopharyngeal** (to the carotid body and pharyngeal plexus) and the **cardiac** (to the cardiac and pulmonary plexuses). The vascular branches ramify on the common carotid and external carotid arteries and their branches. Postganglionic fibres to the dilator pupillae muscle begin in the superior cervical ganglion but their route to the eyeball is uncertain. The middle ganglion gives grey rami to the fifth and sixth cervical nerves. The visceral branches of this ganglion are to the cardiac plexus and the thyroid gland and its vascular branches join the plexuses on the subclavian and inferior thyroid arteries. The grey rami of the inferior ganglion pass to the seventh and eighth cervical nerves, its visceral branch passes to the cardiac plexus, and its vascular branches pass to the subclavian and vertebral arteries.

Thoracic part

There are usually twelve sympathetic ganglia in the thoracic trunk although the first is often fused with the inferior cervical ganglion. Each is connected with the corresponding spinal nerve by a grey and a white ramus. From the upper five ganglia vascular branches pass to the thoracic aorta and its branches and visceral branches to the pulmonary plexuses. The lower seven ganglia give off large visceral branches which unite to form the **greater** (from ganglia 5–9 or 10), **lesser** (from ganglia 10 and 11) and **least** (from ganglion 12) **splanchnic nerves.** These pierce the diaphragm and join the autonomic plexuses in the abdominal cavity. It seems that the splanchnic nerves are made up largely, if not entirely, of preganglionic fibres which have passed through the ganglia of the sympathetic chain without interruption and which synapse with postganglionic neurons in the abdominal autonomic plexuses.

Lumbar and sacral parts

The upper two or three ganglia of the lumbar region connect with the corresponding spinal nerves by white and grey rami communicantes. The remaining lumbar ganglia have grey rami only. The visceral branches of the ganglia are the lumbar splanchnic nerves which travel to the abdominal and pelvic autonomic plexuses and their associated ganglia. Vascular branches pass to the plexus on the abdominal part of the aorta.

Grey rami pass from the sacral ganglia to the sacral and coccygeal spinal nerves, visceral branches pass to the adjacent autonomic plexuses and vascular branches to the plexuses on the pelvic arteries.

Parasympathetic (craniosacral) outflow

The parasympathetic system has no regularly ganglionated chain equivalent to the sympathetic trunk. Instead the ganglia are arranged in an irregular fashion close to the organs being supplied. The preganglionic neurons tend, therefore, to be considerably longer than the postganglionic neurons.

Cranial part

The parasympathetic fibres in the cranial region begin in motor nuclei of the brainstem equivalent to the lateral grey horn of the spinal cord. They leave in cranial nerves III, VII, IX, and X. The parasympathetic fibres in the cranial nerves are also termed general visceral motor to distinguish them from the special visceral fibres to the pharyngeal arch musculature.

A detailed account of the parasympathetic outflow in the cranial nerves is given in Chapter 5.6 and need not be repeated here. The situation can be briefly summarized by stating that the parasympathetic fibres in the oculomotor nerve supply the ciliary body and sphincter pupillae of the eyeball, those in the facial and glossopharyngeal nerves supply salivary and other glands in the head and neck and those in the vagus innervate the respiratory system, heart and the gastrointestinal tract as far as the left flexure of the large intestine. The preganglionic fibres in the oculomotor, facial and glossopharyngeal relay respectively in the ciliary ganglion, in the pterygopalatine and submandibular ganglia, and in the otic ganglion. The corresponding relays in the case of the vagus nerve are found in the autonomic plexuses and the ganglia in, or close to, the organ being supplied.

Sacral part

The gastrointestinal tract below the left flexure and the remaining pelvic viscera receive their parasympathetic innervation through preganglionic neurons which leave the spinal cord in the second to fourth sacral spinal nerves. These connect with the postganglionic neurons in ganglia close to the viscera.

Visceral afferents

Visceral sensory fibres may be divided into two main groups, the **special visceral afferents** concerned with taste (some authors include olfaction as a special visceral sense) and the **general visceral afferents** from the viscera and blood vessels. The pathways for taste are described in Chapter 5.6.

The general visceral afferent fibres convey information which does not usually reach consciousness. They are the peripheral processes of cells located in the sensory ganglia of the same spinal nerves which contribute to the sympathetic efferent outflow and in the ganglia of the glossopharyngeal and vagus nerves. These processes are of various diameters and may be myelinated or unmyelinated. They are distributed with the pre- and postganglionic efferent fibres but pass through the autonomic ganglia without synapse. Thus many visceral afferents leave the spinal cord in the thoracic and upper lumbar regions, their cell bodies being located in the spinal ganglia of the

first thoracic to second or third lumbar spinal nerves. Their peripheral processes pass out through the dorsal roots, spinal nerves, and white rami communicantes to reach the sympathetic ganglia and are then distributed through the visceral and vascular branches. They terminate mostly as unencapsulated endings. The central processes enter the cord through the dorsal roots and end in the grey matter of the thoracic and upper lumbar segments. They connect, either directly or through connector neurons, with the preganglionic visceral efferents of the lateral horn so establishing the pathways for reflex visceral action.

There is a large general visceral afferent component in the vagus nerve. The cell bodies are located in the inferior ganglion of the nerve. Their peripheral processes are widely distributed through the branches of the nerve, the area of supply corresponding broadly with that of the visceral efferent component of the vagus. Their central processes end in the caudal part of the nucleus of the tractus solitarius. There are also general visceral afferents in the glossopharyngeal nerve (from the carotid sinus and body). The oculomotor nerve, and probably the facial nerve as well, contains no visceral afferent fibres despite contributing to the autonomic efferent outflow.

Under certain pathological conditions sensations of pain from the viscera may reach consciousness. Probably the best known example is 'stomach ache' following dietary indiscretions. The pain may be felt in the region of the viscera itself or may be referred to the area of skin which receives somatic sensory fibres from the same segments of the cord. The central pathways followed by these pain impulses are not well understood.

Clinical aspects

One of the main practical reasons for acquiring a knowledge of the structure and functioning of the autonomic nervous system is as a basis for understanding the pharmacology of the many important drugs used in clinical practice that act through their effects upon the sympathetic or parasympathetic efferents or by mimicking their actions.

Diseases of the autonomic nervous system itself are not common although parts of the system may be affected by lesions in adjacent organs. The sympathetic preganglionic fibres passing upwards to the cervical ganglia may, for example, be interrupted by compression of the upper part of the thoracic sympathetic trunk. One cause of such compression is enlargement of the mediastinal lymph nodes as a result of the spread of bronchial carcinoma from the lung. The interruption of the sympathetic fibres produces, on the side of the lesion, (i) constriction of the pupil (miosis) due to paralysis of the dilator pupillae muscle; (ii) drooping of the upper eyelid (ptosis) because of paralysis of the part of levator palpebrae superioris composed of smooth muscle; (iii) absence of sweating (anhydrosis) in the skin of the face; and (iv) slight retrusion of the eyeball (enophthalmos). This group of clinical signs is known as Horner's syndrome and may be the first clinical manifestation of the primary disease.

6

Cranial nerves III to XII

The structure, function, development, and evolution of the ten 'true' cranial nerves have been briefly discussed in Chapter 2.3. It was pointed out there that, according to the classical scheme of head segmentation worked out in the nineteenth and early twentieth centuries, each of these nerves might be thought of as equivalent to either a ventral or a dorsal root of a spinal nerve. As in the spinal region the ventral nerves (oculomotor, trochlear, abducent, and hypoglossal) supply somatic motor fibres to striated, voluntary muscle derived from myotomes or mesoderm equivalent to myotomes. The dorsal nerves (trigeminal, facial, glossopharyngeal, and vagus + cranial accessory), like their spinal counterparts, supply sensory fibres to the corresponding dermatomes and their derivatives. The dorsal nerves, therefore, can be recognized by the fact that they bear sensory ganglia equivalent to the spinal ganglia. There are, however, three major ways in which the dorsal cranial nerves differ from the dorsal spinal roots: (1) the dorsal cranial nerves do not fuse with the corresponding ventral nerves (although it has been postulated that there was an original one-to-one correspondence between dorsal and ventral nerves); (2) the general visceral motor fibres leaving the brain (all parasympathetic) pass in the dorsal cranial nerves—in the spinal region, by contrast, the general visceral motor fibres (mostly sympathetic) leave the spinal cord in the ventral roots; (3) each dorsal cranial nerve has become associated with a specific pharyngeal arch and carries motor fibres to the muscles from that arch. The trigeminal is associated with the first (mandibular) arch, the facial with the second (hyoid) arch, the glossopharyngeal with the third arch, and the vagus + cranial accessory with the succeeding arches. Because the mesoderm of the arches was thought to be of lateral plate (i.e. visceral) origin the nerve fibres supplying the arch muscles were called special visceral motor ('special' because although of supposed visceral origin the muscles are striated and voluntary). It now appears that the myogenic component of the arch mesoderm comes initially from the somitomeres of the anterior head region in which case the term visceral is inappropriate and a better name for these nerve fibres would be branchiomotor. However, the term special visceral motor is still by far the most widely used in human anatomy and, for that reason, is retained here.

It will probably be helpful at this stage to summarize the types of neuron that may be found in the cranial nerves. According to the scheme just propounded, the ventral cranial nerves (III, IV, VI, and XII, should contain somatic motor fibres only. On a similar basis, the dorsal cranial nerves (V, VII, IX, and X + cranial XI) should contain somatic sensory (cutaneous sensation and proprioception), visceral sensory (general visceral sensory and special visceral sensory or taste), general visceral motor (parasympathetic), and special visceral motor (branchiomotor) fibres. There is general agreement with these expectations but a few exceptions occur. In particular the oculomotor contains a general visceral motor component (parasympathetic fibres

to the eyeball) and several of the dorsal cranial nerves are lacking one or more of their components.

The vestibulocochlear nerve probably represents fused components of the facial, glossopharyngeal, and vagus nerves which supplied that part of the lateral line organ in the head region which became, during evolution, the internal ear. It is not described further in this chapter but is dealt with briefly in the section on the auditory pathway in Chapter 5.5 and in Appendix 3.

There is an essential similarity between the functional arrangement of the nuclei of the cranial nerves in the brainstem and of the grey matter in the spinal cord, reflecting the fact that in both of these regions the motor grey areas develop from the basal plates and the sensory areas from the alar plates (p. 59). In order to understand this similarity it is helpful to imagine a series of columns extending into the brainstem from the grey horns of the spinal cord. Each column will then be found to contain nuclei with functions similar to those of the grey horn with which they are in line. Apart from the trigeminal sensory nuclei, however, these nuclei occupy only parts of their respective columns; as can be seen from Fig. 5.36 there are long stretches in between where no nuclei are present.

One column can be considered as extending upwards from the dorsal grey horn. This contains nuclei associated, like the dorsal grey horn itself, with somatic sensory neurons – that is the various sensory nuclei of the trigeminal nerve. A second column ascends in line with the ventral grey horn and contains nuclei in which are found, as in the ventral horn, cell bodies of somatic lower motor neurons – that is the nuclei of the oculomotor, trochlear, abducent, and hypoglossal nerves.

Between the somatic sensory and somatic motor columns are the visceral sensory and visceral motor columns. They occupy the same general position within the brainstem as does the lateral grey horn in the thoracolumbar segments of the cord. In the brainstem region, however, both of the visceral columns are further subdivided into general and special. As would be expected, the sensory visceral columns lie dorsal to the motor visceral columns and within each pair the special column lies further from the midtransverse plane than does the general column. Hence the sequence of visceral columns in a dorsoventral direction is special visceral sensory, general visceral sensory, general visceral motor, and special visceral motor (although it should be emphasized again that the muscles supplied from the last column are probably not of visceral origin).

The special visceral sensory column contains the rostral part of the nucleus of the tractus solitarius. The taste fibres, which are conveyed to the brainstem in the facial, glossopharyngeal, and vagus nerves, end here. The general visceral sensory fibres arriving at the brainstem, principally in the vagus, but also in the glossopharyngeal nerve, terminate in the caudal part of the nucleus of the tractus solitarius. As can be seen from Fig. 5.36 this inclines from the rostral part of the nucleus to lie in the general visceral sensory column. The general visceral motor column contains the superior and inferior salivatory nuclei and the dorsal nucleus of the vagus. The cell bodies of the preganglionic parasympathetic neurons, which are distributed in the facial, glossopharyngeal, and vagus nerves, begin in these nuclei. In the midbrain there is a further general visceral motor nucleus associated with the oculomotor nerve. This, the Edinger–Westphal nucleus, provides preganglionic parasympathetic fibres for the innervation of the eyeball. The special visceral motor column contains the motor nuclei of the trigeminal and facial nerves, for the muscles of the mandibular and hyoid arches respectively, and the nucleus ambiguus from which fibres pass in the glossopharyngeal, vagus, and cranial accessory nerves to the muscles of the remaining arches. Owing to migration during embryonic development the nucleus ambiguus is situated rather more laterally than would be expected on theoretical grounds. Migration also affects the relative positions of some of the other cranial nuclei but the scheme just outlined is sufficiently accurate to provide a useful basis for understanding their general arrangement.

In the pons and upper medulla the dorsoventral arrangement of the columns is disturbed by the presence of the fourth ventricle. The enlargement of the central canal to form the ventricle takes place principally in a dorsal direction so that the grey matter originally located dorsal to the canal is displaced laterally. In other words the columns in the upper part of the medulla and in the pons become arranged in a medial to lateral, rather than a ventral to dorsal, sequence but their order with respect to each other remains unchanged. The position of the columns in this part of the brainstem, as shown in Fig. 5.36, can be related to the sulcus limitans in the floor of the fourth ventricle which represents, just as it does in the spinal cord, the dividing line between the alar and basal plates.

In the following sections of this chapter the emphasis is on the types of neurons in the cranial nerves and their central connections. The peripheral course and distribution of the nerves are described in the chapters on the regional anatomy of the head and neck.

CRANIAL NERVES III, IV, VI, XII

Oculomotor

The oculomotor nerve supplies the extraocular muscles, with the exception of the superior oblique and lateral rectus, and most of levator palpebrae superioris. It also supplies parasympathetic fibres to the sphincter pupillae and ciliary muscle of the eyeball. The somatic lower motor neurons to the extraocular muscles and the levator muscle begin in the **oculomotor nucleus** which is situated ventral to the aqueduct of the midbrain in the central grey matter at the level of the superior colliculus. It is the most rostral of the nuclei in the somatic motor column. The axons from this nucleus run ventrally through the tegmentum of the midbrain, traverse the red nucleus and emerge from the brainstem in the interpeduncular fossa. It appears likely that some of the axons cross the midline to join the oculomotor nerve of the opposite side. As with the other nerves supplying the extraocular muscles, the number of muscle fibres supplied by each nerve fibre (i.e. the motor unit) is very small (about six) so allowing a very precise control of eye movements.

The general visceral motor, or parasympathetic, preganglionic fibres for the sphincter pupillae and ciliary body begin in the **Edinger–**

Westphal nucleus. This is situated close to the rostral part of the main oculomotor nucleus, in the central grey matter. The preganglionic fibres leave the brainstem in company with the somatic motor fibres, pass into the inferior branch of the oculomotor nerve and then into the motor branch to the **ciliary ganglion.** Within the ganglion they synapse with postganglionic fibres which run to the eyeball in the short ciliary nerves.

The oculomotor nucleus has numerous central connections, important amongst which are those with the cerebral cortex (through the superior colliculus and pretectal area), the reticular formation, nuclei controlling the other extraocular muscles, and the vestibular nuclei, for the voluntary control of eye movements, and the coordination of eye and head movements. The Edinger–Westphal nucleus receives afferents from the pretectal area and superior colliculus for reflex responses to light and accommodation.

Trochlear

The trochlear nerve innervates the superior oblique muscle. Its fibres begin in the **trochlear nucleus** which lies in the central grey matter of

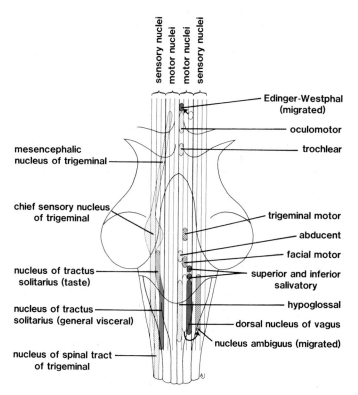

Fig. 5.36. Brainstem in dorsal view to illustrate the arrangement of the motor (right) and sensory (left) cranial nerve nuclei. For clarity the columns are shown in medial to lateral sequence. This is correct for the open medulla but in the closed medulla and midbrain the sequence is ventral (= medial) to dorsal (= lateral). The arrangement shown here is an idealized one based on developmental and evolutionary studies. In fact several of the nuclei change their relative positions to some degree during development. This is especially true for the Edinger–Westphal nucleus and the nucleus ambiguus (cf. Fig. 2.33).

the midbrain at the level of the inferior colliculus. It is immediately caudal to, and in line with, the oculomotor nucleus. The central connections of the nucleus are similar to those of the oculomotor nucleus.

The trochlear nerve is unique in that it is the only cranial nerve which emerges from the dorsal surface of the brainstem and in which all the fibres cross the midline. The fibres leave the trochlear nucleus by running dorsally and medially behind the aqueduct, where they decussate with the fibres from the opposite nucleus, to emerge from the midbrain below the contralateral inferior colliculus.

Abducent

The **abducent nucleus** is situated in the grey matter forming the floor of the fourth ventricle. It is in the same column as the oculomotor and trochlear nuclei and has similar central connections. Fibres from the motor nucleus of the facial nerve loop dorsal to the abducent nucleus to form the **facial colliculus**. The abducent fibres run ventrally through the pons to emerge at the junction of this part of the brainstem with the medulla. The nerve has a long intracranial course (p. 137) before entering the orbit through the superior orbital fissure. It supplies the lateral rectus muscle.

Hypoglossal

The **hypoglossal nucleus** is located in the closed part of the medulla in the ventral part of the grey matter surrounding the central canal. It extends rostrally for a short distance into the open part of the medulla where it lies beneath the hypoglossal triangle in the floor of the fourth ventricle. It is the most caudal of the nuclei in the somatic motor column. Axons from the nucleus run ventrally and emerge from the brainstem as a series of rootlets between the pyramid and olive. These rootlets join together to form two trunks which leave the cranial cavity through the hypoglossal canal and unite just outside the skull. The hypoglossal nerve supplies all the intrinsic muscles of the tongue as well as hyoglossus, genioglossus, and styloglossus.

The hypoglossal nucleus receives afferents mostly from the contralateral corticobulbar tract. It also receives afferents from the sensory nuclei of the trigeminal nerve and the nucleus of the tractus solitarius for reflex tongue movements during chewing and swallowing. Unilateral interruption of the corticobulbar tract causes weakness of the opposite side of the tongue. Damage to the nucleus or the nerve produces paralysis and atrophy of the lingual muscles on the side of the lesion. If the tongue is protruded it deviates to the affected side because of the unopposed action of the normal genioglossus.

CRANIAL NERVES V, VII, IX, X + XI

Trigeminal

The trigeminal is made up chiefly of sensory fibres from the skin of the front of the head, the cornea, the mucous membranes lining the oral, nasal, and paranasal cavities, much of the dura mater, the teeth and their supporting tissues and from proprioceptive endings in many of the muscles of the head and in the temporomandibular joint. It also contains special visceral motor neurons to the muscles derived from the first pharyngeal arch. As it leaves the brainstem the

trigeminal contains no general visceral motor neurons but some of its peripheral branches give passage to such fibres received through communications with the facial and glossopharyngeal nerves.

The trigeminal nerve is attached to the lateral part of the pons by a large **sensory** and a small **motor root** (the latter being in fact not entirely motor). The sensory root is continuous with the **trigeminal ganglion** which is located within the trigeminal cave in the middle cranial fossa. The three divisions of the nerve spring directly from the ganglion. The motor root runs beneath the ganglion to join the mandibular division.

The cell bodies of most of the first-order sensory neurons in the trigeminal nerve are situated in the trigeminal ganglion. The central processes of these cells make up the sensory root of the nerve. In the brainstem the large diameter processes, for discriminative touch, end in the **chief sensory nucleus** of the trigeminal which is located in the dorsolateral part of the tegmentum of the pons (i.e. in the somatic sensory column). Some of the smaller diameter processes for simple touch and pressure also give branches which end in the chief nucleus.

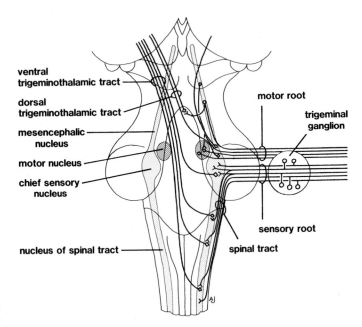

Fig. 5.37. The nuclei and central connections of the trigeminal nerve in dorsal view.

Most of the central processes for simple touch and pressure as well as the small-calibre processes for pain and temperature turn caudally on entering the brainstem to form the **spinal tract of the trigeminal**. This tract descends through the brainstem and into the upper three segments of the spinal cord. Immediately medial to the tract is the **nucleus of the spinal tract** which is continuous rostrally with the chief sensory nucleus and caudally with the dorsal grey horn of the upper part of the cord. It is situated, therefore, in the somatic sensory column. The spinal tract gradually diminishes in a caudal direction as its fibres terminate at successive levels in the nucleus. There is a somatotopic arrangement of the fibres in the spinal tract such that those from the ophthalmic division of the trigeminal run in its ventral part, those from the mandibular division in its dorsal part and those from the maxillary division in its intermediate part.

The spinal nucleus can be divided into three main parts—**caudal**, **intermediate**, and **rostral**. The caudal part has a similar cellular composition to the dorsal grey horn of the spinal cord (laminae I–IV). Most of the processes ending in this part of the nucleus are for pain and temperature. The somatotopic representation of the face in the caudal part of the spinal nucleus has been described as lamellar. If the area of trigeminal innervation on the face is divided into a series of approximately circular zones arranged concentrically around the mouth, then the innermost or circumoral zone (i.e. the lips and adjacent areas) is represented in the uppermost segment of the caudal subnucleus while the remaining zones are represented in successively more inferior segments with the outermost zone (stretching from the lower border of the chin across the posterior parts of the cheeks and the anterior parts of the auricles to the top of the scalp) being represented in the lowermost segment of the subnucleus. This is often referred to as an 'onion-like' representation because the facial zones are arranged rather like the layers of an onion. It is believed to apply to only the sensations of pain and temperature. The intermediate and rostral parts of the nucleus contain numerous small and medium sized cells. The processes ending here are mostly for simple touch and pressure, although the intermediate part is described as also receiving pain fibres from the teeth. The most caudal part of the nucleus receives pain and temperature fibres from the upper cervical nerves, as well as from the trigeminal.

Second-order neurons from the chief and spinal nuclei travel to the ventral posterior nucleus of the thalamus mainly in the contralateral **ventral trigeminothalamic tract**. Smaller numbers of fibres from the chief nucleus travel to the thalamus in the **dorsal trigeminothalamic tract** of both sides. The ventral and dorsal tracts are often referred to together as the **trigeminal lemniscus**. Efferents from the spinal nucleus also connect with the motor nuclei of the cranial nerves for reflex responses to stimulation of trigeminal sensory fibres.

Continuing rostrally from the chief sensory nucleus into the lateral part of the central grey matter of the midbrain is the **mesencephalic nucleus of trigeminal**. The cells in this nucleus are those of pseudounipolar first-order sensory neurons for proprioception and are unusual in that they are located in a central nucleus not in a sensory ganglion. Most of the peripheral processes of these cells leave the brainstem in the motor root of the trigeminal nerve and are distributed through the mandibular division to the neuromuscular spindles in the jaw muscles and to endings in the jaw joint and in the supporting tissues of the lower teeth. A lesser number are believed to travel through the sensory root and the ganglion to be distributed through the maxillary division to endings in the supporting tissues of the upper teeth and palate. In addition, proprioceptive fibres from neuromuscular spindles in the extraocular muscles, and possibly also from spindles in the facial, lingual, and laryngeal muscles, are believed to end in the mesencephalic nucleus in a manner similar to that just described. The central processes of the neurons whose cell bodies are located in the mescencephalic nucleus contact cells in the trigeminal motor nucleus for reflex control of jaw movements and also cells in the reticular formation from which axons pass to the thalamus.

The special visceral motor neurons in the trigeminal nerve begin in the **motor nucleus** of the nerve which is located medial to the chief sensory nucleus. It is the most rostral nucleus in the special visceral motor column. The axons of these cells run in the motor root of the nerve to the mandibular division through which they are distributed to the muscles derived from the mandibular arch (i.e. the muscles of mastication, mylohyoid, anterior belly of digastric, tensor veli palatini, and tensor tympani). The motor nucleus receives afferents from both the ipsilateral and contralateral corticobulbar tracts. It is connected with the sensory nuclei of the trigeminal nerve for reflex responses to stimulation of the area of sensory distribution of the nerve.

Clinical aspects

The importance of the trigeminal nerve in the practice of dentistry has already been sufficiently emphasized. The nerve is also involved in a number of other conditions which, while lying outside the province of the dental practitioner, may be seen in patients attending for dental treatment. The central connections of the trigeminal nuclei may be interrupted in cerebrovascular accidents, such as strokes, although because of the crossed nature of the higher tracts the effects are often difficult to demonstrate. The nuclei may be involved in lesions of the brainstem. If the motor nucleus is damaged there will be paralysis of the muscles of mastication with the result that on opening the mouth the jaw will deviate to the side of the lesion due to the unopposed contraction of the opposite lateral pterygoid muscle.

A particularly unpleasant condition is trigeminal neuralgia in which the victim suffers spasms of violent pain in the area of distribution of one of the divisions of the trigeminal nerve, usually the maxillary. Often the spasm is set off by touching a particular part (the 'trigger' area) of the skin of the face. Its cause is unknown but it is generally believed to operate in the trigeminal ganglion. The pain may be so bad and so frequent that surgery, to interrupt the pain pathway from the affected area, is necessary.

The trigeminal nerve may also be involved in shingles (*Herpes zoster*). This condition is caused by reactivation of the virus which lies latent in sensory nerve ganglia following a previous infection of chickenpox. It causes pain and crops of numerous small lesions on the skin in the area supplied by the ganglia. When it affects the trigeminal ganglion the pain and lesions occur on the face and in the mouth, their exact distribution depending upon which divisions of the nerve are involved. If the ophthalmic division is affected the lesions may occur on the cornea of the eye and may be followed by scarring with permanent impairment of vision.

Facial

The bulk of the facial nerve is made up of special visceral motor neurons to the numerous muscles derived from the second pharyngeal arch. The nerve also contains general visceral motor fibres which are secretomotor to the lacrimal gland, the submandibular and sublingual glands and to the glands associated with the mucosa of the nasal cavity, paranasal air sinuses, nasopharynx, and part of the oral cavity. The largest sensory component is provided by the special sensory fibres from the taste buds on the anterior two-thirds of the tongue and in the palate. There are also a few cutaneous (somatic sensory) fibres from a small area around the external acoustic meatus.

The facial nerve is attached to the brainstem at the junction of pons and medulla by a large **motor** and a small **sensory root**. Since the latter, which is not entirely sensory, emerges between the motor root and the vestibulocochlear nerve it is sometimes referred to as the **nervus intermedius.** The two roots enter the internal acoustic meatus

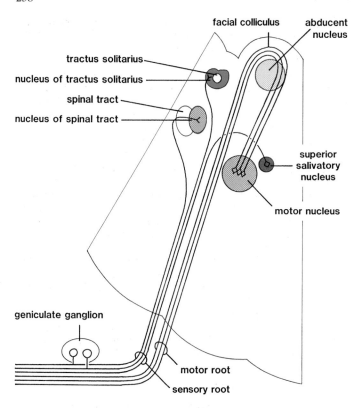

Fig. 5.38. The nuclei of the facial nerve.

in company with the vestibulocochlear nerve. At the bottom of the meatus the roots enter the facial canal and unite. Shortly beyond this point the nerve makes an abrupt turn, the genu, to run posteriorly and then inferiorly across the medial wall of the middle-ear cavity. At the turn the nerve bears the **geniculate ganglion**.

The cell bodies of the first-order sensory neurons in the facial nerve are contained within the geniculate ganglion. The central processes of the taste fibres enter the brainstem through the sensory root and then turn caudally in the **tractus solitarius**, where they are joined by taste and general visceral sensory fibres from the glosso-pharyngeal and vagus. The fibres end in the **nucleus of the tractus solitarius** which lies immediately alongside the tract. The **rostral part of the nucleus** (sometimes known as the gustatory nucleus) receives the taste fibres from the tract and is situated in the special visceral sensory column. The nucleus has numerous connections with the hypothalamus and with the motor nuclei of the cranial nerves, especially the salivatory nuclei and the dorsal nucleus of the vagus, for reflex responses to taste. Fibres from the nucleus project to the ventral posterior nucleus of the thalamus (probably bilaterally), from where third-order neurons pass to the taste area in the lower part of the postcentral gyrus.

The peripheral processes of the taste fibres which join the facial nerve are distributed through the greater petrosal branch to the palate and through the chorda tympani to the anterior two-thirds of the tongue.

The central processes of the cutaneous fibres pass to the brain-stem in the sensory root, enter the spinal tract of the trigeminal nerve

and end in its nucleus. The peripheral processes are distributed to a small area of skin on the auricle and in the external acoustic meatus and to part of the ear drum through communicating branches which leave the facial nerve at its exit from the stylomastoid foramen and pass to the greater auricular and auriculotemporal nerves.

The special visceral motor neurons begin in the **motor nucleus of the facial nerve**. This is situated in the lateral part of the tegmentum of the pons in the special visceral motor column. The axons leave the nucleus in a dorsal direction and then loop around the abducent nucleus in the facial colliculus (Fig. 5.38) to run ventrally to their exit from the brainstem. They constitute the whole of the motor root of the nerve. They innervate the muscles of facial expression (including occipitofrontalis), auricular muscles, stapedius, stylohyoid, and the posterior belly of digastric, all derived from the hyoid arch. The upper part of the motor nucleus receives afferents from the corticobulbar tracts of both sides but the lower part of the nucleus is supplied exclusively if not predominantly, by crossed corticobulbar fibres. The nucleus receives afferents from several other sources including the tectum of the midbrain and the sensory trigeminal nuclei.

The preganglionic parasympathetic neurons commence in the **superior salivatory nucleus**, a collection of cells situated close to the motor nucleus, in the general visceral motor column. Their axons leave in the sensory root of the nerve. Fibres for the lacrimal gland and the glands of the nasal cavity, nasopharynx, paranasal air sinuses, oral surface of the palate, upper lip and upper part of cheek travel in the greater petrosal branch of the facial nerve and synapse in the **pterygopalatine ganglion** with postganglionic neurons which are distributed through the branches of the ganglion. Fibres for the submandibular and sublingual glands and the small glands in the floor of the mouth leave the facial nerve in the chorda tympani, join the lingual nerve and relay in the **submandibular ganglion**. The superior salivatory nucleus receives afferents from the nucleus of the tractus solitarius, the trigeminal sensory nuclei, and the olfactory system and hypothalamus. The part of the nucleus supplying the lacrimal gland (sometimes referred to separately as the lacrimal nucleus) is connected with the trigeminal spinal nucleus for the reflex production of tears in response to corneal and conjunctival stimulation.

Clinical aspects

Facial paralysis is a not uncommon clinical condition which has many causes. Since each cause tends to operate at a specific point along the course of the facial nerve or its central connections it is useful for diagnosis to be able accurately to locate the site of the lesion. In order to do this it is first necessary to distinguish an upper motor neuron (or supranuclear) paralysis from a lower motor neuron (infranuclear) paralysis. The most frequent cause of an upper motor neuron paralysis is interruption of the supranuclear fibres from the motor areas of the cerebral cortex as they travel through the internal capsule on their way to the facial motor nucleus as a result of a stroke. This results in voluntary paralysis of the muscles supplied by the facial nerve on the opposite side to the lesion. Because the upper part of the facial motor nucleus receives both crossed and uncrossed supranuclear fibres the frontalis and orbicularis oculi muscles are spared to a considerable degree. The victim of a stroke involving the supranuclear fibres to the facial nucleus is able, therefore, to wrinkle the forehead and close the eye on the contralateral side despite the fact that the muscles in the lower part of the face on this side show marked voluntary paralysis with drooping of the corner or the mouth and puffing of the cheek.

In a lower motor neuron paralysis of the facial nerve all activity of the muscles supplied by the interrupted fibres is lost and the muscles consequently atrophy. The commonest site for the lesion to occur is in the lower part of the facial canal and is due to compression of the facial nerve as a result of oedema of the tissues lining the canal caused, it is believed, by a viral infection. The resulting facial paralysis is termed Bell's palsy. The victim suffers complete paralysis of all the muscles supplied by the facial nerve, apart from stapedius which is innervated by a branch which leaves the nerve higher up in the facial canal. As well as drooping of the corner of the mouth and puffing of the cheek there is also an inability to close the eye and to wrinkle the forehead on the affected side. There is usually a slow and frequently incomplete recovery of muscle function. If the oedema spreads upwards along the facial canal it will involve the chorda tympani resulting in ipsilateral loss or impairment of taste in the anterior two-thirds of the tongue and of secretion by the salivary glands in the floor of the mouth.

If the lesion is situated proximal to the geniculate ganglion all functions of the nerve are lost. The paralysis will involve stapedius, as well as the other muscles supplied by the facial nerve, resulting in hyperacuity (sounds seeming abnormally loud). There will also be impaired secretion of tears and loss of taste in the palate on the affected side in addition to the features already described as resulting from dysfunction of the chorda tympani. One cause of damage to the facial nerve in this part of its course is a neurofibroma (a variety of tumour) of the vestibulocochlear nerve in the internal acoustic meatus which compresses the facial nerve.

The facial nerve or its branches may be interrupted in the parotid gland or face by trauma (including surgery). Temporary facial paralysis follows the inadvertent introduction of local anaesthetic solution into the parotid gland when attempting to give an inferior alveolar block (p. 178).

Glossopharyngeal

The glossopharyngeal is a complete dorsal cranial nerve containing all the varieties of neuron expected according to the classical theory of cranial nerves outlined at the beginning of this chapter.

General visceral sensory neurons in the glossopharyngeal nerve supply the baroreceptors in the carotid sinus and the chemoreceptors in the carotid body. The cell bodies of these fibres are situated in the **inferior ganglion** of the nerve. Their central processes enter the **tractus solitarius** and end in the **caudal part of its nucleus**. From here connections are made with the vital centres in the reticular formation and with the hypothalamus.

The special visceral sensory fibres supply the taste buds in the posterior one-third of the tongue, including the vallate papillae, and adjacent areas of the pharyngeal wall. Their cell bodies are located in the inferior glossopharyngeal ganglion and the central processes terminate in the **rostral part of the nucleus of the tractus solitarius**.

The glossopharyngeal nerve also contains fibres for touch, pain, and temperature from the posterior part of the tongue, pharynx, and middle-ear cavity and possibly a few cutaneous fibres from the region around the external ear. The cell bodies of these fibres are believed to be situated in the small **superior glossopharyngeal ganglion** and their central processes to pass into the **spinal tract of the trigeminal nerve** to end in its nucleus.

The preganglionic visceral motor fibres in the glossopharyngeal nerve begin in the **inferior salivatory nucleus**. Most pass through the tympanic branch of the nerve, the tympanic plexus and the lesser petrosal nerve to the **otic ganglion**. Here they synapse with postganglionic fibres which pass to the auriculotemporal nerve through a communicating branch and so reach the parotid gland. A few postganglionic fibres run from the otic ganglion to the mandibular division of the trigeminal nerve to be distributed through its inferior alveolar and buccal branches to the small glands in the lower lip and lower part of the cheek. Preganglionic parasympathetic fibres also pass in the pharyngeal branch of the glossopharyngeal nerve to supply the glands in the mucous membrane of the oral and laryngeal parts of the pharynx. These synapse with postganglionic neurons in relay stations in the pharyngeal wall. Parasympathetic secretomotor fibres have been described as passing in the lingual branch of the glossopharyngeal nerve to supply the small glands in the mucosa of the posterior third of the tongue and vallate papillae after relay in small ganglia situated in the lingual mucosa.

The inferior salivatory nucleus lies immediately caudal to the superior salivatory nucleus in the general visceral motor column. It has connections with the nucleus of the tractus solitarius, trigeminal sensory nuclei, olfactory system, and hypothalamus.

The glossopharyngeal nerve supplies the single muscle, stylopharyngeus, derived from the third pharyngeal arch. The special visceral motor neurons to this muscle begin in the rostral part of the **nucleus ambiguus** (see next section).

Vagus and cranial accessory

The cranial accessory can be regarded as a detached portion of the vagus. After a short course, during which it unites briefly with the spinal accessory, it joins the vagus and its constituent fibres are distributed through the branches of the latter nerve. It is convenient, therefore, to describe the two nerves together.

The vagus contains a large number of general visceral sensory fibres which are distributed to the viscera of the thorax and abdomen. It is thus sensory to the respiratory system, the heart and most of the alimentary tract as far as the left flexure of the large intestine. It also supplies the baroreceptors in the aortic arch and the chemoreceptors in the aortic bodies. The cell bodies of these neurons are located in the **inferior ganglion** of the nerve. Their central processes enter the **tractus solitarius** and end in the **caudal part of its nucleus**. Through the connections of this nucleus with the hypothalamus and the vital centres in the reticular formation of the brainstem, these sensory neurons are involved in the reflex control of cardiovascular, respiratory, and alimentary activity.

The few taste fibres in the vagus supply the taste buds on the epiglottis and in the adjacent pharyngeal mucosa. Their cell bodies are in the inferior vagal ganglion and their central processes end in the **rostral part of the nucleus of the tractus solitarius**.

Like the glossopharyngeal nerve, the vagus contains fibres for pain, temperature, and touch. Most of these are from the pharynx, oesophagus, and larynx. Through its auricular branch the vagus nerve also supplies fibres to a small area of skin in the external acoustic meatus and on the auricle and to part of the ear drum. The cell bodies of these neurons are in the small **superior ganglion** of the vagus and their central processes end in the **spinal nucleus of the trigeminal**.

The vagus is the great parasympathetic nerve of the body. It

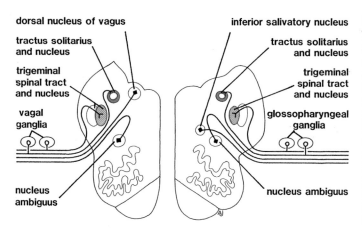

dorsal nucleus of vagus

tractus solitarius
and nucleus

trigeminal
spinal tract
and nucleus

vagal
ganglia

nucleus
ambiguus

inferior salivatory nucleus

tractus solitarius
and nucleus

trigeminal
spinal tract
and nucleus

glossopharyngeal
ganglia

nucleus ambiguus

Fig. 5.39. The nuclei of the glossopharyngeal (right) and vagus (left) nerves.

contains the preganglionic outflow for practically all the viscera in the head and neck, thorax, and abdomen. The only exceptions are the salivary glands and the small glands in the upper parts of the alimentary and respiratory tracts, which are supplied with parasympathetic fibres through the facial and glossopharyngeal nerves, and the large intestine below the left flexure and the pelvic viscera which are supplied by the pelvic parasympathetic outflow. Most of the preganglionic neurons begin in the **dorsal nucleus of the vagus,** a large collection of cells which occupies the general visceral motor column throughout much of the medulla. In the closed part of the medulla it is situated in the central grey matter and in the open part it lies in the floor of the fourth ventricle beneath the vagal triangle. It is in line with and caudal to the salivatory nuclei. The fibres are distributed through the vagus and its many branches and synapse with postganglionic neurons situated in autonomic ganglia or plexuses in or close to the organ being supplied. The dorsal nucleus receives afferents from the hypothalamus, the nucleus of the tractus solitarius and the vital centres in the reticular formation. Through these connections the vagus plays a major role in maintaining an appropriate level of visceral activity.

The vagus and cranial accessory nerves are associated with the fourth and sixth pharyngeal arches (the fifth arch being suppressed). The special visceral motor neurons to the muscles derived from these arches begin in the **nucleus ambiguus**. This is a long column of cells situated dorsal to the inferior olivary nucleus. It migrates somewhat during embryonic development and so lies rather more laterally in the brainstem than might be expected for a special visceral motor nucleus. Fibres from the rostral part of the nucleus enter the glossopharyngeal nerve, those from the intermediate part enter the vagus and those from the caudal part constitute the cranial root of the accessory nerve. The special visceral motor neurons of the vagus and cranial accessory are distributed through the pharyngeal, superior laryngeal, and recurrent laryngeal branches of the vagus to the muscles of the pharynx and soft palate (except the tensor) and to the intrinsic muscles of the larynx. The striated muscle in the upper two-thirds of the oesophagus is also supplied by vagal fibres which begin in the nucleus ambiguus. The nucleus ambiguus receives afferents from the sensory nuclei of the trigeminal nerve and the nucleus of the tractus solitarius. These connections provide the central pathways for the swallowing, coughing, and other reflexes involving the larynx, pharynx, and soft palate.

There is evidence that some or all of the vagal preganglionic parasympathetic fibres supplying the heart begin in the nucleus ambiguus not in the dorsal nucleus.

Spinal accessory

The nature and homologies of this nerve are still disputed. It consists of motor fibres which begin in the lateral part of the ventral grey horn of the first to fifth cervical segments of the cord and supply trapezius and sternocleidomastoid muscles. Probably the most widely held view is that these muscles were originally of pharyngeal arch origin and that the spinal accessory represents a detached part of the vagus. The fact that the motor neurons for the trapezius and sternocleidomastoid first differentiate close to the cells that will eventually form the nucleus ambiguus is quoted as evidence supporting this view. An alternative possibility is that the spinal accessory is the fused ventral roots of a number of cervical spinal nerves and that the muscles it supplies are derivatives of cervical myotomes. The difficulty with this suggestion is identifying the segments which provide the myotomal contributions.

Section 6

Appendices

Appendix 1 Anatomy of intravenous and intramuscular therapy

ANATOMY OF INTRAVENOUS THERAPY

It is often necessary to administer drugs or other preparations directly into the circulating bloodstream. In dentistry the drugs most frequently given in this way are general anaesthetics and related agents. The usual site for such injections is one of the superficial veins on the anterior surface of the upper part of the forearm. These veins are also used for withdrawing blood for laboratory examination. Immediately deep to the superficial veins of this region is the cubital fossa containing several important nerves and vessels. Some knowledge of this region is necessary therefore for the practising dentist.

The cubital fossa

The cubital fossa (Fig. 6.1) is a triangular area on the anterior aspect of the upper part of the forearm. Its medial and lateral borders are formed by two of the flexor muscles in the forearm (pronator teres

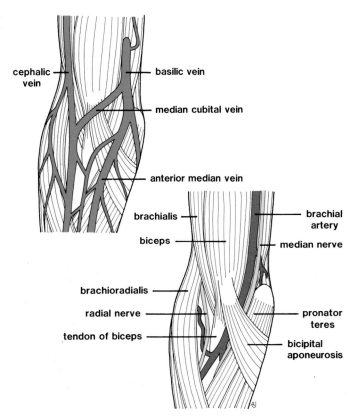

Fig. 6.1. Superficial veins of the anterior surface of the right forearm (above); structures passing through the right cubital fossa (below).

and brachioradialis respectively) while its superior border is an imaginary line joining the two humeral epicondyles (these are projections located on the medial and lateral sides of the humerus just above the elbow joint). The roof of the fossa is formed by the investing layer of the deep fascia of the forearm. The skin covering this region is thin and there are few hairs and the superficial fascia contains little fat. The floor of the fossa is formed by muscle (mainly brachialis, a flexor of the elbow joint). Traversing the fossa are several important structures. From medial to lateral side these are the **median nerve,** the **brachial artery,** the **tendon of biceps brachii,** and the **radial nerve**.

Running in the superficial fascia of the forearm are a number of easily visible veins. They are variable in their arrangement but the most usual pattern is as follows. The **basilic vein** runs along the ulnar border (little finger side) of the forearm and the **cephalic vein** along the radial border (thumb side). They both drain the prominent network of superficial veins on the back of the hand. Just below the elbow the cephalic vein gives off the **median cubital vein** which passes in the superficial fascia across the roof of the cubital fossa to join the basilic vein. It receives a communicating tributary from the deep veins of the forearm as they traverse the cubital fossa in company with the brachial artery. A third vessel, the **anterior median vein,** runs along the midline of the anterior surface of the forearm and drains into the basilic vein or median cubital vein.

The tendon of biceps passes deep into the cubital fossa to be inserted into the tuberosity on the medial surface of the radius. From the medial border of the tendon a broad sheet of connective tissue, the **bicipital aponeurosis,** passes obliquely across the roof of the cubital fossa to mingle with the deep fascia over the muscles on the ulnar side of the forearm. The bicipital aponeurosis thus reinforces the roof of the cubital fossa and intervenes between the median cubital vein, which runs in the superficial fascia across the roof of the fossa, and the brachial artery and median nerve, which traverse the fossa medial to the bicipital tendon.

The median nerve (containing fibres from spinal segments C5 to T2 inclusive) gives muscular branches to most of the flexor muscles of the forearm and thumb muscles and sensory branches to the palmar aspect of the radial side of the hand including the radial 3½ digits. The radial nerve (spinal segments C6 to C8 inclusive) supplies the extensor muscles of the arm and forearm and much of the skin on the back of the hand. The remaining muscles of the forearm and hand and the remainder of the skin of the hand are supplied by the ulnar nerve which does not traverse the cubital fossa.

The brachial artery is the main artery of the upper limb being a continuation of the axillary artery, itself a continuation of the subclavian artery. In the cubital fossa it divides into radial and ulnar branches. These run down their respective sides of the forearm under cover of superficial muscles. A short distance above the wrist they emerge from beneath the muscles and here the radial and ulnar pulses can be felt as the arteries run on the radius and ulna (pulses can be felt wherever a superficial artery crosses bone). The brachial artery and its branches are accompanied by venae comitantes which form the deep veins of the upper limb.

The superficial veins in the region of the cubital fossa are easily seen if pressure is applied around the upper arm by hand or tourniquet while the fist is clenched and released several times, when they become distended with blood.

The bicipital aponeurosis was once known as the Grace Dieu fascia, thanks being given to God that it usually protected deeper structures from the lancet in the once popular operation of blood-letting.

ANATOMY OF INTRAMUSCULAR THERAPY

Several pharmacological preparations are administered by injecting them into a conveniently located, large muscle mass. Probably the most important of these preparations from the dentist's point of view is benzylpenicillin which is used to treat many oral infections. The two muscle masses most frequently chosen for intramuscular injections are the deltoid muscle in the upper arm (Fig. 6.2) and the

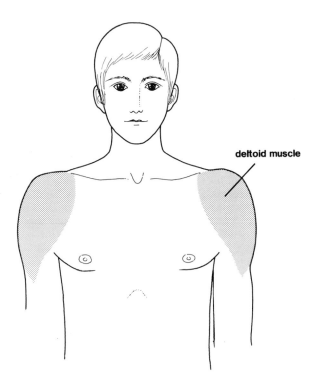

Fig. 6.2. To show the extent of the deltoid muscles.

gluteal muscles in the buttock. There is a potential hazard in injecting into the gluteal muscles arising from the close proximity of the large and important sciatic nerve. For this reason a knowledge of the relationships of this nerve to the gluteal muscles is essential for anyone involved in giving intramuscular therapy at this site.

Gluteal muscles and sciatic nerve

The prominence of the buttock is produced by three large muscles – **gluteus maximus, gluteus medius,** and **gluteus minimus** – and the presence of a large amount of fat in the subcutaneous tissue of the region. Running through the buttock is the **sciatic nerve** which descends into the lower limb and supplies it with many motor and sensory fibres.

Pelvic girdle

The pelvic girdle consists of the two **innominate bones** and the **sacrum**. Each innominate bone has an expanded, blade-like, upper part, the **ilium,** an anteroinferior part, the **pubis,** and a postero-inferior part, the **ischium.** The pubis and ischium together surround the **obturator foramen.** The posterior border of the ischium bears two projections. Pointing medially is the **ischial spine** and below this is the rounded **ischial tuberosity.** Above the ischial spine the posterior border of the innominate bone is deeply concave forming the **greater sciatic notch.** At the junction of ilium, ischium, and pubis is the acetabulum, a large crescentic area which provides the articular surface for the head of the femur. The two innominate bones articulate with each other anteriorly at the **pubic symphysis.** Posteriorly the pelvic girdle is completed by the sacrum.

Gluteus maximus

This is a large, coarse-fibred muscle. It arises from the posterior part of the gluteal (posterolateral) surface of the ilium, from the lateral part of the sacrum and from associated fascia and ligaments. Its fibres slope downwards and outwards across the buttock to be inserted into the iliotibial tract, a strong band of fascia running vertically down the lateral aspect of the thigh to be attached below the knee to the tibia.

The muscle is a lateral rotator and extensor of the hip joint and, through the iliotibial tract, a supporter of the extended knee.

Gluteus medius

Gluteus medius arises from the gluteal surface of the ilium in front of the origin of gluteus maximus. Its fibres run laterally and converge to

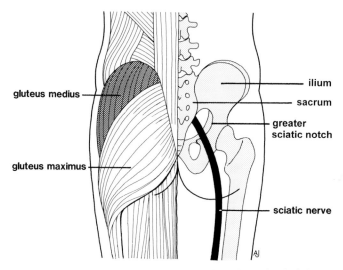

Fig. 6.3. The sciatic nerve in the buttock. The safe area is stippled.

be inserted into the **greater trochanter**, a prominent boss of bone on the lateral aspect of the femur at the junction of its neck and shaft.

Gluteus minimus

This muscle arises from an area on the gluteal surface of the ilium located in front of and inferior to the origin of gluteus medius. It is inserted into the greater trochanter.

Gluteus medius and minimus are abductors of the hip joint. Their more usual action is to prevent adduction of the joint on the weight-bearing side during walking.

Sciatic nerve

The sciatic nerve is formed from the fourth lumbar to the fifth sacral spinal nerves and is the largest peripheral nerve in the body. It passes from the pelvic cavity into the buttock through the greater sciatic notch. It then passes downwards deep to gluteus maximus and enters the hamstring compartment of the thigh. It supplies the hamstring muscles and, through its branches, the muscles of the leg and foot.

The sciatic nerve runs through the lower and inner quadrant of the buttock. Intramuscular injections should always be given, therefore, into the **upper and outer quadrant**, that is into the gluteus medius and minimus muscles. In order that the upper and outer quadrant be correctly defined it is important to remember that the anatomical buttock extends much further in a superior direction than is implied in the non-medical use of the term. The full extent of the buttock and the safe area for injection are shown in Fig. 6.3.

Appendix 2 Development of eye

The eyes are first seen early in the fourth week as **optic vesicles**, bilateral outpushings of the forebrain derived from the **optic grooves** (optic sulci) which were present even before closure of the neural tube (Fig. 6.4). As these vesicles form they become surrounded by sheaths of mesoderm consisting, at least in part, of neural crest cells derived from the vesicles themselves. The vesicles contact the overlying ectoderm and induce it to form **lens placodes**. The lens tissue continues to proliferate and pushes into the vesicle, making it cup-shaped. The mouth of the **optic cup** will eventually form the **pupil**.

The invagination which forms the optic cup is not confined to the centre of the optic vesicle, but also includes part of its ventral surface (Fig. 6.5) and the **optic stalk** which connects the vesicle to the brain. This fold forms the **choroid fissure** which is important as it allows the **hyaloid artery**, a branch of the ophthalmic artery, and its accompanying vein, to gain access to the anterior region of the optic cup and developing lens. During the seventh week the lips of the choroid fissure fuse enclosing the hyaloid vessels within the optic stalk.

While this is happening the ectoderm of the lens becomes folded and invaginated and cuts itself off as the **lens vesicle**, which lies within the mouth of the optic cup. During the fifth week the outer layer of the optic cup becomes pigmented (Fig. 6.6) by melanin produced by neural crest derived cells. When the eye begins to function this outer **pigmented layer** will prevent loss of light and also reflection back to the inner, **neural layer** of the retina. The neural layer of the retina develops in a complex way. Adjacent to the original space between inner and outer layers of the optic cup (the **intraretinal space**, Fig. 6.5) most of the cells differentiate into a layer of photosensitive **rods** and **cones**. Deep to the rods and cones lie further layers of cells which differentiate into bipolar **connector cells** and **ganglion cells**. The ganglion cells sprout axons which emerge onto the inner surface of the retina as **optic fibres** and grow across it towards the optic stalk and thence, surrounding the hyaloid vessels, towards the brain as the **optic nerve**. This apparently clumsy arrangement means that light striking the surface of the retina passes through a mat of axons and several cell layers before reaching the sensitive rods and cones. The **macula** or **blind spot** is the area of the retina corresponding to the optic nerve, which, of course, has no light-sensitive cells.

Shortly before entering the brain the optic nerves of right and left sides unite to form the **optic chiasma**. Here the nerve fibres from the nasal side of each retina cross over the midline to travel to the contralateral side of the brain. The optic pathway proximal to the chiasma (the optic tract) contains, therefore, uncrossed fibres from the temporal side of the ipsilateral retina and crossed fibres from the nasal side of the contralateral retina. The bulk of the fibres end in the lateral geniculate body of the thalamus.

The lens vesicle is transformed into a lens proper by the enlargement of its deeper part, so that the original lumen is displaced anteriorly and later abolished (Fig. 6.6). The cells lying posterior to the lumen become **primary lens fibres** by the loss of their nuclei and the secretion of a transparent protein. **Secondary lens fibres**, which are added as the lens grows, are derived from a simple epithelium which

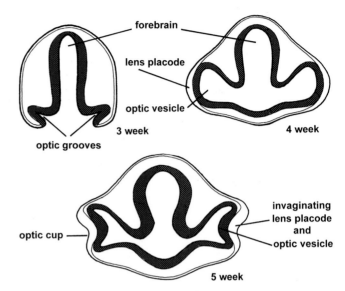

Fig. 6.4. Transverse sections through forebrain region of three-week, four-week, and five-week-old (approximately) embryos.

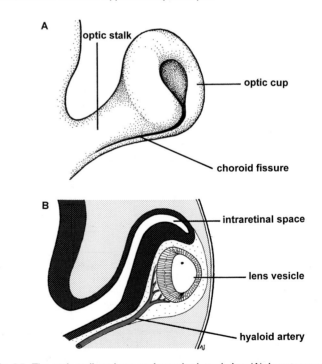

Fig. 6.5. The optic stalk and cup at six weeks: lateral view (A); in anteroposterior section (B).

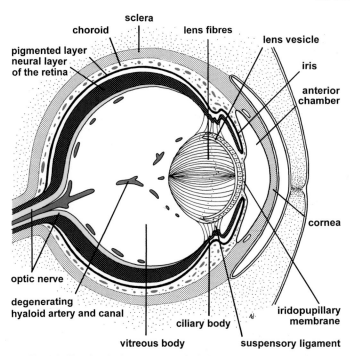

Fig. 6.6. The developing eye at 15 weeks in anteroposterior section.

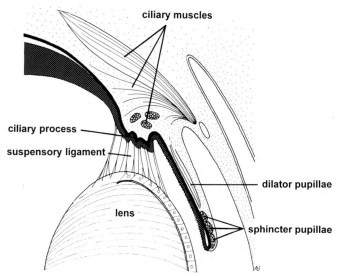

Fig. 6.7. The developing iris and ciliary body.

differentiates from cells on the anterior wall of the lens vesicle. As soon as the lens vesicle is formed it is vascularized by a branch of the hyaloid artery. As the lens matures during fetal life this vascularization atrophies. After degeneration its course is marked in the **vitreous body** (a gelatinous matrix formed from mesoderm which invades the eye via the choroid fissure and lying between the optic cup and the lens vesicle) by the **hyaloid canal**. The hyaloid canal and remnants of the hyaloid vessels can be seen by most people as 'floaters' against a clear sky. The parts of the hyaloid vessels traversing the optic stalk persist within the optic nerve as the **central artery** and **vein** of the retina.

The **choroid, sclera,** and **cornea** are formed during the sixth and seventh weeks from the mesenchymal sheath around the developing optic vesicle. The choroid forms a second pigmented layer over most of the eye, surrounded by the tough connective tissue of the sclera. The choroid is often considered equivalent to the pia and arachnoid mater of the brain: the sclera is equivalent to the dura mater and is continuous with the dural wrapping of the optic nerve.

During the sixth week mesenchyme invades the region between lens and surface ectoderm. A vesicle appears in this mesenchyme, forming the **anterior chamber of the eye**. The mesoderm superficial to this split is continuous with the sclera and, with the overlying ectoderm, forms the cornea. The mesenchyme deep to the split is continuous with the choroid and forms the **iridopupillary membrane**, which disappears in the seventh month of fetal life to form the **pupil**.

Towards the end of the third month the rim of the optic cup around the future pupil, together with the overlying choroid, form a thin circular membrane (Fig. 6.7). The outer pigmented layer of the optic cup gives rise to the pigmented layer of the **iris** and **ciliary body**

and the inner (unpigmented) layer forms the unpigmented layer. In the overlying choroidal mesenchyme **sphincter** and **dilator pupillary muscles** develop from neural crest derived cells. Similarly **ciliary muscles** develop in association with the ciliary body. The lens is attached to the ciliary body by the radially arranged fibres of the **suspensory ligament** which insert into the ciliary process. Through this ligament the ciliary muscle controls the shape of the lens.

Appendix 3 Development of ear

In the adult the ear forms a single unit with two functions, hearing and balance. In the embryo it develops as three parts, the external ear which serves as a sound collector, the middle ear which conducts and amplifies sound and the inner ear which both converts sound into nerve impulses and registers changes in equilibrium. These are most logically dealt with in reverse order.

The inner ear

The first sign of ear development is the formation of ectodermal **otic placodes** opposite the hindbrain at 22 days (Fig. 6.8). Each invaginates to form an **otic vesicle** which differentiates into two parts. The ventral part forms the **saccule** and the **cochlear duct**; the dorsal part the **utricle, semicircular canals**, and the **endolymphatic duct** (Fig. 6.9). The ventral and dorsal parts are joined by the narrow **utriculosaccular duct**. These sets of structures are known collectively as the **membranous labyrinth**. The cavity within the membranous labyrinth contains a fluid, **endolymph**. Later in development (ninth week) the ectomesenchyme around the membranous labyrinth forms the cartilaginous **otic capsule**. The membranous labyrinth thus comes to lie within a similarly shaped cavity in the otic capsule. The membranous labyrinth is separated from the otic capsule by the fluid-filled **perilymphatic space**. In the fourth month the otic capsule begins to ossify to form **the petrous part of the temporal bone**. The membranous labyrinth now lies in a bony cavity, the **bony labyrinth**.

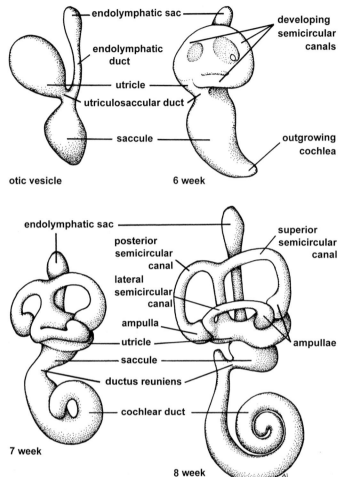

Fig. 6.9. Development of utricle, saccule, and cochlear duct and formation of the semicircular canals from the utricle.

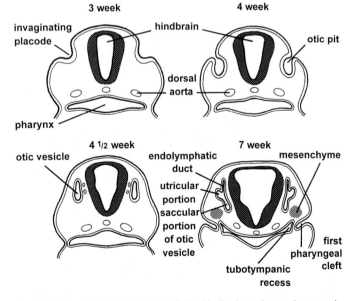

Fig. 6.8. Transverse sections through the hindbrain region at three weeks, four weeks, four and a half weeks and seven weeks approximately.

Saccule and cochlea

In week six the ventral, saccular portion of the otic vesicle begins to form a tubular outpushing, the **cochlear duct** (Fig. 6.9) which grows in a spiral fashion until, by the eighth week it has 2½ turns. The cochlea remains connected to the saccule by the narrow **ductus reuniens**. The perilymphatic space around the cochlear duct increases in size and forms two parts, the **scala vestibuli** and the **scala tympani** (Fig. 6.10) which are visible by 10 weeks. The cochlear duct is now triangular in cross section with three faces, the **vestibular membrane** facing the scala vestibuli, the **basilar membrane** facing the

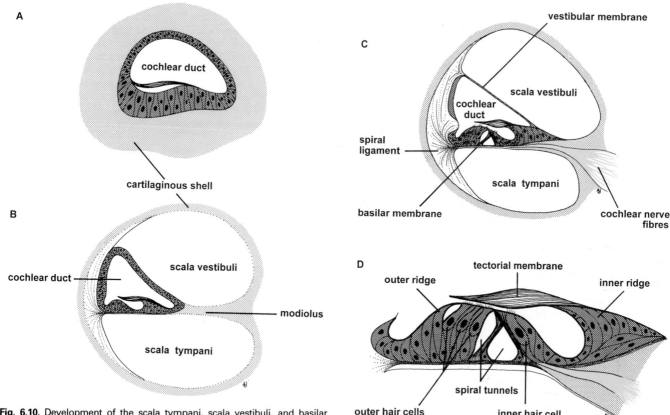

Fig. 6.10. Development of the scala tympani, scala vestibuli, and basilar membrane (A and B); further development of the basilar membrane to form the Organ of Corti (C and D).

scala tympani and the **spiral ligament** connecting the base of the tri-angle to the cartilaginous wall. The apex of the triangle is attached to a process of cartilage between the scalae, the **modiolus**.

The epithelial cells of the basilar membrane now differentiate to form **inner** and **outer ridges**. The outer ridge forms two groups of **hair cells** separated by paired **spiral tunnels** (Fig. 6.10). The inner ridge secretes a gelatinous **tectorial membrane** which overlies both sets of hair cells. The sensory hair cells plus the tectorial membrane constitute the **Organ of Corti** which transmits hearing information to the spiral, or cochlear, ganglion and hence to the cochlear (auditory) fibres of the vestibulocochlear nerve.

Utricle and semicircular canals

The dorsal, utricular part of the otic vesicle (Fig. 6.9) develops flat-tened outpushings during week six. The central parts of the walls of each of these become apposed and eventually disappear leaving the rims as the three semicircular canals, **superior, posterior**, and **lateral**. One end of each canal widens to form an **ampulla**. In each ampulla sensory areas (the **cristae**) develop and transmit information for the maintenance of equilibrium. Similar areas (the **maculae**) develop within the walls of the saccule and utricle. Impulses from cristae and

maculae are transmitted to the vestibular ganglion and thence to the brain via the vestibular fibres of the vestibulocochlear nerve.

The middle ear

The **tympanic cavity** develops from the deeper part of the **tubotym-panic recess**, an evagination of the first pharyngeal pouch (Fig. 6.11), and hence is lined with endoderm. The rest of the tubotypanic recess, connecting the tympanic cavity with the pharynx, persists as the **audi-tory tube**. The **malleus** is derived from the dorsal part of Meckel's cartilage and the **incus** from the pterygoquadrate cartilage (both car-tilages of the first arch); the **stapes** is derived from the cartilage of the second arch. Despite this all develop in a common mesodermal con-densation seen between the tubotympanic cavity and the membra-nous labyrinth towards the end of the second month. The developing ossicles remain surrounded by mesoderm until the eighth month when the tissue between them is removed and the cavity so formed invaded by the endodermal lining of the tubotympanic recess. The three mesodermal ossicles are thus eventually suspended in an endo-derm-lined cavity from endoderm-derived ligaments. The ventral end of the handle of the malleus becomes attached to the **tympanic membrane** (see below) and the footplate of the stapes to the **oval**

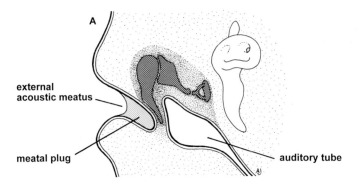

external
acoustic meatus

meatal plug

auditory tube

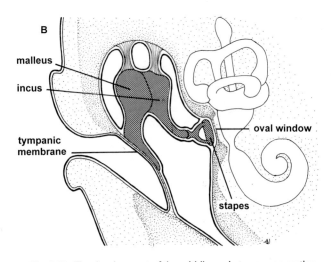

malleus

incus

tympanic
membrane

oval window

stapes

Fig. 6.11. The development of the middle ear in transverse section.

window, a small opening in the bony labyrinth. Vibrations of the tympanic membrane can now be transmitted by the ossicular chain to the membranous labyrinth. These vibrations are transduced in the Organ of Corti in the cochlea into neural impulses transmitted to the brain by the cochlear fibres of the vestibulocochlear nerve. In accordance with their origin the muscle of the malleus (**tensor tympani**) is supplied by the mandibular division of the trigeminal nerve, and that of the stapes (**stapedius**) by the facial nerve.

Expansion of the tympanic cavity continues to form, before birth, the dorsal **tympanic antrum**, and after birth the **air cells of the mastoid process**.

The **external acoustic meatus** develops from the first pharyngeal cleft. During the third month the epithelial cells in the meatus proliferate to produce the **meatal plug**. Later in fetal life this disappears and the floor of the external meatus participates in the formation of the **tympanic membrane**. The latter is complex, consisting of an ectodermal outer layer derived from the external meatus, an endodermal inner layer derived from the lining of the tympanic cavity and an intermediate mesodermal layer.

The external ear

The external ear or **pinna** is formed from six hillocks which lie around the external auditory meatus. Their exact disposition is of little functional importance.

Glossary

Many anatomical terms are derived from Greek and Latin roots. Although some of these are familiar because of everyday derivatives (*canis*, a dog in Latin has given us canine, dog-like, a term also applied to a specific tooth type) others are not.

The following list is composed of an anatomical term, a plural form where this is unusual and in common use, a short explanation or translation, and a mention of the language of origin (G = Greek, L = Latin).

Aditus	Entrance to a cavity (L)	**Condyle**	A knuckle (L)
Ala pl. **alae**	A wing (L)	**Cornu** pl. **cornua**	A horn (L)
Alimentum	Nourishment (L)	**Corona**	A crown (L). Hence coronal pertaining to the crown of the head or any other crown-like structure
Allo-	A prefix meaning different or other (G)		
Alveolus pl. **alveoli**	A cavity or socket (L)	**Coronoid**	Curved (G)
Ampulla	A flask, hence any dilated tube (L)	**Cribriform**	Sieve-like, perforated (L)
Amygdaloid	Resembling an almond (G)	**Crista**	A ridge (L)
Ansa	A loop-like structure (L)	**Crista galli**	A cock's comb (L)
Antrum	A cave (L)	**Cuneate**	Wedge-shaped (L)
Annulus	Diminutive of annus, a ring (L)	**Dendrite**	Tree-like (G)
Aponeurosis	A flat tendon (G)	**Diencephalon**	The ''between'' part of the brain (G)
Arachnoid	Resembling a spider's web (G)	**Diploe**	A fold (G)
Arytenoid	Cup, ladle-shaped (G)	**Dorsum sellae**	The posterior part of the sella (turcica) (L)
Atlas	The first cervical vertebra; named after the Greek god who held up the pillars of Heaven	**Dura**	Hard (L)
		Ectopic	Displaced (G)
Atrium pl. **atria**	A chamber (L)	**Epi-**	A prefix meaning upon (G)
Axon	An axle (G)	**Ethmoid**	Sieve-like (G)
Azygos	Unpaired (G)	**Facet**	Diminutive of facies, face (L)
Bulla pl. **bullae**	A bubble (L)	**Falx**	A sickle (L)
Bursa	A bag (L)	**Fascia** pl. **fasciae**	A bandage (L)
Caecum	A blind pouch (L)	**Fasciculus** pl. **fasciculi**	Diminutive of fascis (a bundle) (L)
Calcarine	Spur-shaped (L)	**Foramen** pl. **foramina**	An opening (L)
Callosum	A beam (L). The corpus callosum is thus a beam connecting the two cerebral hemispheres	**Fornix**	An arch (L)
		Fossa pl. **fossae**	A hollow (L)
Canthus pl. **canthi**	Corner of the eye (G)	**Fovea**	A depression (L)
Carotid	Pertaining to a deep sleep (G). The carotid artery is so called because it was believed that its compression resulted in stupor	**Funiculus** pl. **funiculi**	A cord (L)
		Ganglion	A knot (G)
		Genu	The knee (L). Also used to describe structures bent like a knee. Hence geniculate
Cauda equina	A horse's tail (L)		
Caudal (caudad)	Towards the tail (L)	**Gracile**	Slender (L)
Caudate	Having a tail (L)	**Gyrus** pl. **gyri**	A ring or circle (G)
Cephalic	Towards or pertaining to the head (L)	**Hamulus**	A little hook (L)
Cerebellum	Diminutive of cerebrum (L)	**Hiatus**	A gap (L)
Cerebrum	The brain (L)	**Hippocampus**	A sea horse (G). Hence used to describe the curved structure in the inferior horn of the lateral ventricle
Cervix	A neck (L). Hence cervical		
Chiasma	Two lines crossing (G)	**Hyoid**	U-shaped (G)
Chorda pl. **chordae**	A chord (L)	**Hypo-**	A prefix meaning under (G). Hence hypophysis meaning a downgrowth
Choroid	Resembling the chorion (G)		
Chorion	Outermost layer of zygote (G)	**Incus**	An anvil (L)
Ciliary	Pertaining to or resembling the eyelashes (L)	**Infundibulum**	A funnel (L)
Cinerea	Grey in colour (L)	**Insula**	An island (L)
Cingulum pl. **cingula**	A girdle (L)	**Jugular**	Pertaining to the neck (L)
Claustrum	A barrier (L)	**Lacrimal**	Pertaining to tears (L)
Clava	A stick (L)	**Lacuna**	A pit or hole (L)
Clinoid	Bed-shaped (G)	**Lambdoid**	Shaped like the Greek letter lambda
Clivus	A slope (L)	**Lemniscus** pl. **lemnisci**	A ribbon or band (L)
Colliculus pl. **colliculi**	A small mound (L)	**Lentiform**	Shaped like a lentil or lens (L)
Commissure	A site of joining together (L)	**Leptomeninx** pl.	
Concha pl. **conchae**	A shell (L)	**leptomeninges**	The thin or delicate meninges (G)

Limbic	Pertaining to an edge or border (L)
Lingula	A tongue (L)
Malleus	A hammer (L)
Manubrium	A handle (L)
Mastoid	Breast-shaped (G)
Mater	Mother (L). Hence dura mater, arachnoid mater, and pia mater
meatus pl. **meatus**	A passageway (L)
Mediastinum	Standing between (L)
Medulla	Middle or inner part (L)
Meninx pl. **meninges**	A membrane (G)
Mental	Pertaining to the chin (L)
Mesencephalon	Midbrain (G)
Meso-	A prefix meaning middle or mid (G)
Meta-	A prefix meaning beyond or after (G)
Metencephalon	Hindbrain (G)
Myelencephalon	Middle brain (G)
Mylohyoid	Pertaining to the molar teeth and hyoid bone (G)
Neuron	Sinew or nerve (G)
Nuchal	Pertaining to the neck (L)
Occipital	Pertaining to the back of the head (L)
Ostium	An opening (L)
Pallium	A cloak (L)
Palpebral	Pertaining to the eyelid (L)
Para-	A prefix meaning beyond, against or accessory to (G)
Parietal	Pertaining to a wall (L)
Pedicle	A foot or stalk (L)
Peduncle	Derived from pedicle
Petrous	Rock-like (L). Hence petrosal meaning pertaining to the petrous part of the temporal bone
Physis	A growth (G). Hence epiphysis, metaphysis, hypophysis, etc.
Pia	Tender or soft (L)
Plexus pl. **plexus** or **plexuses**	A network (L)
Plica	A fold (L)
Pons	A bridge (L)
Prosencephalon	The forebrain (G)
Pterion	A wing (G). Hence pterygoid meaning wing-like.
Putamen	A shell (L)
Ramus pl. **rami**	A branch (L)
Raphe (raphé)	A seam (G)
Rectus	Straight (L)
Rete	A net (L)
Rhombencephalon	The hindbrain. The prefix rhomb – means shaped like a kite (G) and refers to the lozenge shape of the posterior brain vesicle
Rima	A chink (L)
Rostrum	A beak (L). Hence rostrad and rostral meaning towards the beak or head

Sagittal	Shaped like an arrow (L). Hence sagittal suture and the sagittal plane named after the suture
Scaphoid	Shaped like a boat (G)
Sella turcica	A Turkish saddle (L)
Septum	A ledge or fence (L)
Sphenoid	Wedge-shaped (G)
Splenium	A band (G)
Splanchnic	Concerning viscera (G)
Squamous	Resembling a scale (L)
Stapes	A stirrup (L)
Styloid	Resembling a pillar (G)
Sulcus	A groove (L)
Suture	A seam (L)
Symphysis pl. **symphyses**	A natural junction (G)
Synapse	A join (G)
Synchondrosis pl. **synchondroses**	A cartilaginous joint (G)
Tectum	A roof (L)
Tegmen and **Tegmentum**	A cover (L)
Tela	A web (L)
Tele-	A prefix meaning at the end or at a distance (G)
Telecephalon	The end or anterior part of the brain (G)
Temporal	Pertaining to time (L). The temporal bone and temple are so called because the hair of the temple is first to turn grey
Tentorium	A tent (L)
Thalamus pl. **thalami**	Inner chamber (L)
Thyroid	Shield-shaped (G)
Trigeminal	Triple (L)
Trochlea	A pulley (L)
Tragus	A goat (L). The tragus of the ear is so called because it bears a tuft of hairs like a goat's beard
Tuber pl. **tubera**	A protuberance (L)
Tuberculum and **tubercle**	Diminutives of tuber
Tympanum	A drum (L)
Uncus	A hook (L). Hence uncinate
Uvula	Little grape (L)
Vaginal	Resembling a sheath (L)
Vagus	Wandering (L)
Velum	A veil-like covering (L)
Vena comitans pl. **venae comitantes**	An accompanying vein (L)
Ventricle	A cavity (L)
Vomer	A ploughshare (L)
Xiphoid	Sword-like (G)
Zygoma	A bar (G). Hence zygomatic

Index